INFECTIOUS FUTURES

Reflections, Visions, and Worlds through and beyond COVID-19

Publish by Tamkang University
Graduate Institute of Futures Studies, Tamsui, Taipei, Taiwan 251
Email: info@jfsdigital.org

ISBN: 978-0-6454283-3-9

INTRODUCTION

SENSING
& SENSEMAKING

FUTURES STUDIES RESPONDS TO THE PANDEMIC

REGIONAL AND NATIONAL RESPONDS STUDIES

WILDCARDS ARE OUR TEACHERS IN A CO-CREATIVE COSMOS

Jose Ramos

August 1st, 2021. The clinic was unusually full of people. A few twenty-somethings in football uniforms, many middle aged and a few older people. The hallway, normally empty except for the occasional watercooler, was packed with people. Every few minutes a doctor or nurse would call out a name. After a few minutes my name was called. Inside the room a man and woman in medical gear took my disclosure form, pulled out a needle and asked me to reveal my upper left arm. Without delay the needle was in and it was done. My wife De Chantal followed a few minutes later. We were told to wait in the clinic lounge for 15 minutes to make sure there were no allergic reactions to the vaccine. The 15 minutes gave me some mental reflection time.

It was just over 18 months ago that a pandemic turned the world upside down. International travel was virtually shut down. Economies were roiled. Over the ensuing months strict lockdowns after lockdowns in every country were imposed. In some cases stay at home orders confined people for weeks without end. In Melbourne and the state of Victoria curfews and a travel radius of 5 km were imposed. Daniel Andrews, the head of the state government here, was nicknamed "Dictator Dan".

With time the true cost of the pandemic was born out. Millions have died and continue to die. Many more people who survived have continued to experience serious lasting effects on their health. Millions more have lost jobs and livelihoods. Stress levels increased and mental health suffered. Loved ones have been unable to visit each other because of travel restrictions, even while the virus threatens.

I've been in the futures studies field for two decades now. In 2000, one of my first teachers, Oliver Markley, taught me and my classmates in Houston about wildcards - low probability high impact events. For most social democracies, we've lived in a *belle epoche*, a period of relative peace and prosperity. Wildcards were an interesting idea. But for this middle-class suburbanite, they remained an idea, not a lived experience. But in many other countries, people have lived through epic disruptions. In the former Soviet Union, people experienced economic disintegration when the union collapsed and was followed by West-led economic shock therapy. In the Middle East, it was the Arab Spring, and the US-led War on Terror. To use an analogy, historical change is a little like the movements of tectonic plates that have created mountains and seas through the eons. Usually change is slow, but sometimes there are earthquakes and volcanic eruptions, and depending on where you are it can become violent and dangerous.

Histories and futures provide us with an opportunity to understand the deeper patterns of change: recorded, empirical, narrativized, imagined, or hypothetical. It can pull us out of our day-to-day sleep walk, and allow us to understand the contours of where we have come from and where we may go. Indeed, this is more than just positioning ourselves on a timeline. Where do our personal stories and broader social change intersect? Our world is experiencing fundamental transitions and transformations. Seeing the pandemic unfold, so many of our hearts have broken open to the collective suffering and challenges we have seen and felt. The world-totality which may have been abstract has reached into our hearts like the root systems of trees, binding us into a new feeling entity. The futures, an abstraction for too long, now calls forth many with bellowing song, asking for new thinking, new strategies, new methods, new narratives and new selves. How can we answer the call of these Epic Times?

Parker Palmer (2009) talks about the importance of giving people space to discover themselves, their sense of purpose. This does not happen very well when we try to solve the purpose problem for others, giving other people what we feel their purpose should be. As Jung (1958) pointed out, a collective loss of purpose is in fact a type of collective unconscious which calls forth that great "leader" that fills this void for others, as cults of personality such as with Adolph Hitler did. We see this threat today. But we also see an awakening of consciousness and purposefulness in its great variety - we feel it. It is not a sole monolithic purpose but an ecology of meaning.

Paolo Freire (1973) argued popular transformation means transforming alienated subjectivity into historically contextualized subjectivity – 'temporal conscientization' (Ramos 2005). Whereby we understand the era in exhaustion and the era that wants to emerge. Such that we may participate in the dramatic unfolding of new worlds. The pandemic has been, and continues to be, such a moment in time that casts light and shade on the contours of Time, giving us conceptual leverage. This then allows us to choose. In our new awakenings of purpose, what futures will we live for, stand for, fight for, and die for?

Will we help to create the new world which W.I. Thompson (1985) called eudaemonic planetization? Where we understand ourselves as intimately interconnected and co-constituting, human and non-human, mind and matter, radicals and reactionaries, the spiritual and the banal. Or will we inhabit split selves, magnifying our contradictions - vanity billionaires in space alongside the reality of a world in crisis? In this anthology are many perspectives that offer temporal conscientisation - that bring meaning, purpose and connectedness to our cosmic journey. They help to stitch our hearts into tapestries of world-making. Hegemonic and unconscious futuresperpetuate only when we fail to search for alternatives. This anthology provides us with a cornucopia of narratives that bring new meaning and purpose to the Epic Times in which we live.

Deep discovery is beyond conventional categories and words. It requires experience and experimentation, it is a journey. The pandemic has challenged dualistic thinking. Don't like governmental power? Government has been critical in protecting people or in failing to protect them. Believe in freedom of speech? How about anti-vaxxers on social media? The pandemic shifts us toward non-binary modes of thinking. The biomedical model produced the vaccine that was injected in me today. But it was the public health and health promotion models that bridged the education and outreach gap. It was my men's group that helped keep me partially sane during a 15 week lockdown, and meditation and therapy that is helping me recover. This new world gives space for an ecology of knowledges, that embraces science, experience, experimentation, testimonial, and just what works for people.

As I write this the Delta strain runs rampant in many parts of the world, creating havoc and pain. It is worth taking a step back and reflecting on the ontogeny of variants. Delta is with us because we allowed COVID-19 to run experiments in millions of people, each time offering an opportunity for mutation. Delta was born of a variety of these experiments, iterative and slow until it found a new "success" formula (Kupferschmidt 2021). Of course we don't consider Delta a success in human terms, but we should learn from the mutational process that we are seeing. What is COVID-19 saying about how we need to experiment and mutate as societies and as a global community?

This brings us to the creative domain of methodological hybridity - mutant futures - where I hope we can use this Overton

Window to create new approaches to futures that support humanity's capacity to navigate change. Our Epic Times call for transgressive creativity, new thinking that can be the basis for bold experiments and breakthrough innovation. Each of these essays brings us into the space of the liminal, the creative and mutant interplay. We can use this thinking to seed a flourishing of new approaches that will support the societal navigation of our biggest challenges.

COVID-19 reminds us that we live in a co-creative universe that we are still learning about. To this day there is still no conclusive understanding of the origin(s) of viruses, how they first emerged and why they exist (e.g. the Progressive, Regressive and Virus-First Hypotheses) (Wessner 2010). We are only beginning to understand the role that viruses have played in the evolutionary web of life (Villarreal, 2008). Our experience of the disruption and pain wrought by this wildcard is born from the interplay between human ignorance and an active and creative cosmos. We did not fully understand the nature of the threats and issues, and we underappreciated the agentic complexity of our world. We are all learning. Perhaps these existential questions about viruses can help us to reframe viruses from "parasitic enemies" into something else, something bigger, that we and it are part of?

So our futures depend on how well we can learn from COVID-19. How can we use this as an opportunity to prepare us for change, to sensitize us to the variety of issues we need to learn about? How can we learn and dance with a co-creative cosmos rather than react and struggle against it? How can we turn COVID-19 into an, albeit painful, teacher, who can show us new paths toward collective health, wellbeing and solidarity? And how can we create the new methods and systems of anticipation that can protect us in years to come? These are some of the formidable questions and challenges we apply ourselves to in this anthology.

REFERENCES

Freire, P. (1973). *Education for Critical Consciousness*. Seabury Press.

Jung, C. G. (2012). *The Undiscovered Self*. Routledge and Kegan Paul.

Kupferschmidt, K. (2021, August 19). New SARS-CoV-2 variants have changed the pandemic. What will the virus do next? *Science | AAAS*. https://www.sciencemag.org/news/2021/08/new-sars-cov-2-variants-havechanged-pandemic-what-will-virus-do-next

Palmer, P. J. (2009). *A Hidden Wholeness: The Journey Toward an Undivided Life*. John Wiley & Sons.

Ramos, J. (2005). Futures Education as Temporal Conscientisation. *Social Alternatives*, 24(4), 25-31.

Thompson, W. I. (1985). *Pacific Shift*. Sierra Club Books.

Villarreal, L. P. (2004). Are Viruses Alive?. *Scientific American*, 291(6), 100-105.

Wessner, D. R. (2010) The Origins of Viruses. *Nature Education* 3(9), 37.

INFECTED BY THE FUTURE

Sohail Inayatullah

I was infected by the future through science fiction. I was in 9th grade at the International School of Islamabad taking a class in English literature. To spur us to read, our teacher Gordon Lindsay suggested strongly we read a book or two a week. For some this seemed over the top, and while this was initially true for me, once I discovered the works of Isaac Asimov, Ray Bradbury, Robert Heinlein, Eugene Zamyatin, Michael Crichton and others, there was no stopping. But why the fascination with science fiction? Our family's frame of reference was questioning the Western development model where particularly during dinner we would have robust discussions on imperialism and colonialism. The underlying narrative was that something was wrong with the world. It was unfair, not right. Science fiction, however, challenged me and shifted the discourse from conventional international relations to unconventional universal possibilities. It created a temporal distance from current affairs so that I could see the present as a particular reality, a fragile victory of one possible world over other presents and futures.

But perhaps my most vivid memory of the future was in my last year of high school at the International School of Kuala Lumpur. Our social studies teacher, Frank Shephard showed us a short video clip directed by Alvin Toffler. In that clip, a couple romantically walks through a forest. They sit to have a picnic. A soft melodious tune plays in the background. Finally, the camera moves from their backs to their faces. It is then we see that they are not humans but robots enjoying a day out at the park. This scene jarred me. It was later through the work of Michel Foucault (1984) and Michael Shapiro (1992) that I understood why. They had made the present remarkable. They had challenged our views of romance and of nature, forcing us to see ourselves and others differently.

By the time, I was a university student at the University of Hawaii, taking classes in Futures Studies was an easy segue. I was fortunate that the University had an established Futures Studies program led by James Dator. From him, we learned methods and tools and began to see the future not just as the realm of the fantastic but as worlds we could design and create (Dator, 1980). The world shifted from "it is not fair to we can create "the future we wish for".

Futures Studies also demanded we did not slide into worlds we did not want. Dator introduced us to numerous methods: three were critical. First was alternative futures or scenarios. This was the process of imagining different worlds so we could distance from the present. This was not the disinterest of the empirical sciences but the epistemological shift to changing horizons so we could better challenge the present and thus anticipate possible futures. Second was the work of Graham Molitor (2004) who suggested that while most focused on current problems and some on trends, the futurist needed to focus on emerging issues: low probability but high impacts events and processes. We need to use the future to reduce risks and increase opportunities, he argued. Lastly was visioning, the inner and outer process of visualizing desired futures, moving away from the world-as-given to the world-as-imagined.

The future for me had moved from the impossible of science fiction to the structured process of creating alternative and preferred futures. The infection had grown.

But not everyone was pleased. One of my professors strongly suggested that I was on the wrong path. The field he remarked, over and over, was "a can of worms". It was best that I leave and study more conventional areas of knowledge. The upheavals suggested by futurists in the 1970s - limits to growth, climate change, a world after capitalism, space travel, the human genome project, the end of American dominance, a world governance system, partnership economics - were unlikely, indeed, silly to ponder on.

I did not change disciplines. Indeed, clearly, he was wrong. The future from being a fascination for many has now shifted to what Anita Hazenburg at INTERPOL suggests a capability one must have (Sheraz, 2019; Vettorello, 2021). The rate of change, moving to what the Asian Philosopher P.R. Sarkar calls the galloping jump – epoch making eras, (Sarkar, 1987 p. 55) requires a futures focus. Studying the future is not just about understanding the structure of social and physical reality but about enhancing personal agency, our ability to shape time and space, to make a difference, to take personal and collective responsibility.

While many of the possibilities suggested by futurists decades ago have not occurred, we have seen the fall of the Berlin wall, the emergence of the Internet, The Asian Financial Crisis, the rise of Al-Qaeda and Daesh, SARS, the Global Financial Crisis, Fintech, the peer-to-peer revolution, the shift toward renewables, the hegemonic shift to China and East Asia, or the rise of fascism in previously democratic nations, COVID-19, and now the return of the Taliban. This is a dramatic period in human history. COVID-19 has accelerated this shift moving futurists from alchemists sitting in basements to being "front line" conceptual workers using foresight to help governments, international agencies, businesses, and individuals make sense of a changing world, indeed, to help make the transition to a sustainable and transformative world.

And how has COVID-19 infected the future? While the essays in this book discuss the politics, the scenarios, the warnings, and the disasters, there have been weak signals of possible pivots to a different future. Over the past year and a half, I have found individuals wishing to gain clarity on what is next, when will it be over, they ask? Some national governments understanding that this is the time to not just focus on the immediate firefighting but seriously take the long-term into consideration have accelerated 2050-2070 projects. One has focused on moving from GDP as the foundational measuring stick of progress to Well-being as the new national indicator. International development agencies have begun to see the crisis as a possible doorway to begin preparing for climate change, arguing that many more pandemics are on the way. Other groups have asked for help to understand the rise in conspiracy theorists. Many businesses have expressed a need to shift their core organizational metaphor, change how they see reality, so they can optimize and become ready for the next wave of change. Those who were caught out, surprised by COVID-19, wish to ensure they are ready for the next pandemic or crisis. Still others have understood that done well, the future and Futures Studies, can become institutionalized in their organization. All have been clear: the future has become infected. This can be a nasty and sinister experience, or this can begin a love affair with the possibility of creating a far better world.

To avoid the former and enhance the possibility of the latter, in our work, we do our best to help organizations and individuals move through various stages of futures thinking (Inayatullah, 2021). In the first, they are focused on "this is not fair, why has this occurred to me, to us". In the second, they seek to reduce risks from emerging issues: possible financial failures, pandemics, geo-political upheavals, demographic shifts, and new technologies. The goal is to avoid used futures, stranded assets, and psychic sunk costs. In the third, using alternative futures, we use scenarios to imagine and create new products and processes, indeed, new worlds. In the fourth stage, we focus on directionality, where do we wish to go, whom do we wish to become, what is our image of our preferred future? In the fifth stage, we make the vision real, to make the future not a pipedream but a tangible new reality. We go from the future to the present and create pathways. In this sixth, we go deeper and move to narrative, the underlying meaning system that supports the entire empirical edifice. We create stories that help in the transformation process. Finally, we move toward inner work, we transform our selves so we can become the future we wish to see. The journey thus starts out with individual and collective powerlessness, moves toward collective clarity and a culture of foresight, and concludes with personal mastery and then aligning the personal with our shared futures. In the latter stages, new ideas infect. This occurs at the intellectual level but as Sarkar suggests at the very deep unconscious, the microvita level of reality (Sarkar, 1987). Futures thinking thus intends to create interpretive frames that change who we were, who we are and who we can become.

We hope the essays that follow infect you with our enthusiasm for Futures Studies. We hope you can use the insights from these essays to help create a transformed world where we co-evolve with nature, technology, and spirit and the virus of the future infects us in transformative ways.

REFERENCES

Dator, J. (1980). Emerging issues Analysis. Honolulu: The Hawaii Judiciary.

Foucault, M. (1984). *The Foucault Reader*. Ed. Paul Rabinow. New York: Pantheon Books.

Inayatullah, S. (2021). *From Anticipation to Emancipation*. Monograph No. 1. Tamsui: Tamkang University.

Molitor, G. (2004). *The Power to Change the World: The Art of Forecasting*, Potomac: MD, Public Policy Forecasting.

Sarkar, P.R. (1987). *Microvitum in a Nutshell*. Kolkata: Ananda Marga Publications.

Sarkar, P.R. (1987). *Prout in a Nutshell,* Vol. 17. Kolkata: Ananda Marga Publications.

Shapiro, M. (1992). *Reading the Postmodern Polity: Political Theory as Textual Practice*. Minneapolis, MN: University of Minnesota Press.

Sheraz, U. (2019, 25 October). Exploring the future of INTERPOL and Policing: an interview with Anita Hazenburg. *Journal of Futures Studies*. Retrieved from https://jfsdigital.org/2019/10/25/exploring-the-future-of-interpol-and-policing-an-interview-with-anita-hazenberg/

Vettorello, M. (2021, 15 June). Anita Hazenburg: Police Futures. *Journal of Futures Studies*. The Briefing Today. Retrieved from https://jfsdigital.org/2021/06/21/thebriefingtoday/.

SENSING & SENSE MAKING

NEITHER A BLACK SWAN NOR A ZOMBIE APOCALYPSE:

The Futures of a World with the COVID-19 Coronavirus

Sohail Inayatullah & Peter Black

31 March, 2020

Our colleague Louis Zheng from the Shanghai FuturistCircle suggested that no one had predicted COVID-19 Coronavirus. "Is it a black swan?" he asked.[1]

Our response was that this is not a black swan, as a black swan event is defined as being unpredictable, a total surprise. The reason this coronavirus is not a black swan is that the emergence of another coronavirus was predicted by many working in the emerging infectious diseases (EIDs) field. Indeed, we argue that we need to be getting ready for the next "Corona".

1. The increasing rate of EIDs is well recorded in the scientific literature (Morse 1995).

2. Many agreed for some time that the most likely severe EIDs would be caused by RNA viruses as these have high rates of mutation (Cleaveland et al. 2001) and would emerge from animals. This simply reflects the recognition that more than 70% of recent EID events have their origins in animals (they are zoonotic) (Woolhouse and Gowtage-Sequeria 2005) with most originating principally from wildlife (Jones et al. 2008).

3. Coronaviruses were high on the list of likely candidates for causing an EID event. Severe Acute Respiratory Syndrome (SARS) emerged in 2003, Middle East Respiratory Syndrome (MERS) in 2012 – both caused by novel coronaviruses (Ge et al. 2013, Fan et al. 2019).

4. Bats as a likely source of viruses causing EIDs have also been well

recognized in the scientific literature (Olival et al. 2017).

5. Research on both SARS and zoonotic avian influenza identified infection spillover pathways that most often included 'wet markets' where live animals are frequently sold and slaughtered on site. In the case of zoonotic influenza, the spread of the virus to people was from poultry at live bird markets (i.e., wet market). For SARS, the initial spillover event occurred at a wet market containing wildlife when people were exposed to civets that were shedding the SARS coronavirus (Webster 2004). Although there has been work in trying to change wet markets (FAO 2015) and in some countries stop wet markets—especially where many species, including wildlife mix—this change has been difficult due to a range of social, economic and cultural factors. We anticipate in the short run these factors will reduce in importance, but insofar as "culture eats strategy for breakfast," they are likely to return without global institutional and cultural shifts.

All the above was known before COVID-19, so people working in the EID space were not surprised. The exact timing of emergence was not predicted, but nonetheless, the emergence of a novel coronavirus associated with wet markets containing wildlife was not unexpected at all (Fan et al. 2019).

Foresight, of course, is not about exact timing – that is market investment and stock trading. This is about creating the capacity to anticipate tomorrow's problems and act today. Thus, the seeds of this COVID-19 pandemic, the weak signals, have been present for a decade or more.

CULTURE EATS STRATEGY FOR BREAKFAST

Why then with this information are we now in the middle of a pandemic? Colleagues in the People's Republic of China (PRC) suggest that: Firstly, "it is related deeply to the Chinese eating culture – preference for fresh meat from animals butchered at the counter". Secondly, the memories of food crises in China remain. Third, there continues to be a level of mistrust of the government. For example, "residents have little knowledge of the frozen meat-producing process due to the lack of information transparency, thus, some ignore the regulations of the live animal ban in the wet markets." They are bounty hunters, focused on wealth creation, irrespective of the costs to the overall society.

Furthermore, many from rural areas live in the ancient episteme where the "liveness" of the animal leads to greater health as one is "eating" life. Thus, the initial lack of response speed can be explained not just by a culture where informing supervisors equates with a fear of losing one's job – but because parts of China live in different times. An ancient worldview, a communist worldview, and now a globalist worldview. Certainly, since the initial issue of transparency emerged, China's response has been robust and dynamic. The speed of virus spread has been dramatically reduced, giving the rest of the world a chance to mitigate.

Social problems emerge, or are difficult to address, where there are varying perspectives each often in tension with others. Interests and strategies are at locked horns or drawing the carriage in different directions.
This is illustrated in the Causal Layered Analysis (Inayatullah and Milojević, 2015) below. Six meta-perspectives are critical – the views from those who sell in wet markets; the views of those in the political bureaucracy (this helps explain the rise of COVID-19 in China early on in the outbreak and Iran, for example); the current strategy of slowing down the virus the Medieval; the Pharma perspective; the Market; and of course, the Citizen.

CLA	Wet market	Political bureaucracy	Public health	Pharma	Economic	Citizen
Litany	Continued wet markets	Information about disease not shared	Slow down the virus so systems can survive	Enlist medical and health systems to create the cure	Economic indicators – recession on the way	Fear and panic

System	Jobs in tension with the need to eliminate them. Outside of the law.	Job – fear of reprisal from those above	Quarantine, Social distancing, Surveillance, Lockdown, Flatten the curve. Use apps and Artificial Intelligence [AI]	Find the vaccine. Vaccinate all. Using new technologies to speed up solutions	Profits and interconnected systems cause downward pressure. Uncertainty driving market volatility.	Citizens looking for direction. Leaders uncertain of how to balance the economy and public health.
Worldview	Economic – wealth accumulation	Political – authoritarian	Medieval- Safety	Pharmaceutical – plus AI plus to some extent public health	Capitalist – markets	Citizen prefer flatter systems, but search for expertise
Myth/ metaphor	"Bounty hunters" "Show me the money"	"The big man"	"Breaking the chain of infection" "Slow down the fire"	"Silver bullet"	"Where to hide" – "opportunities everywhere"	"Whom do I trust"

Thus part of the challenge of a global response is that there are multiple worldviews operating, all with different interests.

While CLA helps us to understand the varying perspectives, scenarios help us address alternative trajectories.

WHAT THEN ARE THE SCENARIOS?

Based on the hundreds of articles, we see at least four possible futures.[2]

Zombie Apocalypse (CDC 2020). This future emerges because of the mutation of the virus plus xenophobia plus panic. Uncertainty leads to continued market crashes. Supply chains, tourism, travel, and conferences are all disrupted. A severe and long term recession, if not depression, results. Failure to act leads to a number of regime changes, as in Iran and the USA, to begin with. Wherever there are system stresses, they break. This is certainly how the future feels to many. The memory of earlier plagues remains at the inter-generational level. Fear and panic rule.

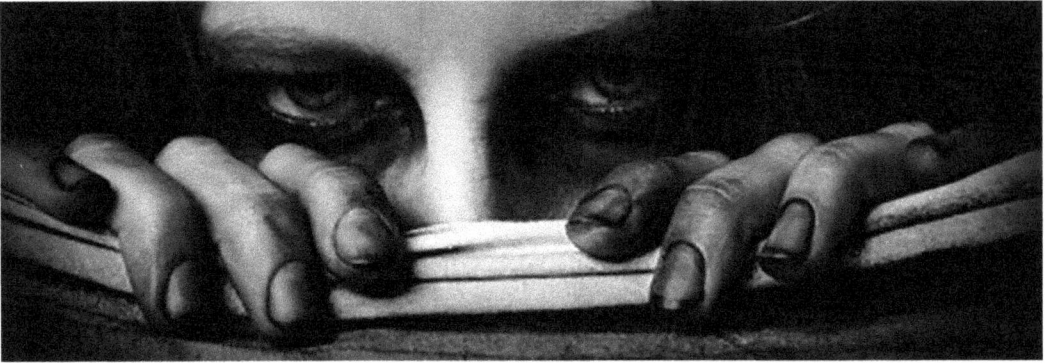

Image from https://www.cdc.gov/cpr/zombie/index.html

The Needed Pause. Efforts are made in most countries to 'flatten the curve' to help health systems cope. In the future, COVID-19 becomes just another winter flu – dangerous as it is for the elderly, those with underlying medical conditions and those who smoke. It is, however, solved and routinized within a year. Big Pharma sees the money-making opportunity and by 2021 a vaccine is available. In the meantime, the frenetic pace of everything slows down, with multiple benefits to the planet and personal health. Greenhouse gas emissions fall, for starters. Over-touristed cities like Venice get a break. Localization heals. People focus on their inner lives. More and more people meditate. For a short period, working from home becomes the norm. However, states still do not support employees in this process as trust is a factor. Thus, after the pause, back to business as usual. We slowed down in order to speed up again.

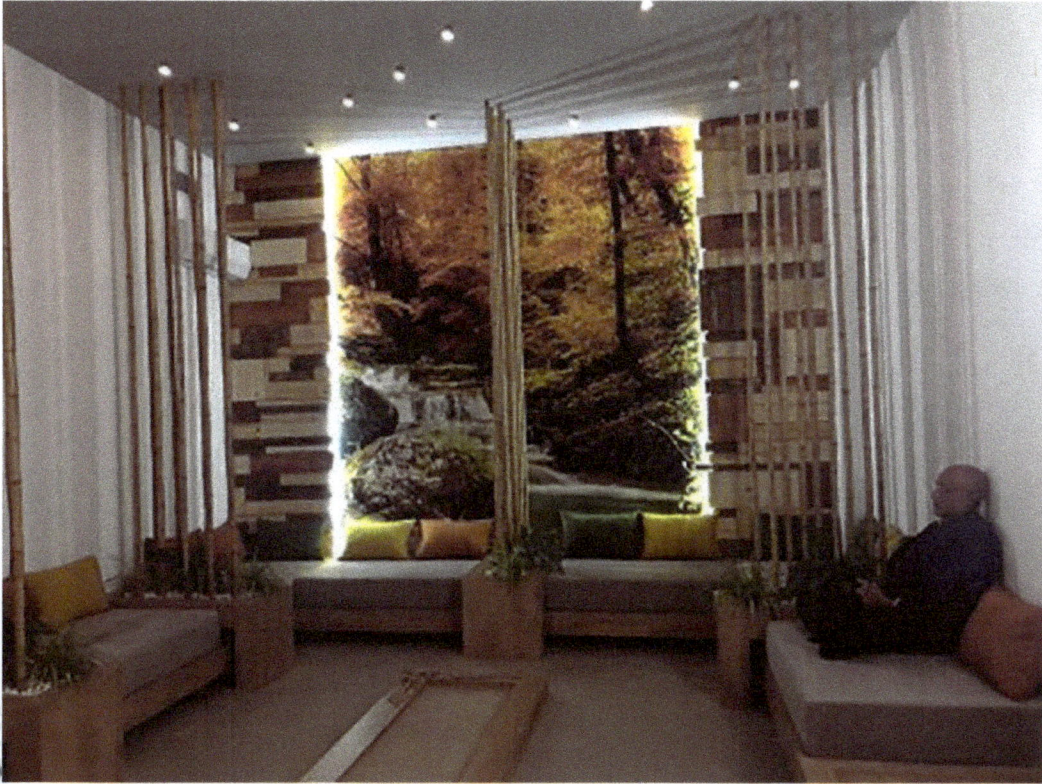

Global Health Awakening. Large AI companies, science, start-ups, and public health expertise come to the rescue. We truly enter the digital fourth wave era – genomics plus artificial intelligence (AI) help monitor and then prevent. The five 'p' health model – prevention, precision, participation, partnership, and personalization become the norm. There is a breakthrough after breakthrough with innovation (real-time detection, health monitoring using big data) cascading through the system. While the virus began in China, the nation leads in innovation as it is forced to adapt. Toynbee's creative minority via open-source science and technology lead the way. Working from home booms as new relationships between employer and employee are created. Universal basic income is supported as the strength of a society is based on how we treat the weakest; not how we glorify the strongest. Young people are no longer the future, but the present. This is the disruption that truly creates the fourth industrial revolution. Along with external innovation, there is inner innovation – a social revolution. Evidence-based science and technology inform public policy; not the whims of particular leaders. The insights from fighting COVID-19 are applied to climate change. There is a dramatic shift to plant-based diets. It is business transformed, social mutation,[3] not back to usual. There are, however, concerns about privacy.

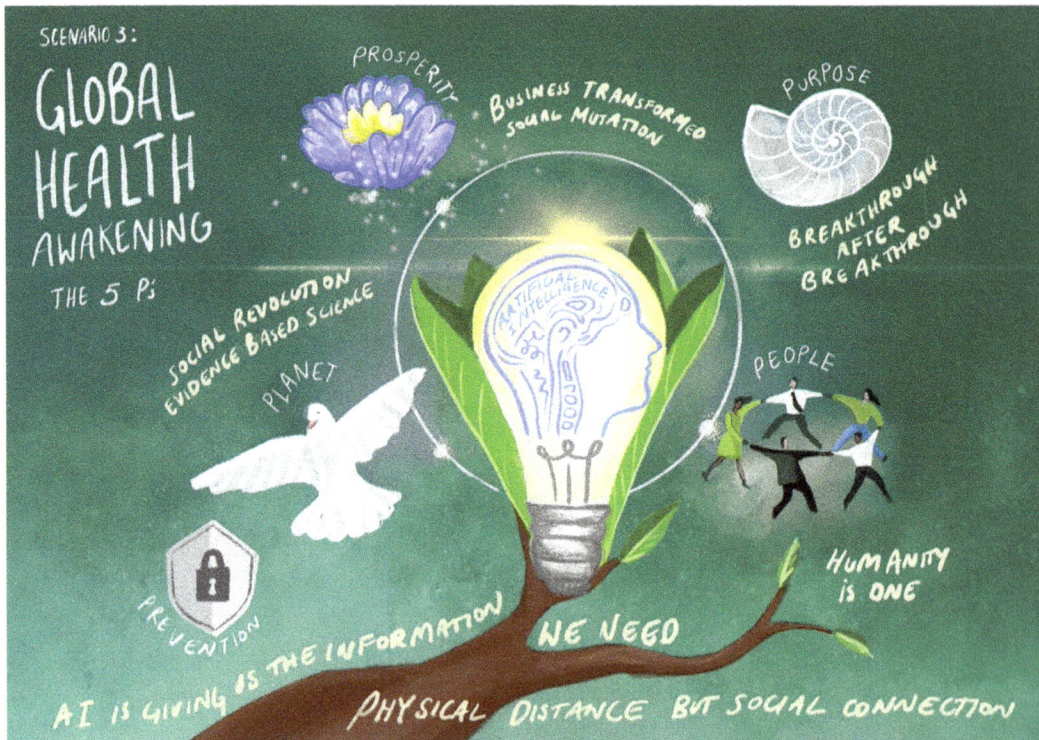

SCENARIO 3:
GLOBAL HEALTH AWAKENING
THE 5 P's
PROSPERITY
BUSINESS TRANSFORMED SOCIAL MUTATION
PURPOSE
BREAKTHROUGH AFTER BREAKTHROUGH
SOCIAL REVOLUTION EVIDENCE BASED SCIENCE
ARTIFICIAL INTELLIGENCE
PEOPLE
PLANET
HUMANITY IS ONE
PREVENTION
AI IS GIVING US THE INFORMATION WE NEED
PHYSICAL DISTANCE BUT SOCIAL CONNECTION

Illustration: Charmine Sevil

The Great Despair. Not an apocalypse, not a depression, no magic – just a slow and marked decline of health and wealth. Walls appear everywhere. The World Health Organization and others try to contain, but the virus repeatedly slips in and infects the bodies, minds, and hearts of all. Back to the European Middle Ages. The efforts to address fail. The least connected to globalization fare the best. The vulnerable are forgotten. Inter-generational memory of past pandemics inform.

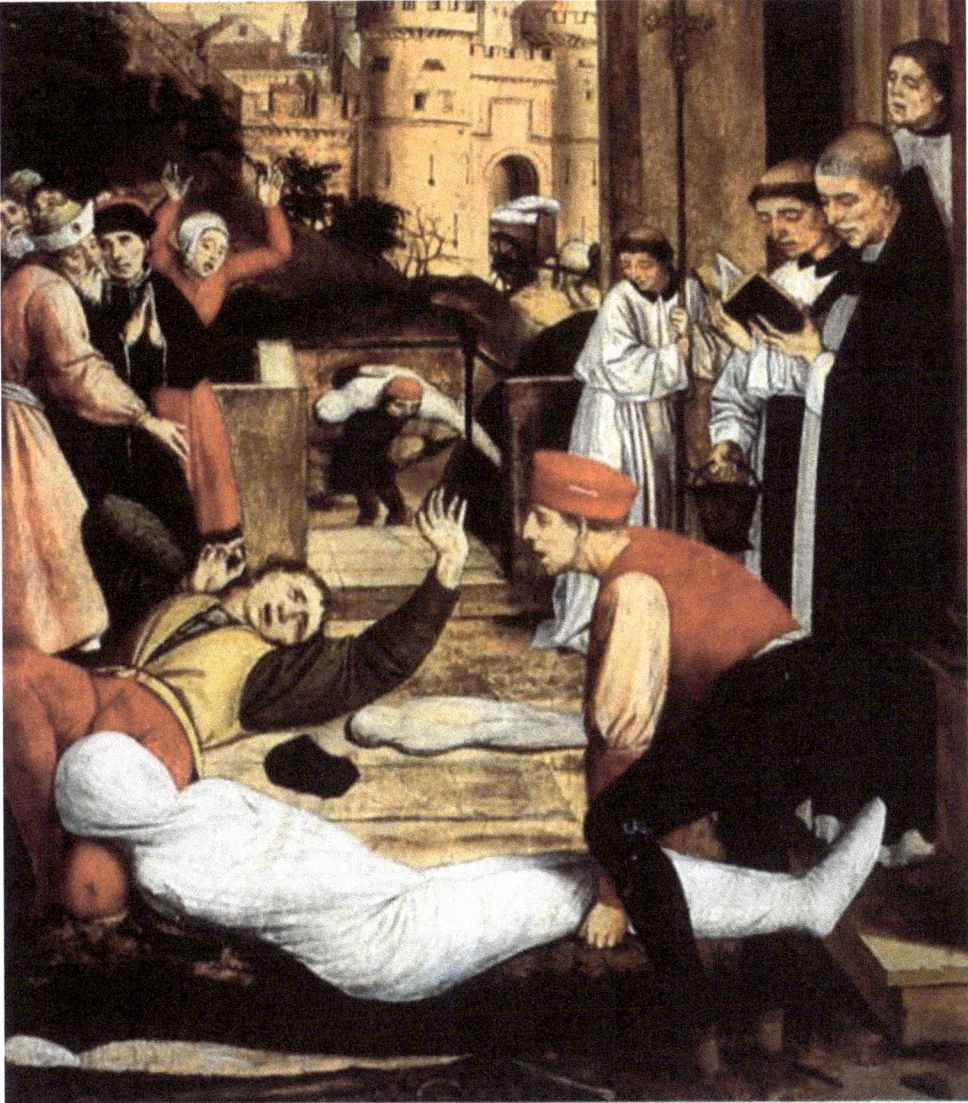

Saint Sebastian Interceding for the Plague Stricken. Josse Lieferinxe, 1497–1499, The Walters Art Museum

Depending on one's worldview the future looks very different. Certainly, the first scenario represents emotional fears. The Needed Pause and Global Health Awakening are based on breakthroughs in science and technology by Big pharma and Tech with varying levels of individual and social intervention. The Great Despair represents a failure to wisely act.

CONCLUSION & NEXT STEPS

To prevent the next outbreak, **first,** a global ban on wet markets and trade in wildlife with real help to transition sellers so they are not impoverished. This is a huge undertaking as both the number of people involved in the wildlife trade and its global economic value are enormous. China's wildlife industry alone is valued at $74 billion USD. However, the cost to China of this outbreak will be many times larger than this, even if only taking account of losses associated with tourism and consumer spending (South China Morning Post 22 and 24 February 2020 as cited in Machalaba and Karesh 2020).

However, there are potential barriers: Even though banning wildlife trade may make economic sense, there could be a cultural backlash – 'Why should I have to live without access to the foods that make me strong. This is the West dictating too much about my lifestyle!'

Irrespective of the success of banning the wet markets and trade in wildlife, the economic costs of this COVID-19 pandemic will be debated and analyzed in great detail. The argument will most likely be made to invest in the same strategies that were suggested post-SARS, and the influenza H1N1 pandemic of 2009 — strategies that were only partially funded and implemented. That is, there will be a support to continue with the status quo and steady the ship by ensuring countries can all meet the International Health Regulations and 'manage' the next epidemic or pandemic challenge.

Second, there should be increased interest in detecting disease, even earlier, especially in areas of increased risk of emergence and disease spillover. This will likely support full investment in new technologies such Next Generation Sequencing (NGS), Big Data, AI and AI combined apps that can detect diseases.

Third —and critically—will be the increased investment in real prevention strategies that acknowledge that the majority of zoonotic pathogens have emerged as a result of changes to food production, agriculture, land use and contact with wildlife (Allen et al. 2017). This could result for example, in the creation of buffer zones between wildlife and human settlements, or cost-benefit studies of new agricultural projects and land-use change that take into account increased EID risk, such as COVID 19. Even more fundamentally, real prevention strategies will mean re-thinking the current "more, more, more" development model. Taking an Eco-health view, we argue that Nature strikes back. Always.

In conclusion: this crisis is a health crisis but, of course, it is much more. It is about leadership and governance, about what type of world we wish to live in. It is a test of the creation of a planetary civilization, working together to solve problems. If we do not succeed, the next 'Corona' is just around the corner.

AUTHORS

Sohail Inayatullah, UNESCO Chair in Futures Studies, Sejahtera Centre for Sustainability and Humanity, Malaysia, Professor, Tamkang University, Taiwan and Associate, Melbourne Business School, the University of Melbourne. sinayatullah@gmail.com. www.metafuture.org

Dr. Peter Black, One Health Foresight Consultant and Veterinary Epidemiologist peter@essentialforesight.com www.essentialforesight.com

Special thanks to Russell Clemens for copy editing the manuscript

REFERENCES

Allen, T., Murray, K.A., Zambrana-Torrelio, C., Morse, S.S, Rondinini, C, Di Marco, M., Breit N., Olival,K.J., and Daszak,P. (2017) Global hotspots and correlates of emerging zoonotic diseases. *Nature Communications 8,* Article 1124. https://doi.org/10.1038/s41467-017-00923-8

Centre for Disease Control and Prevention. (2020) *Zombie Preparedness*. https://www.cdc.gov/ cpr/zombie/index.htm

Cleaveland S., Laurenson, M.K., Taylor, L.H. (2001) Diseases of humans and their domestic mammals: pathogen characteristics, host range and the risk of emergence. Philosophical Transactions of the Royal Society B Biological Sciences,356 (1411), 991-999. https://doi.org/10.1098/rstb.2001.0889

Fan, Y., Zhao, K., Shi, Z.-L. and Zhou, P. (2019) Bat Coronaviruses in China. *Viruses*, 11 (3), 210. https://doi.org/10.3390/v11030210

Ge, X., Li, J., Yang, X., Chmura, A.A, Zhu G., Epstein, J.H., Mazet,J.K., Hu, Zhang, W., Cheng, P., Zhang, Y., Luo, C., Tan, B., Wang, N., Zhu, Z., Crameri, G., Zhang, S., Wang, L., Daszak, P and Shi, Z.-L. (2013) Isolation and characterization of a bat SARS-like coronavirus that uses the ACE2 receptor. *Nature* 503, 535–538 https://doi.org/10.1038/nature12711

Jones, K., Patel, N., Levy, M., Storeygard, A., Balk, D., Gittleman, J.L. and Daszak, P. (2008) Global trends in emerging infectious diseases. *Nature* 451, 990–993. https://doi.org/10.1038/nature06536

Inayatullah, S. & Milojević, I. (2015). CLA 2.0: Transformative Research in Theory and Practice. Tamkang University Press.

Machalaba, C. and Karesh, W.B. (2020, March 6) Fight Pandemics Like Wildfires With Prevention and a Plan to Share the Costs, *Foreign Affairs* https://www.foreignaffairs.com/articles/2020-03-06/fight-pandemics-wildfires

Morse SS. (1995) Factors in the Emergence of Infectious Diseases. *Emerging Infectious Diseases* 1(1):7-15. https://doi.org/10.3201/eid0101.950102

Olival, K.J., Hosseini, P.R., Zambrana-Torrelio, C., Ross, N., Bogich T.L. and Dszak, P. (2017) Host and viral traits predict zoonotic spillover from mammals. *Nature* 546, 646–650 (2017). https://doi.org/10.1038/nature22975

Leng, S. (2020, February 22) Coronavirus: China's economy lost US$196 billion in January, February, says ex-IMF official. *South China Morning Post* https://www.scmp.com/economy/china-economy/article/3051909/covid-19-likely-slash-us185-billion-chinas-economy-january

Xie, E. (2020, February 24) China bans trade, eating of wild animals in battle against coronavirus.*South China Morning Post*. https://www.scmp.com/news/china/article/3052151/china-bans-trade-eating-wild-animals-battle-against-coronavirus

Webster, R.G. (2004) Wet markets—a continuing source of severe acute respiratory syndrome and influenza? *The Lancet*, 363, Issue 9404, 17 January 2004, 234-236. https://doi.org/10.1016/S0140-6736(03)15329-9

Woolhouse, M., & Gowtage-Sequeria, S. (2005). Host Range and Emerging and Reemerging Pathogens. *Emerging Infectious Diseases*, 11(12), 1842-1847. https://doi.org/10.3201/eid1112.050997

United Nations Food and Agriculture Organization (2015) *Biosecurity guide for live poultry markets*. FAO Animal Production and Health Guidelines No. 17. http://www.fao.org/3/a-i5029e.pdf.

NOTES

1.Personal email. February 10, 2020

2.These are best used as points of departure, to capture uncertainty and create alternative futures

3.To use the words of Satya Tanner. Facebook post. March 6, 2020.

LET'S TAKE BOLD ACTION ON HEALTH TO AVOID FUTURE PANDEMICS

Susann Roth & Najibullah Habib

20 mar. 2020

T he COVID-19 pandemic could be an opportunity to take a more holistic approach to health and well-being, invest in health systems and in resilient supply chains.

Viruses that cause new diseases like COVID-19 are unpredictable. Their impact depends partly on population dynamics, partly on demographics and behavior, and of course on the nature of the virus itself. We don't know the virus well enough to know what it will do next, or to say with certainty how we can best protect high-risk groups.

What we do know is that bold actions are needed to contain and defeat this and future pandemics. Dealing with risk factors driving infections requires strong leadership, quick decisions based on scientific evidence, and the full cooperation of national and local governments, as well as people.

Based on our experience, the impacts of national responses to epidemics are often short-lived. Over time, the crisis fades and we forget what it takes to establish fast emergency response capacity, strengthen health systems and ensure population health for the long-term.

This needs to change, particularly in Asia and the Pacific which faces a confluence of risk factors including environmental degradation, climate change, air pollution, cross-border threats, urbanization, population density, global air travel, and trade.

Long-term solutions will only emerge if we expand our understanding of infectious disease risks. So let's look at three important risk factors that drive infections.

The first and most important is a person's overall health. How strong is one's immune system? It is the first line of defense against infectious agents. In cities across the region, air pollution takes a toll on our respiratory system's ability to respond effectively to infectious agents.

Unhealthy living conditions, stress and sleep deprivation weaken people's immune systems and well-being. In addition, rising levels of non-communicable diseases caused by bad diet and unhealthy habits such as smoking and excessive alcohol consumption contribute to poor health, making the population even more vulnerable to infectious diseases like COVID-19.

Second, the likelihood that people will infect each other. This is driven by the virulence of the contagion but also more importantly by behavior. In this region, we often have densely populated urban areas which bring together many people who can infect each other. Trying to manage human interaction leads to social distancing, banning of air travel, closing of borders.

Will these drastic measures be worthwhile considering the harm they can bring, especially on the poor? Will more people suffer from bankruptcy rather than from illness as a result of the containment measures? We don't know yet.

Third, infections can multiply in health care facilities without interventions such as infection prevention and control through personal protective equipment, isolation, decentralized COVID-19 testing and proper triaging of patients. Many hospitals particularly in developing Asia do not follow international best practices in this regard, and global supplies of personal protective equipment are overstretched. Hence, the people you need most in a pandemic – doctors, nurses and health care workers – will fall ill first. This puts already weak health systems at risk of collapsing and failing to provide essential services.

Countries in Asia have valuable lessons to share. These include expanded testing of the population for COVID-19 at no cost in order to help authorities track the progress of the disease and determine whether health interventions are working.

Travel restrictions and strict quarantines, applied rigorously, have been proven to slow the disease and flatten the curve to prevent health services from being overburdened.

Some Asian countries have independently-managed public health bodies that report directly to the top leadership of the country to ensure quick action and reduce red tape. Emergency procurement mechanisms and market protection to allow the fast purchase of goods and even advanced market commitments for vaccines are other important tools. Transparent communication of risks and frequent updates to the public bolster people's confidence in the government's response.

These are important responses, but in the long run we need deeper policy shifts to ward off future outbreaks. We can start with these:

- **Get back to basics.** Take a holistic view of population health and not just medical care. We need clean air in our cities, the promotion of healthy lifestyles, the reduction of harmful food choices and policies that foster wellbeing to prevent people from falling ill in the first place. We need to invest in high quality health care which focuses on health promotion and disease prevention, as well as decentralized and cost-effective primary health care.

- **Manage the confluence of risks**. Risks are multiplying as our world is increasingly interconnected through travel, trade and tourism. Evidence-based management of epidemics using scenario planning and risk assessments can help. The economic impact hits the most vulnerable: daily-wage workers, factory workers, small business owners, gig economy workers, and the self-employed. Coordinated approaches by multiple actors such as the government, private sector and civil society, can help manage the multitude of risks.

The COVID-19 pandemic is an unfolding global crisis. But it is also an opportunity to take a more holistic approach to health and well-being, invest in health systems and in resilient supply chains for the long-term benefit of all.

NOTE

This essay was originally published at the Asian Development Bank Blog on 20 March 2020
https://blogs.adb.org/blog/lets-take-bold-action-health-avoid-future-pandemics

COVID-19 BOTH IS AND IS NOT A BLACK SWAN (AND THAT'S OK):

Futures within and Beyond a Time of Crisis

John A. Sweeney

03/23/2020

We were **warned**

This was the title for a March 18, 2020 article in *The Atlantic* outlining the many and varied warnings about the "next plague" put forward by numerous analysts, futurists, government agencies, journalists, public intellectuals, and researchers. (Alexander 2020; Gates 2015; Yong 2018). Friedman's piece focuses squarely on the United States and its responsiveness capacity for such an outbreak, which, as the article notes, was intentionally dismantled in recent years. Why any government would intentionally weaken its capacity for responding to such a crisis might come as more than curious given the aforementioned warnings, say nothing of the recent anniversary of the Spanish Flu, but with regards to the crises facing the United States, of which there are many, the thin line between comedy and tragedy becomes most apparent when one considers a October 2019 simulation run by the Center for Strategic and International Studies (Brannen and Hicks 2020). With an extremely prescient focus on the effects of a highly-contagious novel coronavirus, this exercise raised a number of critical areas of concern: the need for early action; diminishing trust in institutions; and the need for meaningful international cooperation. None of these, say nothing of the "pandemic playbook" left by the Obama Administration, were taken into consideration (Knight 2020).

Few individuals have been as outspoken about the catastrophic risks associated with a pandemic than Bill Gates, whose foundation works extensively on public health issues. In a TED talk, which has been viewed over 28 million times on YouTube, Gates highlighted the imminent and existential threat of "not missiles, but microbes" (Gates 2015). In spite of the many and varied presentations, reports, scenarios, simulations, and workshops focused on the next outbreak, none of these prognostications predicted "the" future. This is not, however, an indictment of *futures* (herein used as an umbrella term for futures studies, strategic foresight, anticipation, etc.). Quite the contrary: the lack of ability for futures to "predict" is not a bug but rather its most prominent feature. While there continues to be a great deal of uncertainty, particularly concerning the many crises spurred by the pandemic, one thing has become crystal clear: futures does work. But, not in the way that some, if not many, want or think it should.

Futures (again, broadly defined) approaches and practices succeeded in helping many people think through some potential effects, engage with and navigate the uncertainties inherent to an exceedingly complex crisis, and create critical and creative learning for how one might enable certain futures and disable others. This last point is especially evident in contexts where early action and mitigation measures were implemented. Take Taiwan, whose pandemic response plan boasted 124 unique action items (Aspinwall 2020). Learning lessons from the 2002-2004 SARS outbreak, the Taiwanese government created a National Health Command Center, which was tasked with leading responses by coordinating communication and action between local, regional, and central authorities (Wang et al. 2020). Interestingly, a 2015 European Commission analysis of lessons for policy-makers pointed out that while there have only been a few foresight activities linked directly to policy-making in Taiwan, the more than two decade history of teaching futures at Tamkang University, which was integral in organizing the Asia-Pacific Futures Network, has led to an "infiltration" of futures at a systemic level (Cuhls et al. 2015). Correlation is not the same as causation, and there is another "c" word worth considering: culture. The case of Taiwan emphasizes the critical importance of diffusing futures as a capacity/capability within government and beyond, which is to say that for futures to have an impact, it must become an aspect of culture itself. Emphasizing perspective (Taiwan as an island) and context (proximity to high-risk outbreak areas), Taiwan forged a forward-looking culture who took the necessary steps to prepare for what might lie ahead. Furthermore, Taiwan's pandemic response highlights the importance of hindsight, learning lessons from the past, which raises a question: what learning will be passed forward from our current crisis?

If one learning gets passed forward, it must be that the world is not beholden to our imaginings of it, whether historical, contemporary, and/or speculative. In spite of a novel coronavirus-driven outbreak being widely anticipated, futures ought (and must) continue to refrain from positioning itself as a "predictive science," which has long been pointed out and continues to be a foolhardy enterprise (Slaughter 1998). From spotting emerging issues to mapping trends and challenging assumptions to illuminating blindspots, futures is ultimately a learning process by which we come to realize that we do not and cannot have control over "the" future. Taking this point further, and as enshrined within Dator's "Laws" of the Future, it is still very much the case that "the" future does not exist, which is why exploring alternative futures is an absolute necessity (Dator et al. 2015). And, rather than condemning us to ignorance, this contention contains a truth bathed in hope. Were "the" future to exist, then it would be something beyond our ability to shape; *our* future would be a mere inevitability. If one operates from the assumption that "the" future does not exist, then agency to take action and shape the future is not only possible; it becomes a constitutive aspect of our humanity, especially within a time of crisis.

BOTH/AND

During the early days of the pandemic a question began to circulate across numerous social media profiles: was the COVID-19 pandemic a black swan? In early March, the influential venture capital firm, Sequoia, sent out a note, which was later published publicly, entitled "Coronavirus: The Black Swan of 2020." Outlining a few of the probable, but also cascadings, effects of the pandemic, Sequoia likened the pandemic to the 2008 Financial Crisis but also encouraged its Silicon Valley-minded partners to "Stay healthy, keep your company healthy, and put a dent in the world" (Sequoia 2020). As the outbreak bloomed into a full blown pandemic, many, if not most, futurists were quick to point out that the coronavirus pandemic was "not" a black swan. Given the aforementioned warnings, reports, simulations, and various other engagements aimed at anticipating just such an event, the pandemic did not put a (conceptual) dent in the world, especially when one considers the ongoing and growing impacts of our collective climate emergency. However, amongst the global futures community (again, broadly defined), an uneasy consensus began to emerge. Even Taleb, whose namesake book arguably catapulted the metaphor to widespread recognition, delivered a verdict: COVID-19 was indeed "not" a black swan (Avishai 2020). Although Taleb's definition of what constitutes a black swan has changed over time, which has led to the advent of gray and even, more recently, "white" swans, the black swan metaphor remains the most popular metaphoric marker [Taleb 2007]. Black swans, according to Taleb, have three core attributes:

- Must be considered an outlier
- Must have an extreme impact
- Must be retrospectively predictable

One of the main challenges of the black swan metaphor has to do with the ease with which it is invoked. Indeed, "black swan" has become an all-too-common placeholder for any and all surprises, which is to say that Taleb's somewhat technical three-part definition does not always get referenced. Another challenge in using this metaphor as a universal construct is that Taleb's criteria are provided independent of perspective and context, which is to say that the simple question *"for whom?"* not merely complicates using the black swan metaphor; it explodes the binary thinking underlying such a question. Explicitly, the question is premised on the false assumption that everyone not only sees the same thing but sees it in the same way. Rather, the question "for whom might Covid19 be a black swan?" opens up a space to explore the complexities and contextualities of a global event from a variety of perspectives while paying attention to the role and importance of context. Implicitly, the either/or question positions, even if indirectly, futures as an activity centered on predicting/forecasting "the" future, which is certainly not the case. And, perhaps more importantly, this is not the conversation that futurists should want to have, drive, and/or promote.

As the title for this piece suggests, I propose a *both/and* position in order to counter the assumptions underlying the question itself, which is an approach inherent to Narrative Foresight. A brief reflection on the particulars of this approach is merited as Narrative Foresight has developed into a robust area of futures research and practice that blends "empirical, interpretive, critical, and action learning modes" [Milojević and Inayatullah 2015, 152]. As a hybridized and, perhaps most importantly, living pedagogy, Narrative Foresight not only deepens the ways with which futures can and might be analyzed, created, and envisioned; it facilitates critical and creative thinking for framing and reframing both alternative and even preferred futures.

The critical importance of story as a means not only to frame but also reframe is actually something that Taleb himself noted in the prologue of *The Black Swan: the impact of the highly improbable,* although the book takes on the "narrative fallacy" head on and lambasts the power of storytelling. In a passage worth quoting in full, He confesses:

> The philosopher Edna Ullmann-Margalit detected an inconsistency in this book and asked me to justify the use of the precise metaphor of a Black Swan to describe the unknown, the abstract, and imprecise uncertain— white ravens, pink elephants, or evaporating denizens of a remote planet orbiting Tau Ceti. Indeed, she caught me red handed. There is a contradiction; this book is a story, and I prefer to use stories and vignettes to illustrate our gullibility about stories and our preference for the dangerous compression of narratives. You need a story to displace a story. Metaphors and stories are far more potent (alas) than ideas; they are also easier to remember and more fun to read. If I have to go after what I call the narrative disciplines, my best tool is a narrative. Ideas come and go, stories stay (2007, xxvii).

Taleb fails to divine a critical insight delivered by Narrative Foresight: "narratives of the future can also be used to disrupt these attempts to colonise through surfacing problematic assumptions in order to explore alternative scenarios and then move toward preferred futures" (Milojević and Inayatullah 2015, 160). This is perhaps the greatest point of derivation between Narrative Foresight and Taleb, although the latter shares the former's disdain for prediction and all it assumes/ entails. If one calls the very question (was the coronavirus pandemic a black swan?) into question through a Narrative Foresight lens, then the contention that Covid19 both is and is not a black swan becomes the most reasonable, rigorous, and responsible point of view. Let me explain.

REASONABLE, RESPONSIBLE, & RIGOROUS

A *both/and* point of view is *reasonable* in the sense that it is quite unreasonable to universalize a single metaphor without taking into account perspective and context. Metaphors are not immutable Platonic forms but, as noted above, meaning-giving and sense-making lenses from which to reflect and see anew. Given that the story behind the black swan metaphor is itself a lesson in the importance of perspective and the natural limits of our contextual awareness, it is reasonable to suggest that all metaphors have inherent limits, not in what they might help us *imagine* but rather in how they might help us *define*. Reflecting on the metaphors we use to frame and reframe should instill an abiding sense of hubris for the language employed to make sense of complex phenomena as well as possibilities for what might lie ahead. One of the key aspects of futures/foresight work is to call into question what is obvious (normal as well, and more on that below), to test the limits of what is (and is not) reasonable, and to widen one's scope of awareness such that one considers a greater range of potentialities.

A *both/and* point of view is rigorous in that it allows, daresay demands, for a more complex, and arguably more useful, framing of the pandemic and its cascading effects. The process by which come to understand possibilities for the future(s)—whether we are scoping out an area/sector/issue to explore or engaging in the practice of horizon scanning—is one that requires us to engage not just with a single trend or emerging issue but rather to consider how possibilities and potentialities are embedded within a variety of systems and influenced by a range of factors and forces. As such, it is essential not just to "see" something but to understand how one "sees" it, which is why multiple metaphors are useful to frame and reframe trajectories for phenomena to mutate as well as reorient our perceptions about such phenomena. This has led some, myself included, to employ and ultimately support a "menagerie" approach to framing both trends and emerging issues (Sardar and Sweeney 2016). Situating the pandemic as a black swan, grey rhino, black elephant, black dog, and/or black jellyfish has nothing to do with "getting it right" but rather generating further insights by taking on and conceptualizing possibilities through divergent perspectives (Wucker 2016; Camacho 2018; Serra del Pino et al. 2020). Indeed, one person's black swan can and might be another's gray swan, and vice versa. Conceptual framings and reframings that enliven, rather than collapse, possibilities by emphasizing perspective and context is a means to enhance the rigor with which futures, both alternative and preferred, are imagined, which is essential during a time of crisis.

A *both/and* point of view is responsible in the sense that futurists must do all they can to keep the future(s) plural, even and perhaps especially during times of crisis. Perhaps the futures field has become too beholden to the black swan metaphor. This is not to say that the metaphor itself does not have value, but the repeated and widespread invocation of it during the early days of the pandemic points toward what Riel Miller calls the "poverty of the imagination" (Miller 2018). Perhaps the most impoverished, if not irresponsible, imaginings for what might lie ahead are those seeking for things to go back to "normal," which many have noted was part, if not the whole, of the problem (Lichfield 2020; Roy 2020). As such, those engaging in futures work must take on the responsibility of imagining truly alternative futures, including and especially those that delve into the complex potentialities emanating from our all-too-postnormal times.

Encapsulating this contention and highlighting the impoverishing contagion that infects imaginings of the future, Dator argues, "Declarations about The Future are full of references to 'most likely futures,' 'least likely futures,' 'probable futures,' 'worst case scenarios,' 'wild cards,' 'black swans,' and a myriad of other metaphors, all of which are based on the assumption that there is a 'normal future' compared to which all other futures are deviations" (Dator 2016). A *both/and* point of view does not make Dator's contention that there is "no normal future" any less terrifying, or stupefying for that matter, for those yearning for the familiarities of our pre-pandemic world. But, it does provide a means to imagine futures within and beyond a time of crisis that are not beholden to the conditions and currents that facilitated and accelerated the COVID-19 pandemic as well as its accompanying impacts and implications, and that's ok.

LOOKING BACK / FORWARD: JUNE 2021 REFLECTIONS

Taking the opportunity to look back, both on the original piece and this edited version, which was initially drafted in late 2020, one thing has become clear: the turn to identify the COVID-19 pandemic as a black swan, or not, had much more to do with epistemological, if not ontological, comfort than any sort of form of theoretical provenance, which raises some critical questions: can the trappings of simplistic framings be avoided, especially in times of abject crisis? From a practitioner's perspective, how can one balance communicating efficacy (futures/ foresight "works") without engendering a false sense of assurity (e.g. predictive science)? Are clients prepared to hear the truth? Of course, these are perennial questions and not necessarily particular to our current moment, although there is an intensity to them that is precisely felt given how things have unfolded and continue to play out.

In the 15 months since this piece was originally published online, the U.S. has done an "about face" as vaccination rates have grown exponentially, and concerns remain about reaching herd immunity nationally and the Delta variant, which is not only more transmissible but also appears to be more virulent making some vaccines less effective (Elamroussi 2021; Sheikh et al. 2021). With that said, the U.S. appears to be at the precipice of "managing" the crisis in a way that would have seemed (to some) unthinkable just a short time (if not a Presidential Administration) ago. What can and might constitute a black swan (and for whom) can change rapidly. Consider the January 6th attack on the U.S. Capitol, which likely struck many as a black swan, although there have been plentiful pontifications on the weaponization of social media and imminent violence rooted in Trump's vitriolic rhetoric (Sweeney 2015; Editorial Board 2020).

Taking the above into consideration, one absolutely crucial question comes to the fore: is there anything that Jim Dator is wrong about? The presumptions underlying simplified applications of the black swan concept are rooted in a litany of anticipatory assumptions about the future that are not ok.

AUTHOR

John A. Sweeney, Al-Farabi Kazakh National University. Westminster International University in Tashkent

REFERENCES

Alexander, B. (2020, March 10). Coronavirus and the World: How Futurists Have Been Working on This Kind of Thing for Years. *Bryan Alexander*. https://bryanalexander.org/futures/coronavirus-and-the-world-how-futurists-have-been-working-on-this-kind-of-thing-for-years/

Aspinwall, N. (2020, April 9). Taiwan Is Exporting Its Coronavirus Successes to the World. *Foreign Policy*. https://foreignpolicy.com/2020/04/09/taiwan-is-exporting-its-coronavirus-successes-to-the-world/

Avishai, B. (2020). The Pandemic Isn't a Black Swan but a Portent of a More Fragile Global System. *The New Yorker*. https://www.newyorker.com/news/daily-comment/the-pandemic-isnt-a-black-swan-but-a-portent-of-a-more-fragile-global-system

Brannen, S., and Hicks, K. (2020). We Predicted a Coronavirus Pandemic. Here's What Policymakers Could Have Seen Coming. *POLITICO*. https://www.politico.com/news/magazine/2020/03/07/coronavirus-epidemic-prediction-policy-advice-121172

Camacho, J. [@j_camachor] (2018, August 11). After the #19S earthquake in CDMX, I was trying to make sense of it based on @CPPFS's "Menagerie of postnormal potentialities." But I realized that it was a whole different animal: a #BlackDog, a 'known known' with dire consequences due to negligence. [Thumbnail with link attached] [Tweet]. *Twitter*. https://twitter.com/j_camachor/status/1028030724081897472.

Cuhls, K., European Commission, Directorate-General for Research and Innovation, and Innovation Research and Science Policy Experts (RISE). (2015). *Bringing Foresight to Decision-Making Lessons for Policy-Making from Selected Non-European Countries*. Luxembourg Publications Office.

Dator, J.A., Sweeney, J.A., and Yee, A.M. (2015). *Mutative Media*. Springer International Publishing.

Dator, J. (2016). No Normal Future. *MISC*. https://miscmagazine.com/no-normal-future/.

Editorial Board. (2020, December 9). The Danger Is Growing That Trump's Lies about the Election Will Lead to Violence. *Washington Post*. https://www.washingtonpost.com/opinions/the-danger-is-growing-that-trumps-lies-about-the-election-will-lead-to-violence/2020/12/09/cf71d6f0-3a61-11eb-9276-ae0ca72729be_story.html

Elamroussi, A. (2021, June 19). US Coronavirus: The US Marks a Vaccine Milestone, but One Expert Warns That the Coronavirus Delta Variant Has a Worrying Impact on Patients. *CNN*. https://edition.cnn.com/2021/06/19/health/us-coronavirus-saturday/index.html

Friedman, U. (2020, March 18). We Were Warned. *The Atlantic*. https://www.theatlantic.com/politics/archive/2020/03/pandemic-coronavirus-united-states-trump-cdc/608215/

Gates, B. (2015, April 3). The Next Outbreak? We're Not Ready [Video]. *YouTube*. https://www.youtube.com/watch?v=6Af6b_wyiwl

Knight, V. (2020, May 15). Obama Team Left Pandemic Playbook for Trump Administration, Officials Confirm. *PBS NewsHour*. https://www.pbs.org/newshour/nation/obama-team-left-pandemic-playbook-for-trump-administration-officials-confirm

Lichfield, G. (2020, March 17). We're Not Going Back to Normal. *MIT Technology Review*. https://www.technologyreview.com/2020/03/17/905264/coronavirus-pandemic-social-distancing-18-months/

Pearce, K. (2019, November 6). Pandemic Simulation Exercise Spotlights Massive Preparedness Gap. *The Hub*. https://hub.jhu.edu/2019/11/06/event-201-health-security/

Roy, A. (2020, April 3). The Pandemic Is a Portal. *Financial Times*. https://www.ft.com/content/10d8f5e8-74eb-11ea-95fe-fcd274e920ca

Sardar, Z., and Sweeney, J. A. (2016). The Three Tomorrows of Postnormal Times. *Futures* 75:1–13.

Sequoia. (2020, March 5). Coronavirus: The Black Swan of 2020. *Medium*. https://medium.com/sequoia-capital/coronavirus-the-black-swan-of-2020-7c72bdeb9753

Serra del Pino, J., Jones, C., and Mayo, L. (2020, May 5). The Postnormal Perfect Storm Part 2. *Post Normal Times*. https://postnormaltim.es/insights/postnormal-perfect-storm-part-2

Sheikh, A., McMenamin, J., Taylor, B., and Robertson, C. (2021). SARS-CoV-2 Delta VOC in Scotland: Demographics, Risk of Hospital Admission, and Vaccine Effectiveness. *The Lancet* S0140673621013581.

Slaughter, R. (1998). The Knowledge Base of Futures Studies. In D. Hicks and Slaughter, R. (Eds.), *World Yearbook of Education 1998: Futures Education*. Routledge.

Sweeney, J. A. (2015). Infectious Connectivity: Affect and the Internet in Postnormal Times. In J. Winter and R. Ono (Eds.), *Futures of the Internet*. Springer International Publishing.

Sweeney, J. A. (2020, March 23). Hot Take v2.0: Why Covid-19 'Is and Is Not' a Black Swan, Futures/Foresight, and a New/Old Metaphor. *Medium*. https://medium.com/@aloha_futures/hot-take-v2-0-why-covid-19-is-and-is-not-a-black-swan-futures-foresight-and-a-new-old-metaphor-424ff59ddddb

Taleb, N. N. (2007). *The Black Swan: The Impact of the Highly Improbable*. 1st ed. Random House.

Wang, J.C., Ng, C.Y., and Brook, R.H. (2020). Response to COVID-19 in Taiwan: Big Data Analytics, New Technology, and Proactive Testing. *JAMA*. https://doi.org/10.1001/jama.2020.3151

Wucker, M. (2016). *The Gray Rhino: How to Recognize and Act on the Obvious Dangers We Ignore.* First edition. St. Martin's Press.

Yong, E. (2018, August 15). The Next Plague Is Coming. Is America Ready? *The Atlantic.* https://www.theatlantic.com/magazine/archive/2018/07/when-the-next-plague-hits/561734/

THREE SCENARIOS FOR THE FUTURE OF EDUCATION IN THE ANTHROPOCENE

Kathleen Kesson

12 abr. 2020

We have entered the Anthropocene — a new era in geological history — a phase of planetary development in which human impacts on the Earth may cause or have caused irreversible damage. We are witness to "the great acceleration" in which geothermal, biological, ecological, and atmospheric changes threaten to bring about irreparable changes in the planetary ecosystem, and by extension, our social and economic systems. Every day brings news of wildfires, drought, floods, conflicts, hurricanes, locusts, extinctions, and the latest, a Coronavirus pandemic, which has managed to shut down many of the global systems we rely on for survival.

Humans (GR: *ánthrōpos*) have been blamed for the tragic despoliation of our Earth. It is not humans in general, however, but a specific human civilization that has driven the processes of resource extraction, labor exploitation, capital accumulation, and what we can only call "ecocide." While historically, empires have come and gone and laid waste in countless ways to people and planet, the current modern era of industrialization/capitalism, paralleling a centuries-long narrative of conquest, genocide, plunder, slave labor, and economic imperialism has created the conditions of this new age that some scholars suggest we more rightly call the "Capitalocene" (see Moore, 2016).

Given the climate and other ecological crises, the rise of authoritarian/totalitarian governments, and the general breakdown of multiple systems, there is an urgent need to create new, nimble configurations of communities, ecologies, and learning centres to respond to the uncertain and rapidly changing environment. The education (not necessarily "schooling") of young people is at the heart of the future; it is only through education that a "new human" might emerge, capable of enacting the mindset and behaviors that might create a livable world. Education alone, however, absent substantial changes in culture, thinking and behavior, is incapable of bringing about the fundamental changes necessary to survival.

I offer here three scenarios for the future of education, each of them tied to various components of a dominant governing ideology. Each Scenario is accompanied by structuring metaphors as well as a dominant "binding quality." The notion of a binding quality comes to us from an ancient Indic episteme; it is said that consciousness and matter operate in three fundamental modes: sattva (sentient), rajah (mutative), and tamah (static), collectively known as gunas in Sanskrit. Understanding the gunas is a complex philosophical matter; I use them here metaphorically, to describe the predominant energy of each Scenario. I have drawn largely on the comprehensive projections of P.R. Sarkar (1992; 1999) for the vision of the future portrayed in Scenario 3, though it must be said that the various components of this vision are emerging from multifarious directions and under different appellations at the present time.

Futures thinking is an uncertain art. It is likely that the future of humanity will include dimensions of each Scenario; in fact, the present moment contains all of them, though Scenario 2 dominates because of the globalization of the economy and hegemonic forms of culture. I believe, however, that the survivability of humanity is dependent on learning the lessons of the multiple current crises we face, and figuring out how to navigate through complexity, chaos and the general breakdown of systems to facilitate the self-organized, positive evolutionary outcomes highlighted in Scenario 3.

An important caveat: When considering the "Big Picture," generalizations are unavoidable. These scenarios are mapped in very broad strokes, and we must remember that the map is not the territory. Details, diversities, exceptions, and contradictions certainly need to be taken into consideration.

SCENARIO 1: REGRESSION/DEVOLUTION

I start with the grimmest of the forecasts, in order to disabuse us of the modernist notion that history is an inevitable trajectory of progress, of increasing individual freedom and rights, of economic growth, constantly improved standards of living, and the capacity of positivist reason and logical thinking to solve all human problems. As in the aftermath of the Roman Empire or perhaps more vividly, in modern dystopian films, societies can deteriorate rather swiftly.

In European history, the years between 500-1250 AD are usually considered the "Dark Ages." After the fall of the Roman Empire, and due to many factors including ineffective leadership, economic failures, internal struggles for power, external invasions, and yes — climate change — the western territories of the Roman Empire entered a long period of decline. Historians disagree on many of the details, though there is a general consensus that it was a period of breakdown and change of the social and economic infrastructures. Schools were closed, and illiteracy spread. Travel and trade were restricted, epidemics wiped out huge populations, and conflict was prevalent.

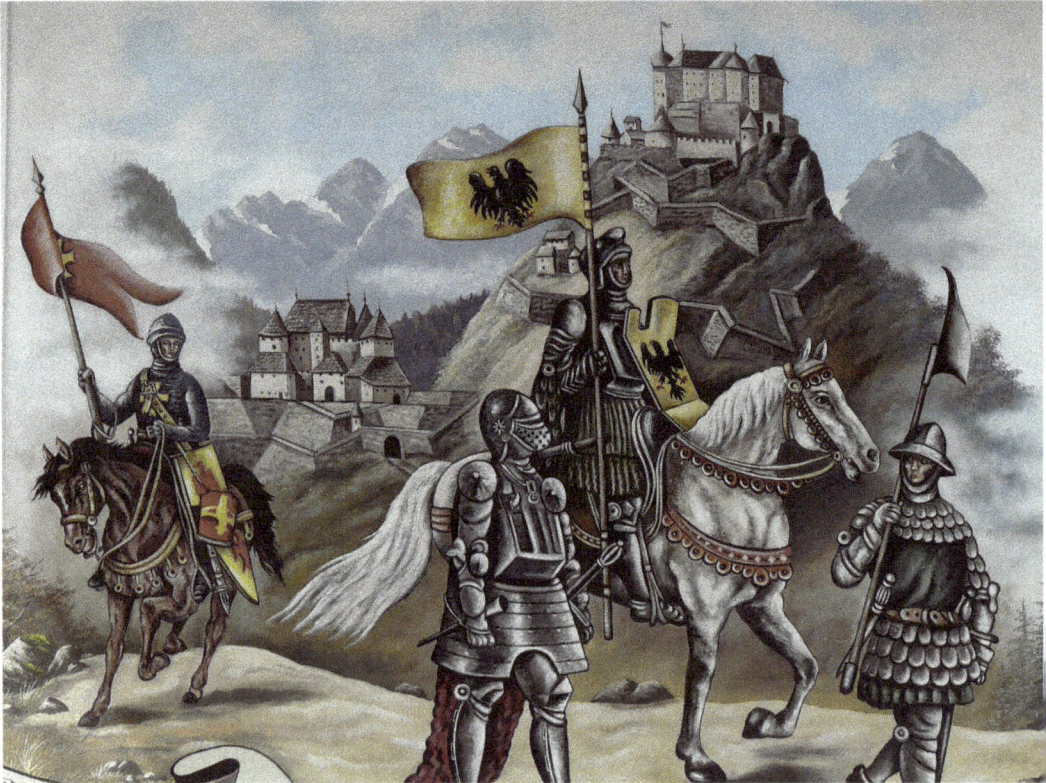

Hans Braxmeier | Pixabay

While our modern era may seem to have little to do with the European Medieval period, it's altogether possible that we (at least in the "West") are living through the deterioration of an empire begun in the European colonial period and culminating in late capitalism and the economic imperialism that is an essential component of the globalized economy. This world-historical empire has been engaged in endless wars throughout its reign, has deep internal fractures and multiple external pressures, not least from other empires. Most important, as noted above, the bio-systems upon which life depends, and upon which so much of its wealth was created, are deteriorating.

In times of collective stress such as the current pandemic, it is tempting to withdraw, to retreat from the forward flow of life and pull into individual and social cocoons, burrow into the past. That tendency is currently exacerbated by the pandemic related strictures to isolate, to distance ourselves from the social world. Should these tendencies persist after the disease is brought under control, we could see a "devolution." In such a regressive move, we are likely to see rising xenophobia, racism, religious prejudice, sexism, strong borders, and ever-increasing economic inequality.

Scenarios and metaphors	Worldview/ Philosophy	Power	Social/ Economic organization	Ecological perspective	Knowledge	Education Institutions	Spirituality
Regression/ Devolution Binding quality: Tamah (static) Contraction, decay, degeneration, ignorance, death and inertia.	Pre-Humanist submersion in forces thought to be beyond human control. Recycling of medieval ontologies and philosophies. People concerned with their own immediate land, clan, family and social group.	Power/over-exerted through superstition and propagation of false ideas; patriarchal structures control behavior, social life, and education.	Provincial, feudal, mostly dispersed rural populations. Centralization of (weak) control in urban centres. Subsistence economy for the masses; wealth flows upward—vast inequalities.	Nature as a force to be feared. Attempts to exert dominion over nature. The exploitation of natural resources benefits the few.	Past knowledge valued over experimental, new knowledge. Knowledge distribution restricted as a form of social control.	Knowledge production concentrated in centres of power. Private teachers/ schools for the wealthy. Survival skills adequate for the general population.	Traditional/ orthodox/ dogmatic; power centralized in the clergy. Metaphysical beliefs grounded in irrationality and superstition—emphasis on domination and control of thought.

SCENARIO 2: STATUS QUO/BUSINESS AS USUAL

Thinking optimistically, we're unlikely to sink into the miasma of Medieval Europe, but young people who have not lived through a Depression, or an epidemic, or a war on their own territory cannot be blamed for fearing that this is the "end of the world as we know it." This pandemic, however, and the economic dislocations, the social isolation, the fear and uncertainty that it has brought, while perhaps not the apocalypse many fear, may be a harbinger of the future. It is human nature to want to "get back to normal" following a crisis of great magnitude, to restore a sense of equilibrium and stability. But what if "normal" forms of social, economic, and ecological behaviors are themselves at the root of the crisis? Astute observers of our current modernist trajectories, including a majority of the scientific community, warn us that we are now living through a transition period, which, depending on collective decisions we make in this next decade, have the potential to transform the conditions of life as we know it on Planet Earth, and not for the better. If we continue the rate of petroleum extraction, fossil fuel burning, deforestation, unrestrained consumption, pollution, and so much more, it is clear that humanity is in for a century of increasingly deadly wildfires, droughts, floods, ocean acidification, pandemics, rising sea levels, and massive extinctions on a scale heretofore unimagined. If current power relations persist, and we do not affect a deep reordering of our economic system, power structures, worldview and ways of thinking, if we merely tinker with existing conditions while hoping to achieve what could only be a "false equilibrium," elites will prosper while our life systems continue to degrade and masses of people suffer. The kind of thinking that has created the multi-faceted crises we face is unlikely to help us solve them, but humans may not, in this Scenario, demonstrate the will or the capacity to radically transform their thinking and their behaviors, or challenge the existing power structure.

Scenarios and metaphors	Worldview	Power	Social/ economic organization	Ecological perspective	Knowledge	Education institutions	Spirituality
Status quo/ Business as usual Binding quality: Rajah (mutative) Pulsation, change, growth, movement, restlessness and activity.	Secular. Mainstream rejection of spirituality based on widespread materialistic worldview. Man is seen as the pinnacle of creation. Humanistic emphasis on individualism, independence, personal autonomy.	Power/ over-exerted through economic domination and hegemonic media; Power/ with only mythology of democratic capitalism. Dramatic concentration of wealth; oligarchical rule.	Increasing inequalities. The illusion of a relatively prosperous (if shrinking) "middle class" sustains myths of growth and progress.	Humans are seen as separate from nature (dualism). Nature understood as a resource to be exploited for profit.	Conventional, hierarchically organized. Positivist thinking dominates. Scientific and technological advances are double-edged (i.e., air travel creates mobility + air pollution, greenhouse gases and rapid spread of disease). Sifting and sorting mechanisms maintain inequities of race, ethnicity, gender, and social class.	Increasing concentration of influence over standards and curriculum in the interest of global economic competition. Higher education commodified, fewer young people have access. Western forms of education spread globally, resulting in loss of languages, local cultures and epistemes.	Mostly secular. Fundamentalisms operate at the fringe, often with major impacts on systems (re 9/11). Commodified "new age" practices amongst middle classes are oriented towards individual well-being.

SCENARIO 3: EVOLUTION/REVOLUTION

The current crisis has brought into sharp relief the injustice and unsustainability of socio-economic systems that value profits over human needs and the well-being of the planet. It is possible that this moment in time could signal a great awakening, the tipping point that pushes us into creative new ways of thinking about what it means to be human and how we should live our lives. What if the present moment were a space of 'liminality' - a moment between what has been and what will be? A space between the 'what was' and the 'next.' A space of transition, a season of waiting, during which we collectively question where we have been and where we are going. A space in which we reconceptualize the entire edifice the mental and the material structures that have brought us to the current crossroads in our evolution.

In Scenario 3, we find the courage to design and implement new economic structures that serve the welfare of the whole of humanity, not just the elite few. We begin to understand our essential embeddedness in nature and explore how to cultivate relations of harmony and reciprocity with the "more-than-human-others" with whom we share the planet. And perhaps most important, we overcome the false notion that matter and spirit occupy independent realms, separated by an impassable abyss. We begin to understand that the purpose of life is not the mere accumulation of material goods, or the acquisition of political power, or even the development of a brilliant intellect, but the unification of body, mind and spirit in the quest for spiritual enlightenment.

Unlike the "tinkering" referred to in Scenario 2, Scenario 3 represents a radical paradigm shift, an evolutionary transformation of consciousness, values, and human behavior. Education has a core role to play in that it is young people who will carry the present into the future. A philosophy of Neohumanism (Sarkar, 1999), in which we reconsider the fundamentals — the nature of human beings, the nature of knowing, what we value, and how we are to live — asks us to rethink the purposes of education. Rather than educate so that a tiny sliver of people rise to the top of the global income chain, a Neohumanist education would prepare all people for the art of living well on a fragile and sacred planet. It would emphasize not just academic achievement and high test scores, but shift the focus to fostering compassion, community, empathy, imagination, insight, friendship, creativity, communication, justice, practicality, pleasure, courage, humor, wisdom, introspection, transcendence, ethics, service, and the ability to live well within the carrying capacity of our ecosystems. It would tear down the walls that have separated school and community and invite local and intergenerational knowledge and traditional ways of knowing into conversation with modern empirical science and technological know-how. Importantly, Neohumanism would welcome our inner lives into education and foster multiple epistemologies (embodied knowing, intuitional knowing, narrative knowing, aesthetic knowing, mythic knowing). Adults and young people together would plant gardens and reinvigorate forests, clean up our waterways, and regenerate the soil. We would "rewild" our children and ourselves so that we might begin to understand the vital part we all play in a living web of interconnection, a web that encompasses not just humans, but the eight million other species with whom we share the planet. Only with such an educational process might we "elevate humanism to universalism, the cult of love for all created beings of this universe" (Sarkar, 1999, p. 7).

Scenarios and metaphors	Worldview	Power	Social/economic organization	Ecological perspective	Knowledge	Education Institutions	Spirituality
Evolution/ Revolution Binding quality: Sattva (sentient) Awareness, purity, happiness, sensitivity, expansion and lightness.	Human life an integrated whole encompassing the material and spiritual worlds. Neohumanism: the liberation of the intellect and the expansion of mind. Emphasis on interdependence of all species. Resilient local cultures, universal, inclusive outlooks.	Power/ with radical democracy, people organized to resist domination. Co-creation of new systems that serve the whole. Gender partnership, full inclusion. Moral leadership based in service replaces corruption and self-interest. Cooperative global governance regulates international affairs.	Progressive Utilization Theory (Prout) — Social equality fostered through worker's cooperatives, caps on wealth accumulation, food sovereignty, gift and sharing economies, the rights of all people for a decent job, housing, food, health care and education, and the protection of biodiversity and natural habitats. (see Sarkar, 1992).	Deep connection and sense of interrelatedness of all species; humans learn to live in balance with the ecosystem and practice reciprocity. All living beings accorded moral standing and rights.	Integration of modern science/ technology and ancient wisdom and indigenous perspectives. Epistemological pluralism. Elimination of dogma. Knowledge balanced between introversial and extroversial.	Schools take on new role as centers of resource, connections, healing, community building, mentorship. Self-organizing learning groups form around real life problems and issues. Eco-versities. Decolonizing pedagogies.	Transformative, new understanding of human potential and the cosmic dimensions of individual life. Pragmatism and contemplative practice exist in mutual harmony (subjective approach/objective adjustment); intuition and rationality complement each other.

Scenario 3 is not a pipe dream. In this present crisis, multitudes of people are acting selflessly to care for others and serve the greater good. Heroic health workers are struggling to mitigate suffering without adequate resources. Teachers are working to reinvent schooling so that children might stay connected to their peers and engaged in learning. Regular folk are creating mutual aid societies, ensuring that those who are sick, disabled, or elderly are not forgotten. In many places, small organic farms are beginning to supply much of the local food. Young people are inclined towards egalitarian socio-economic formations, and they are willing to challenge the status quo and struggle for the future of their planet. People the world over are awakening to spiritual wisdom. We are making the road by walking.

The world right now is in a state of chaos – a "far-from-equilibrium" state. Chaos is unpredictable and destabilizing, and small inputs can have huge effects, illustrated by the compelling image of the fluttering wings of the butterfly in the Amazon, causing a cyclone in China.

But chaos theory also teaches us that systems re-organize, often in surprising new ways. A far-from-equilibrium state is a liminal space; liminality is described by one author as "the sacred space where the old world is able to fall apart, and a bigger world is revealed." [Rohr, 1999]. Will we find the courage to allow this dissolution, in order to make way for the world we hope to create? Or will we eagerly seek the status quo, business as usual, or worse, regress into barbarism? I believe that we are in the thick of what may come to be understood as the "great transition" – the death of an old era and the birth of the new. Such a birth is not accomplished painlessly, but with extraordinary labor. Those of us who share the values of Scenario 3, who hold a Neohumanist vision of human potential and a social vision of a just, ecological and joyful Earth home (Prout) share a responsibility to be midwives to this birth. Systems demand that we evolve and adapt. The butterfly effect reminds us that small actions can have big impacts. Our small collective actions, mindfully taken, could have important collective impacts, so let us proceed with Scenario 3 as consciously and compassionately as we can.

AUTHOR

Kathleen Kesson is Professor Emerita, LIU-Brooklyn, and is the former Director of the John Dewey Project on Progressive Education at the University of Vermont and Director of Education at Goddard College. She currently lives in Barre, Vermont and is actively engaged in the work to make Vermont schools more equitable, sustainable, and joyful. Her latest book is Unschooling in Paradise. You can read other writings by her as well as an excerpt from this book at https://www.kathleenkesson.com

REFERENCES

Moore, J. (2016). *Anthropocene or capital scene? Nature, history, and the crisis of capitalism*. PM Press.

Rohr, R. (1999). *Everything belongs: The gift of contemplative prayer*. The Crossroad Publishing Company.

Sarkar, P.R. (1992). *Proutist Economics: Discourses on economic liberation*. Ananda Marga Pracaraka Samgha.

Sarkar, P.R. (1999). *The liberation of intellect: Neo-Humanism*. 4th edition. Ananda Nagar. Ananda Marga Publications.

PANDEMICS

*Lessons Looking Back
From 2050*

Fritjof Capra & Hazel Henderson

03-17-20

Imagine, it is the year 2050 and we are looking back to the origin and evolution of the coronavirus pandemic over the last three decades. Extrapolating from recent events, we offer the following scenario for such a view from the future.

As we move into the second half of our twenty-first century, we can finally make sense of the origin and impact of the coronavirus that struck the world in 2020 from an evolutionary systemic perspective. Today, in 2050, looking back on the past 40 turbulent years on our home planet, it seems obvious that the Earth had taken charge of teaching our human family. Our planet taught us the primacy of understanding of our situation in terms of whole systems, identified by some far-sighted thinkers as far back as the mid-nineteenth century. This widening human awareness revealed how the planet actually functions, its living biosphere systemically powered by the daily flow of photons from our mother star, the Sun.

Eventually, this expanded awareness overcame the cognitive limitations and incorrect assumptions and ideologies that had created the crises of the twentieth century. False theories of human development and progress, measured myopically by prices and money-based metrics, such as GDP, culminated in rising social and environmental losses: pollution of air, water and land; destruction of biological diversity; loss of ecosystem services, all exacerbated by global heating, rising sea levels, and massive climate disruptions.

These myopic policies had also driven social breakdowns, inequality, poverty, mental and physical illness, addiction, loss of trust in institutions — including media, academia, and science itself — as well as loss of community solidarity. They had also led to the pandemics of the 21st century, SARS, MERS, AIDS, influenza, and the various coronaviruses that emerged back in 2020.

During the last decades of the 20th century, humanity had exceeded the Earth's carrying capacity. The human family had grown to 7.6 billion by 2020 and had continued its obsession with economic, corporate, and technological growth that had caused the rising existential crises threatening humanity's very survival. By driving this excessive growth with fossil fuels, humans had heated the atmosphere to such an extent that the United Nations (UN) climate science consortium, IPCC noted in its 2020 update that humanity had only ten years left to turn this crisis situation around.

As far back as 2000, all the means were already at hand: we had the know-how and had designed efficient renewable technologies and circular economic systems, based on nature's ecological principles. By 2000, patriarchal societies were losing control over their female populations, due to the forces of urbanization and education. Women themselves had begun to take control of their bodies and fertility rates began to tumble even before the turn of the twenty-first century. Widespread revolts against the top-down narrow economic model of globalization and its male-dominated elites led to disruptions of the unsustainable paths of development driven by fossil fuels, nuclear power, militarism, profit, greed, and egocentric leadership.

Military budgets that had starved health and education needs for human development gradually shifted from tanks and battleships to less expensive, less violent information warfare. By the early 21st century, international competition for power focused more on social propaganda, persuasion technologies, infiltration and control of the global internet.

In 2020, the coronavirus pandemic's priorities in medical facilities competed with victims in emergency rooms, whether those wounded by gun violence or patients with other life-threatening conditions. In 2019, the nationwide US movement of schoolchildren had joined with the medical profession in challenging gun violence as a public health crisis. Strict gun laws gradually followed, along with rejection of gun manufacturers in pension funds' assets crippling the gun lobby and, in many countries, guns were purchased back by governments from gun owners and destroyed, as Australia had done in the 20th century. This greatly reduced global arms sales, together with international laws requiring expensive annual licenses and insurance, while global taxation reduced the wasteful arms races of previous centuries. Conflicts between nations are now largely governed by international treaties and transparency. Now in 2050, conflicts rarely involve military means, shifting to internet propaganda, spying and cyber warfare.

By 2020, these revolts exhibited all the fault lines in human societies: from racism and ignorance, conspiracy theories, xenophobia and scapegoating of "the other" to various cognitive biases — technological determinism, theory-induced blindness, and the fatal, widespread misunderstanding that confused money with actual wealth. Money, as we all know today, was a useful invention: all currencies are simply social protocols (physical or virtual tokens of trust), operating on social platforms with network effects, their prices fluctuating to the extent that their various users trust and use them. Yet, countries and elites all over the world became enthralled with money and with gambling in the "global financial casino," further encouraging the seven deadly sins over traditional values of cooperation, sharing, mutual aid, and the Golden Rule.

Scientists and environmental activists had warned of the dire consequences of these unsustainable societies and retrogressive value systems for decades, but until the 2020 pandemic corporate and political leaders, and other elites, stubbornly resisted these warnings. Previously unable to break their intoxication with financial profits and political power, their own citizens forced the re-focus on the well-being and survival of humanity and the community of life. Incumbent fossilized industries fought to retain their tax breaks and subsidies in all countries as gas and oil prices collapsed. But they were less able to buy political favors and support of their privileges. It took the global reactions of millions of young people, "grassroots globalists," and indigenous peoples, who understood the systemic processes of our planet Gaia — a self-organizing, self-regulating biosphere which for billions of years had managed all planetary evolution without interference from cognitively-challenged humans.

In the first years of our twenty-first century, Gaia responded in an unexpected way, as it had so often during the long history of evolution. Humans' clear-cutting large areas of tropical rainforests and massive intrusions into other ecosystems around the world, had fragmented these self-regulating ecosystems and fractured the web of life. One of the many consequences of these destructive actions was that some viruses, which had lived in symbiosis with certain animal species, jumped from those species to others and to humans, where they were highly toxic or deadly. People in many countries and regions, marginalized by the narrow profit-oriented economic globalization, assuaged their hunger by seeking "bush meat" in these newly exposed wild areas , killing monkeys, civets, pangolins, rodents and bats, as additional protein sources . These wild species, carrying a variety of viruses were also sold live in "wet markets," further exposing ever more urban populations to these new viruses.

Back in the 1960s, for example, an obscure virus jumped from a rare species of monkeys killed as "bush meat" and eaten by humans in West Africa. From there it spread to the United States where it was identified as the HIV virus and caused the AIDS epidemic. Over four decades, they caused the deaths of an estimated 39 million people worldwide, about half a percent of the world population. Four decades later, the impact of the coronavirus was swift and dramatic. In 2020, the virus jumped from a species of bats to humans in China, and from there it rapidly spread around the world, decimating world population by an estimated 50 million in just one decade.

From the vantage point of our year 2050, we can look back at the sequence of these viruses: SARS, MERS, and the global impact of the various coronavirus mutations which began back in 2020. Eventually, such pandemics were stabilized, partly by the outright bans on "wet markets" all over China in 2020 . Such bans spread to other countries and global markets, cutting the trading of wild animals and reducing vectors, along with better public health systems, preventive care and the development of effective vaccines and drugs.

The basic lessons for humans in our tragic 50 years of self-inflicted global crises — the afflictions of pandemics , flooded cities, burned forestlands, droughts and other increasingly violent climate disasters — were simple, many based on the discoveries of Charles Darwin and other biologists in the nineteenth and twentieth centuries:

- We, humans, are one species with very little variation in our basic DNA.

- We evolved with other species in the planet's biosphere by natural selection, responding to changes and stresses in our various habitats and environments.
- We are a global species, having migrated out of the African continent to all others, competing with other species, causing various extinctions.

Our planetary colonization and success, in this Anthropocene Age of our twenty-first century, was largely due to our abilities to bond, cooperate, share and evolve in ever larger populations and organizations.

Humanity grew from roving bands of nomads to live in settled agricultural villages, to towns, and the mega-cities of the twentieth century, where over 50% of our populations lived. Until the climate crises and those of the pandemics in the first years of our 21st century, all forecasts predicted that these mega-cities would keep growing and that human populations would reach 10 billion by today, in 2050.

Now we know why human populations topped out at the 7.6 billion in 2030, as expected in the most hopeful scenario of the IPCC, as well as in the global urban surveys by social scientists documenting the decline of fertility in Empty Planet (2019). The newly aware "grassroots globalists", the armies of school children, global environmentalists and empowered women joined with green, more ethical investors and entrepreneurs in localizing markets. Millions were served by microgrid cooperatives, powered by renewable electricity, adding to the world's cooperative enterprises, which even by 2012 employed more people worldwide than all the for-profit companies combined. They no longer used the false money metrics of GDP, but in 2015 switched to steering their societies by the UN's SDGs, their 17 goals of sustainability and restoration of all ecosystems and human health.

These new social goals and metrics all focused on cooperation, sharing and knowledge-richer forms of human development, using renewable resources and maximizing efficiency. This long term sustainability, equitably distributed, benefits all members of the human family within the tolerance of other species in our living biosphere. Competition and creativity flourish with good ideas driving out less useful ones, along with science-based ethical standards and deepening information in self-reliant and more connected societies at all levels from local to global.

When the coronavirus struck in 2020, the human responses were at first chaotic and insufficient, but soon became increasingly coherent and even dramatically different. Global trade shrunk to only transporting rare goods, shifting to trading information. Instead of shipping cakes, cookies and biscuits around the planet, we shipped their recipes, and all the other recipes for creating plant-based foods and beverages; and locally we installed green technologies: solar, wind, geothermal energy sources, LED lighting, electric vehicles, boats, and even aircraft.

Fossil fuel reserves stayed safely in the ground, as carbon was seen as a resource, much too precious to burn. The excess CO_2 in the atmosphere from fossil fuel burning was captured by organic soil bacteria, deep-rooted plants, billions of newly planted trees, and in the widespread re-balancing of the human food systems based on agro-chemical industrial agribusiness, advertising and global trading of a few monocultured crops. This over-dependence on fossil fuels, pesticides, fertilizers, antibiotics in animal-raised meat diets, all were based on the planet's dwindling freshwater and proved unsustainable. Today, in 2050, our global foods are produced locally, including many more overlooked indigenous and wild crops, saltwater agriculture and all the other salt-loving (halophyte) food plants whose complete proteins are healthier for human diets.

Mass tourism, and travel in general, decreased radically, along with air traffic and phased-out fossil fuel use. Communities around the world stabilized in small- to medium-sized population centers, which became largely self-reliant with local and regional production of food and energy. Fossil-fuel use virtually disappeared, as already by 2020 it could no longer compete with rapidly developing renewable energy resources and corresponding new technologies and upcycling of all formerly-wasted resources into our circular economies of today.

Because of the danger of infections in mass gatherings, sweat shops, large chain stores, as well as sports events and entertainment in large arenas gradually disappeared. Democratic politics became more rational, since demagogues could no longer assemble thousands in large rallies to hear them. Their empty promises were also curbed in social media, as these profit-making monopolies were broken up by 2025 and now in 2050 are regulated as public utilities serving the public good in all countries.

The global-casino financial markets collapsed, and economic activities shifted back from the financial sector to credit unions and public banks in our cooperative sectors of today. The manufacture of goods and our service-based economies revived traditional barter and informal voluntary sectors, local currencies, as well as numerous non-monetary transactions that had developed during the height of the pandemics. As a consequence of wide-spread decentralization and the growth of self-reliant communities, our economies of today in 2050, have become regenerative rather than extractive, and the poverty gaps and inequality of the money-obsessed, exploitive models have largely disappeared.

The pandemic of 2020, which crashed global markets, finally upended the ideologies of money and market fundamentalism. Central banks' tools no longer worked, so "helicopter money "and direct cash payments to needy families, such as pioneered by Brazil, became the only means of maintaining purchasing power to smooth orderly economic transitions to sustainable societies. This shifted US and European politicians to create new money and these stimulus policies replaced "austerity" and were rapidly invested in all the renewable resource infrastructure in their respective Green New Deal plans.

When the coronavirus spread to domestic animals, cattle, and other ruminants, sheep and goats, some of these animals became carriers of the disease without themselves showing any symptoms. Consequently, the slaughter and consumption of animals dropped dramatically around the world. Pasturing and factory-raising of animals had added almost 15% of annual global greenhouse gases. Big meat-producing multinational corporations became shorted by savvy investors as the next group of " stranded assets", along with fossil fuel companies Some switched entirely to plant-based foods with numerous meat, fish, and cheese analogs. Beef became very expensive and rare, and cows were usually owned by families, as traditionally, on small farms for local milk, cheese, and meat, along with eggs from their chickens.

After the pandemics subsided, and expensive, vaccines had been developed, global travel was allowed only with the vaccination certificates of today, used mainly by traders and wealthy people. The majority of the world's populations now prefer the pleasures of community and online meetings and communicating, along with traveling locally by public transport, electric cars, and by the solar and wind powered sailboats we all enjoy today. As a consequence, air pollution has decreased dramatically in all major cities around the world.

With the growth of self-reliant communities, so-called "urban villages" have sprung up in many cities — re-designed neighborhoods that display high-density structures combined with ample common green spaces. These areas boast significant energy savings and a healthy, safe, and community-oriented environment with drastically reduced levels of pollution.

Today's eco-cities include food grown in high rise buildings with solar rooftops, vegetable gardens, and electric public transport, after automobiles were largely banned from urban streets in 2030. These streets were reclaimed by pedestrians, cyclists and people on scooters browsing in smaller local stores, craft galleries and farmer's markets. Solar electric vehicles for inter-town use often charge and discharge their batteries at night to balance electricity in single-family houses. Free-standing solar-powered vehicle re-charger units are available in all areas, reducing the use of fossil-based electricity from obsolete centralized utilities, many of which went bankrupt by 2030.

After all the dramatic changes we enjoy today, we realize that our lives are now less stressful, healthier, and more satisfying, and our communities plan for the long-term future. To assure the sustainability of our new ways of life, we realize that restoring ecosystems around the world is crucial, so that viruses dangerous to humans are confined again to other animal species where they do no harm. To restore ecosystems worldwide, our global shift to organic, regenerative agriculture flourished, along with plant-based foods, beverages and all the saltwater -grown foods and kelp dishes we enjoy. The billions of trees that we planted around the world after 2020, along with the agricultural improvements gradually restored ecosystems.

As a consequence of all these changes, the global climate has finally stabilized, with today's CO_2 concentrations in the atmosphere returning to the safe level of 350 parts per million. Higher sea levels will remain for a century and many cities now flourish on safer, higher ground. Climate catastrophes are now rare, while many weather events still continue to disrupt our lives, just as they had in previous centuries. The multiple global crises and pandemics, due to our earlier ignorance of planetary processes and feedback loops, had widespread tragic consequences for individuals and communities. Yet, we humans have learned many painful lessons. Today, looking back from 2050, we realize that the Earth is our wisest teacher, and its terrible lessons may have saved humanity and large parts of our shared planetary community of life from extinction.

AUTHORS

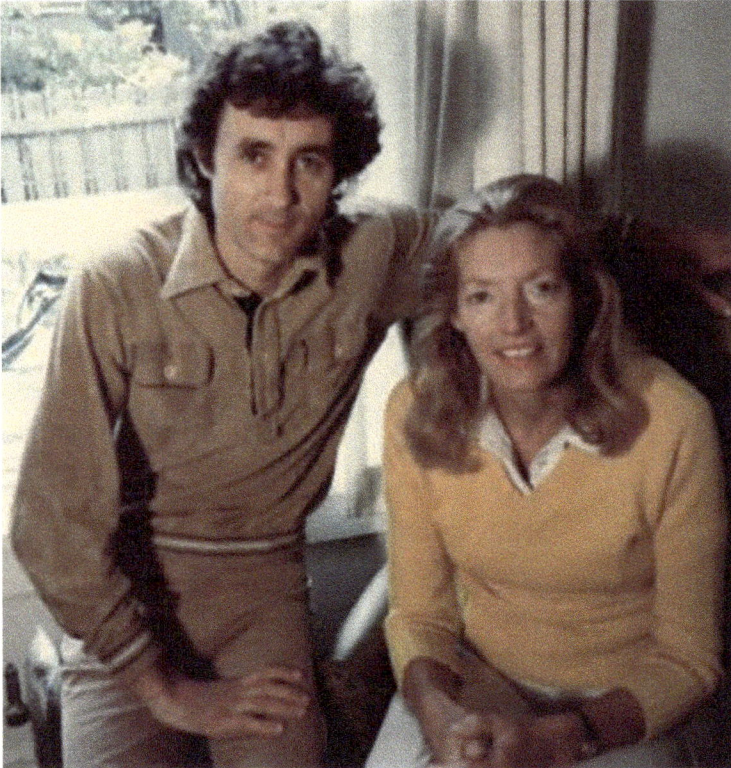

Fritjof Capra and Hazel Henderson
University of California, Berkeley, CA
1982

Fritjof Capra, Ph.D., physicist and systems theorist, is the author of several international bestsellers, including The Tao of Physics (1975) and The Web of Life (1996). He is coauthor, with Pier Luigi Luisi, of the multidisciplinary textbook, The Systems View of Life. Capra's online course (www.capracourse.net) is based on his textbook.

Hazel Henderson, D.Sc.Hon., FRSA, futurist, systems and science-policy analyst, is author of "The Politics of the Solar Age" (1981, 1986) and other books, including "Mapping the Global Transition to the Solar Age" (2014). Henderson is CEO of Ethical Markets Media Certified B. Corporation, USA (www.ethicalmarkets.com), publishers of the Green Transition Scoreboard ®, and the forthcoming textbook and global TV series "Transforming Finance."

COLLECTIVE INTELLIGENCE TO SOLVE THE MEGACRISIS

William E. Halal

MAy 1st 2020

The coronavirus is a stark reminder of the devastating damage that could be inflicted by cyberattacks, superbugs, freak weather and a variety of other threats. These wild cards are in addition to the existential challenge posed by climate change, gross inequality, financial meltdowns, autocratic governments, terrorism and other massive problems collectively called the Global MegaCrisis.

For a prominent example, Peter de Menocal, director of the Center for Climate and Life, warned: "The tragedy and inconvenience we've seen from this pandemic pale in comparison to what's in store from climate change." (New York Times, April 24, 2020)

I sense the world is so frightened by the Coronavirus disaster that people are searching for new solutions. They seem ready to break from the past that is no longer working. Climate change is starting to bite, for instance, and there is a growing consensus that the status quo is no longer sustainable.

I have studied this dilemma for decades, and I think it can be best understood as a transition to the next stage of social evolution. The Knowledge Age that dominated the last two decades is fading into the past as AI automates knowledge, forcing us to move beyond knowledge and develop a global consciousness able to resolve the MegaCrisis.

Yes, I know this is a bold claim, but that is how the shift to a world of knowledge looked 40 years ago. When computers filled rooms, I recall telling people that we were entering a world of personal computers. The typical response was "Why would anyone want a personal computer?"

Just so, today's post-factual era illustrates how the smart phone, social media, and autocrats like Trump have moved public attention beyond knowledge and into a world of values, emotions and beliefs. Now the challenge is to use these new powers of social media to shape a global consciousness or face disaster. While this may seem impossible, that is always the case before major upheavals. Nobody thought the USSR would collapse up until its very end.

In fact, the Business Roundtable's recent announcement that businesses should move beyond the bottom line to include the interests of all stakeholders is revolutionary. It has now been promulgated by the World Economic Forum and other influential bodies.

The gravity of this change is such that business is now being told to help resolve the climate crisis. Larry Fink, who runs the biggest investment firm in the world (Black Rock), directed the companies he owns to help address climate costs in their operations; within days, many firms announced climate abatement plans. This historic shift in consciousness could make corporations models of cooperation for society at large.

In short, I think the world is heading toward some type of historic shift in consciousness, a collective epiphany, a code of global ethics, a spiritual revolution, a political paradigm shift or a new mindset. Without a consciousness based on global unity, cooperation and other essential beliefs, there seems little hope. And with a shift to global consciousness, it all seems possible.

TOWARD A GLOBAL CONSCIOUSNESS

I sent the above background information to readers of my newsletter at BillHalal. com and asked them to provide short "solutions" to the MegaCrisis. The twelve statements we received are noted briefly in this analysis. This is hardly a scientific survey, but it does represent a collection of forward ideas by some of the best thought leaders in the world. Here's my quick analysis of what each has to offer, followed by what we can learn collectively.

The central theme running through these diverse statements is that the governing ideas inherited from the industrial past are outdated and heading toward disaster. It is a collapse of today's reigning "materialist" ideology of Capitalism, economic growth, money, power, self-interest, rationality, knowledge, etc. These values remain valid and useful, of course, but they are now badly limited. Prevailing practices in the US, as the most prominent example, are failing to address the climate crisis, low wage employee welfare, universal health care, women's rights, political gridlock, aging infrastructure and other social issues that lie beyond sheer economics.

For instance, **Ruben Nelson**, Executive Director, Foresight Canada, sees this as the passing of today's "modern techno-industrial" civilization. While he is not hopeful about a solution, he does think what's needed is a "wise, integral, and meta reflexive form of consciousness." In other words, rather than thinking of economic growth, "The only way to grow, is UP."

A penetrating view is provided by **Sohail Inayatullah**, UNESCO Chair in Futures Studies, Sejahtera Centre for Sustainability and Humanity, Malaysia, and Professor, Tamkang University. Sohail digs beneath the layers of these continuing crises to probe into the underlying causes. Sohail finds that we need a "Gaian re-balance by moving to a world with a quadruple bottom line: Prosperity, Purpose, People, and Planet. A new Renaissance is needed – the transformation of self and society, home and plant."

This could become a "Collapse of Capitalism" roughly equivalent to the "Collapse of Communism" in the 1990s, and it stems from the same fatal flaw – failure to adapt to a changing world. Communism could not meet the complex demands of the Information Revolution, and now Capitalism seems to be failing to adapt to a unified globe threatened by pandemics, climate change and the other threats making up the MegaCrisis.

Jim Dator, University of Hawaii, is dismayed by attitudes favoring economic growth over cultural and ecological values. "The only way forward is through the imminent self-destruction of dominant values, behavior and institutions, with the hope that a million phoenixes rise from the ashes ... the countless tsunami that we must learn to surf with pleasure and pain."

Hazel Henderson, Futurist and CEO of Ethical Markets Media, offers guides to avoid a collapse of the Internet under heavy loads caused by the virus crisis. "Now that everyone and every organization on the planet is going virtual ... the question is on everyone's lips: 'Will the coronavirus break the internet?' We at Ethical Markets are using some simple rules... politeness and consideration for essential users and public information can help assure that the internet can continue to be the vital backbone of our lives for the foreseeable future.

Jose Cordeiro, Vice-Chair, HumanityPlus and Director, Venezuela, The Millennium Project, shows how this crisis presents both threats and opportunities. "We are currently living in a MegaCrisis, which implies MegaDanger but also MegaOpportunity to move forward together as one global family in our small planet. Such statements from prominent futurists are compelling. The coronavirus crisis has brought these failings of the present global order on vivid display now for all to see, and it has also raised hopes for structural changes. Similar ideas can be found running through common exchanges on the web and other media.

The big question remaining is, "What should be the new vision, values, principles, and policies?" At the risk of appearing pedantic, I integrate what has been learned above and my forthcoming book, **Beyond Knowledge**, to outline five principles of what I consider "global consciousness."

> 1. **Treat the planet and all life forms as sacred.** The Fermi Paradox notes that no other civilizations have been detected after decades of SETI searching. This rarity of life reminds us what a miracle plant Earth really is, and that we are responsible for its well-being.

The primary role of Nature is stressed in Peter King's vision of life in a Nature-centric society. Peter is an environmental Consultant and formerly with the Asian Development Bank. He urges us to be "Guided by the natural wisdom of Earth's ecosystems, we would find abundant energy, food, medicines, water, jobs, economic growth and a more satisfying lifestyle. To avoid dangerous tipping points, we must move forward into a visceral and directly experienced relationship with Nature."

> 2. **Govern the world as a unified whole.** Nations remain the major

players in this global order, but they should be lightly governed by some type of global institution like the UN and other international bodies. Individuals should continue to be loyal to their nations and local institutions, but they should also accept their role as global citizens.

David Passig, Professor at Bar-Ilan University, Israel, finds two phases that could unfold from the coronavirus. "The first phase will disrupt the present idea behind globalization as mutual collaboration based on voluntary respect and common interests. The second will establish the idea of 'entanglement' as symbiotic undetachable ties with enforced collaboration that respects mutual dependency on each other."

3. **Manage markets to serve human and social needs.** Free enterprise is the basis of society, and the good news is that business is on the verge of becoming cooperative. The Business Roundtable announcement that all stakeholders should be treated equally with investors seems a historic breakthrough. This move to a quasi-democratic form of enterprise could set a new standard for collaborative behavior and human values throughout modern societies. One of the benefits of a tragedy like this crisis may be a loss of faith in the status quo and an urge to cooperate. I see it everywhere, and it is a blessing in disguise emerging out of chaos.

Julio Millan, President of the World Future Society, Mexico, thinks "The mega-crisis ... is showing us that we have been leading the wrong model: it is not about individual gains, but about the common welfare. ... to behave like good citizens and understand what it means to do things for our community, to be empathetic to our neighbors, and to create better societies. Our concern now should be what are we going to do when the liberal order, to which we are so accustomed, falls? We are in a historical moment because after the pandemic our preconception of the world is going to change: we are entering a new era.

Amy Fletcher, for example, urges us to listen to those who have no public voice as they often have good answers. Amy is an Associate Professor of Political Science, The University of Canterbury, Christchurch New Zealand. She is concerned with how this crisis highlights the failures that are prolonging the pain. She advises us to "listen to those voices who do not have a platform and speak truth to power. The role of the futurist is to facilitate those who do not have power because the answers we need may lie with them."

>4. **Embrace diversity as an asset**. Rather than becoming a uniform pallid bureaucracy, a unified world should embrace the wondrous diversity of cultures and individuals. Working across such differences poses a challenge, naturally, but differences are also a source of new knowledge, talents and human energy.

Michael Lee, futurist and author wonders if we can realize the potential of diverse races: "We could be facing unemployment and poverty on a scale that will dwarf the impacts of the financial crisis of 2008-9. Will the epoch of wars and empires, which have engulfed history and caused more death and grief than I have the stomach to calculate, finally be over? Can we come together as one human race, black, white, yellow, brown and all the beautiful shades of human skin, to focus on the one reason why we're all here in the first place: to use our fleeting lives for the total, ethical upliftment of human civilization?"

Dennis Bushnell suggests a "back-to-the-land" scenario, for instance, which would encourage a far richer diversity. Dennis is Chief Scientist, NASA Langley. He envisions a provocative possibility in which people become self-sustaining on a small plot of land while connected seamlessly to the entire world on tele-everything. Dennis concludes that all problems would disappear – "no pandemics, no energy crisis, no climate change, no financial mess, no job losses, etc. But one must think big to see this solution."

>5. **Celebrate life.** Any society needs frequent opportunities to gather together in good spirit, enjoy differences and commonalities, and to simply celebrate the glory of life. The World Olympics Games, for instance, are special because they provide a rare feeling of the global community. We could witness an online flowering of celebratory events over the coming years to nourish the global soul.

Fadi Bayoud, a consultant from the UAE, offers his visión of a preferable future:

"beautiful as a priceless piece of art where spirituality drives human relationships. Science is respected and governments invest more in scientific research ... Education becomes free and foresight oriented ...The economy becomes shared and sustainable ... The countryside and Nature are a source for spiritual, psychological, and somatic healing. Energy production is sustainable. Individual households produce their own energy needs ... where rivers and lakes are a source of pure and clean water. Health paradigm shifts to prevention."

SHAPING CONSCIOUSNESS

This is only one small study, of course, but I hope it provokes thinking toward a widely held vision for planet Earth at a time of crisis. A historic change in consciousness is hardly done overnight, and the obstacles posed by the status quo are formidable.

But the Information Revolution provides a powerful method for shaping consciousness by using the Internet and public media. Think of the explosion of ideas, hatred and forbidden desires released by billions of people blasting into loudspeakers like Facebook and Twitter. Anybody can use the media to shape public opinion instantly, for better or worse. We are awash with the wildly diverse views of actors, TV stars, politicians, athletes, ordinary people with heart-breaking stories, cute kids doing smart things and influencers like Kim Kardashian.

The task we face is to shape a unified consciousness out of this morass of differences to solve the global crises that loom ahead. Today's threats to reason is challenging us to counter wrongheaded beliefs and to provide more attractive visions, such as the principles for global consciousness outlined here.

I suggest the place to begin is by discussing these ideas as widely as possible, and to shape public opinion roughly along these lines. I would like to invite comments, suggestions, and contributions by contacting me at Halal@gwu.edu.

AUTHOR

William E. Halal, PhD is professor emeritus of management, technology, and innovation at George Washington University, with degrees from Purdue and UC Berkeley. He has published 7 books and hundreds of articles, consults to corporations and governments, and is a frequent speaker, once substituting for Peter Drucker. Halal is founder of The TechCast Project and also co-founded the Institute for Knowledge & Innovation. He received the 1977 Mitchell Prize for his article "Beyond the Profit-Motive," and was cited by the Encyclopedia of the Future as one of the top 100 futurists in the world. His article, "Through the MegaCrisis," was awarded Outstanding Paper of 2013 by Emerald Publishing. Bill's latest book can be seen at www.BeyondKnowledge.org.

MINIMISING CONFLICTS AMIDST THE COVID-19 PANDEMIC

Ivana Milojević

"The challenge of the COVID-19 pandemic is that ...[a]t times such as these, our stress levels become higher and our difficult emotions seem to surface more readily. This not only leads to more conflicts, it leads to more unresolved conflicts."[1]

"As a rise in family violence due to the coronavirus crisis is set to strain an already critically overstretched social support system, some abusers are reportedly using COVID-19 as a psychological weapon."[2]

"We could be facing multiple famines of biblical proportions within a short few months ... the world is not only facing "a global health pandemic but also a global humanitarian catastrophe."[3]

"COVID-19 has brought wealthy nations to their knees. What will happen when the virus breaks out in a war zone?[iv] ... the impact [may]be unpredictable and potentially catastrophic.[4]

"As the coronavirus sweeps the world, it hits the poor much harder than the better off. One consequence will be social unrest, even revolutions."[5]

"COVID-19 is fuelling conflict: New ways will be needed to make peace."[6]

05 / 15 / 2020

The headlines above suggest the critical importance of enhancing our conflict resolution capacities. As COVID-19 races around the world, we can anticipate further increases in conflicts. Indeed, psychologists and humanitarian organizations (such as WHO[7], the Red Cross[8], Beyond Blue[9]) have already posted some helpful guidelines as to how to defuse intra- and inter-personal conflicts. Developing mental resilience along these recommendations is critical because it is our response to the pandemic rather than the virus itself that will cause conflicts. And while, at this stage, we cannot fully control the virus's spread and its impact on the economy, there are still actions we can do to minimize conflict. Even in situations of protracted social conflict, the outbreak is opening up a variety of 'new and unexpected scenarios', making a whole range of strategies, impossible before the pandemic, possible today (Garrigues, 2020).[10]

Exploring our options for the futures of conflict is linked to how and why conflicts arise in the first place. However, the causes and mechanisms of conflict differ. There are several specific areas over which conflicts tend to arise. They include: information, resources, relationships, structures, and values. Furthermore, there is intrapersonal/inner conflict. Negative economic, social, and health impacts of the 2020 pandemic are already expected to be huge.[11,12] Fuelling existing and emerging conflicts will only make matters worse. Epidemics and pandemics have historically been known to change the course of history. At times, the change was positive, for example: improvement in hygiene practices, redistribution of wealth, improved individual and social relationships in the aftermath, and even "the end of chattel slavery" (Snowden, 2020)[13] in some parts of the world. How damaged, or, alternatively, how well we come out of this one, will depend on many factors, including how we negotiate numerous conflicts ahead. Smart and workable strategies to minimise, manage and even transform the conflict for the better, will significantly influence our future lives and worlds.

INFORMATION

To start with, conflicts often arise in relation to insufficient information. Addressing conflicts about information is one of the easiest ways to prevent and ease the conflict. Policy makers and government agencies, reputable media, ethical individuals, organisations, and various experts all have a role to play in providing timely, accurate, and transparent information. This should help with finding the right balance between underestimating ['I/we will certainly not get it'] and overestimating ['we are all doomed'] the threat from the virus. Gathering facts and clarifying confusion makes a significant contribution to the easing of rising tensions – tensions that commonly bring fear, superstition, magical thinking, and conspiracy ideation into the open. This is always important, but it is especially critical nowadays (i.e., with the prevalence of 'false/fake news' and the 'doubling-down' of ideological positions), to rely on scientific, evidence-based and reputable sources of information. Governments, social media, and all of us can make a positive contribution in that regard. It can also be helpful to have a guiding metaphor or tagline to enable a focused strategy. For example, a helpful saying to address conflict related to insufficient or false information could be: 'Accurate information, timely shared' or 'Information Hygiene'.

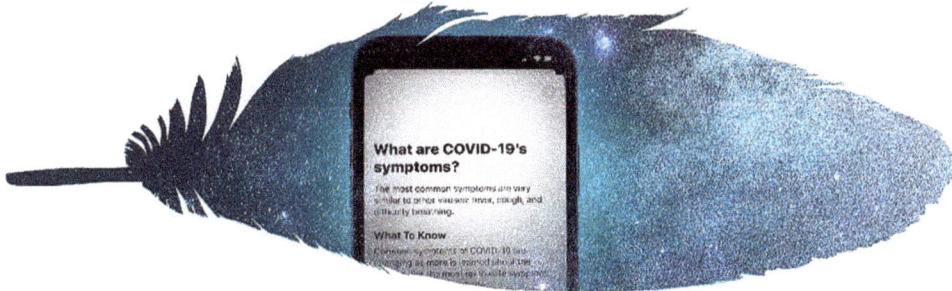

RESOURCES

Another common source of conflict is the scarcity of resources. We have seen 'the battle over respirators' increasingly becoming a source of international conflicts, corruption, and weakening previously friendly ties between nations (e.g. the US versus Germany or France and Germany versus Italy). At the community level, the police needed to intervene when 'battles over toilet paper rolls' in supermarkets manifested in physical violence.

Three key developments work in relation to conflicts over scarce resources. First, conflict decreases when the need for the resources dissipates, or individuals anticipate that there is no restriction, i.e., there are positive expectations of the future. This will likely happen if the need for respirators and other necessities – either due to virus containment or prevention/the invention of a cure or even fair rationing – diminishes. The race to find a workable vaccine and/or cure is already occurring and should be further encouraged and enabled. Fair rationing is currently ad-hoc, dependent on the goodwill of businesses and sporadic government measures. These measures should be made systemic, ongoing, and predictable. Uncertainty feeds into the existing and creates new conflicts. As much as possible, uncertainty should be reduced.

Another common strategy is to provide more of the resources that are currently scarce. In the context of the COVID-19 pandemic that means producing more respirators and other necessities (i.e., products needed for hygiene and protection such as disinfectants, masks, and so on). As is already happening in some places (i.e., distillers producing hand sanitizers or clothing factories producing face masks) this means reevaluating current production priorities and/or repurposing existing production capacities. Local/national/global bodies coordinating such efforts could become invaluable.

The third strategy focuses on the fair sharing and allocation of resources. We usually deal with the lack of resources better than we do with uncertainty or (real or perceived) injustice in how resources are distributed. Clear and fair rules based on community needs and legal and ethical frameworks would go a long way in making this type of conflict dissipate. These rules and strategies should focus on people's needs rather than wants; i.e., sharing what is needed, as opposed to free-market principles that enable panic buying.

A helpful guiding metaphor or saying for addressing conflicts related to the scarcity of resources could be: 'There is enough for all – solidarity' or 'equitable/ fair sharing'.

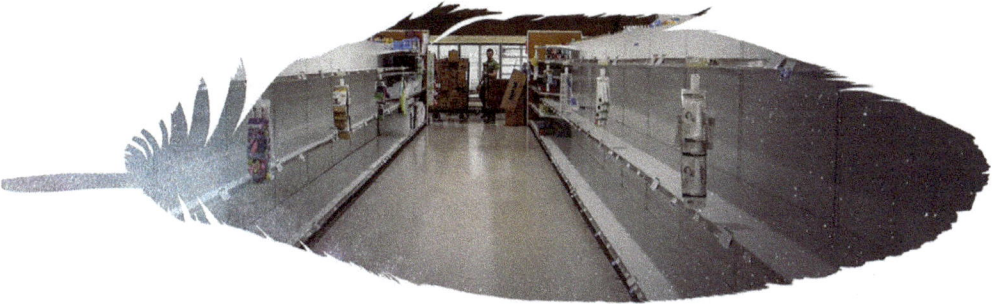

Mick Haupt, Unsplash

RELATIONSHIPS

Yet another common source of conflict is over relationships. We are already witnessing considerable damage done to interpersonal relationships because of people's tendency to overreact and/or become more selfish when fear and panic strike. Also dangerous is the 'blame game' – accusations as to who has or may contract the virus from whom, who is (ir)responsible and who is excessively cautious/'over the top', who has done something similarly irresponsible in the past, and so on. These tensions will introduce some destructive elements to the existing differences between people and communities which would otherwise not cause many problems. Alternatively, if problems do arise due to these differences, they would (in calmer times) find relatively easy solutions. So what we all need to watch for is the possibility of the breakdown of personal relationships, and do our best to avoid stereotyping and scapegoating – both are very common practices amongst humans, especially during times of stress. The best antidote here is to not 'other' individuals and communities, but to turn our thinking around – from judgment and exclusionary/excessive self-focus to a compassionate view and concern for others. That is, other people can be seen as very similar to me/us, with the same fears, concerns and needs. This mental practice helps avoid 'the worse of humanity' which often manifests during times of conflict.

A helpful guiding metaphor for addressing conflicts related to relationships could be: 'Everyone is me' or 'We are all in this together'.

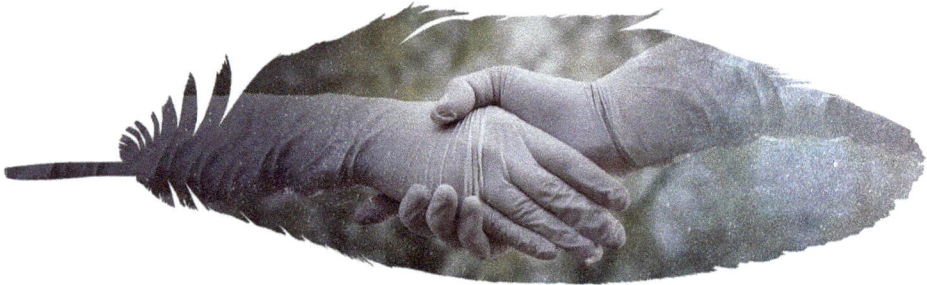

Filip Filkovic-philatz, Unsplash

STRUCTURE

Conflicts about structure are related to access to power or resources, as well as to different amounts of respect and decision-making authority that are given to groups and individuals (Kraybill, 2001)[14]. We have created a very unequal world, where structural injustices determine that the well-being and even lives of certain groups of people are endangered. During crisis situations, the system ensures that those 'on the top' have higher chances of survival and a higher quality of life. Those at 'the bottom' face the opposite. For example, all over the world, the system of patriarchy ensures that women and children in situations of domestic violence will suffer violent conflict and abuse even more during the COVID-19 pandemic. Indeed, reports about the increased rate of domestic violence during lockdowns and other restrictive measures are multiplying (e.g. OHCHR,[14] Graham-Harrison et al. 2020,[15] Murray & Young, 2020,[16] Kelly, 2020[17]). As economically difficult and stressful situations are known to increase this type of violence, systemic countermeasures are absolutely necessary. Other protective measures are also needed for millions of people who are currently losing their jobs and incomes, those already unemployed and homeless, refugees and low-income foreign workers. Structural measures are needed to address the possibility of being evicted, deported or not being able to afford the basics – for this reason welfare payments, universal basic income or aid need to be enhanced. If these measures are not put in place, we could expect a rise in violent conflict, criminality and the number of preventable deaths. Ideally, the COVID-19 pandemic can provide an opportunity to address the world's unequal systems and structures and create more equitable and fair societies. It is also an opportunity to provide much-needed support to the struggling health sector and health workers. In place of the 'survival of the fittest' and 'dog eats dog' the guiding metaphor could be 'global fairness', 'equitable societies – better for all' or 'flattening the inequity curve'.

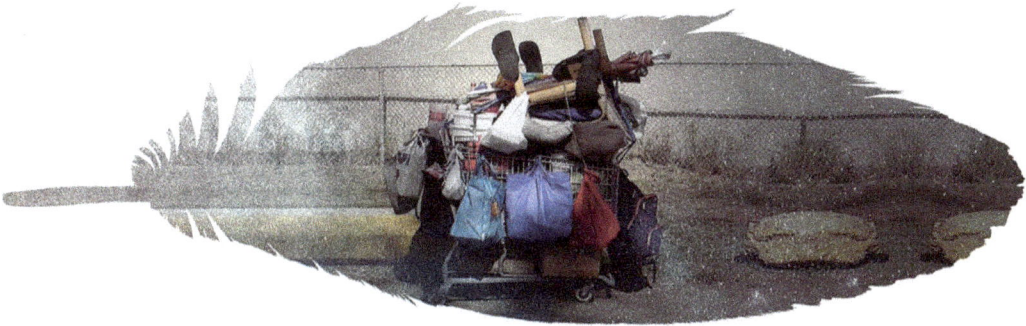

Rusty Gouveia, Pixabay

VALUES

Conflicts over relationships and structure can be difficult to resolve due to our common insular and myopic views based on short-term thinking. Even harder is resolving conflicts involving values. For example, the rush to create a workable vaccine may be motivated by values which focus on profit or national interest (such as the US president's offer[18] to purchase exclusive access to coronavirus vaccine being developed by a German company) versus those that focus on altruism and the long-term greater good. Yet another value position is based on certain religious beliefs ('God decides what happens') versus values based on rational/

secular beliefs ('Humans are in charge'). Values and beliefs are commonly formed based on certain previous life experiences or ideological and faith positions. We can expect a shift in personal values (i.e., 'It is important to shake peoples' hands when we first meet them' towards 'social-distancing') based on new experiences, whereas others might solidify even further (i.e., various faith positions). For example, the anti-vaxxer position is unlikely to shift, even if a reliable vaccine becomes available and the illness caused by the coronavirus (SARS-CoV-2) becomes more visible in their community. Discourses about 'Big Pharma', 'natural' immunity and the 'benefits' of the virus eliminating the old or sick members of the community will most likely continue acting as a cognitive 'shield' that prevents personal values and beliefs from being undermined by external reality. The best strategy so far invented here is to allocate a separate sphere of influence for each set of values – rational/secular/evidence-based/ scientific to the realm of the state and government and policy-making vis-à-vis religious beliefs to the realm of the spiritual and psychological. Moreover, there will be an ongoing discussion in relation to privacy issues and individual freedom vis-à-vis public safety. Individualistic and liberal communities and societies will struggle more with the coming restrictions than collectivist and rules-based authoritarian societies. The helpful guiding metaphor will thus depend on the context: i.e., 'In Government/Our Leaders (or Scientists and Health Workers) We Trust' or 'Community Mobilizes'.

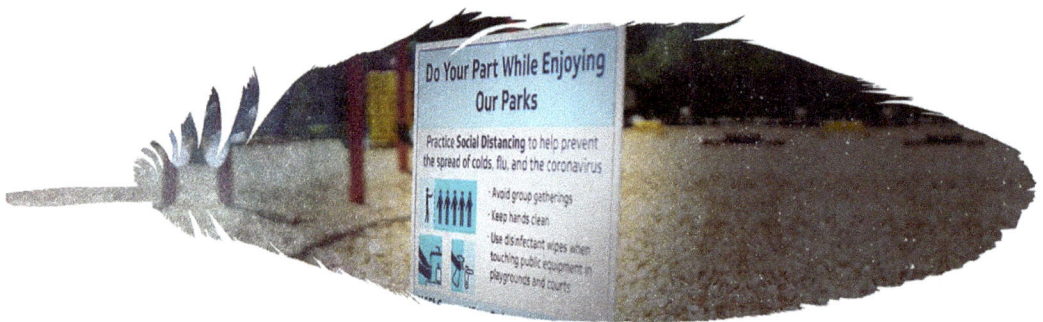

Jordan Hopkins, Unsplash

INTRAPERSONAL

Certainly, the inner, intrapersonal conflict will also skyrocket. 'Should I exercise in a closed area?', 'Should I go visit such and such?', 'Should I travel to XYZ?', 'How much food should I stock up on?', 'Do I have enough toilet paper?', 'How long will this last?', 'How will I make ends meet?, 'Is XYZ financial decision smart or stupid?', 'What will happen to the others if I get sick', 'How will I cope if I get ill?', etc. The main conflict will be between our 'rational' self and our 'fearful/ panicky' one, as well as between our 'inner extrovert' and 'inner introvert'. The best strategy so far invented in this regard is to practice 'watching one's own thoughts' (i.e., mindfulness, cognitive behavioral therapy, critical thinking) and to attempt to distance ourselves a bit from them. Once we gain that small distance, we can then try to investigate what each sub-personality has to offer. Perhaps some sort of balance between rationality and fear should inform our actions? For example, we can take some precautions such as washing our hands and channel our fearful self (subpersonality) into vigilance over that specific set of actions related to personal hygiene. Another specific set of actions we can take based on our fearful self is to be vigilant about sources of information and double-check whether they are coming from reputable sources – information hygiene. On the other hand, our rational self (sub-personality) can assist us in preventing overreactions and making rash decisions based on emotions. Striking a balance between the two will, once again, go a long way in addressing our inner conflicts. Thus, one may choose to see themselves as assets rather than imaging these selves as opposing sides in a battlefield.

Another common inner conflict is between 'control' and 'letting go'. Once again, balancing insights from these different types of mental processes is critical. The key is to direct time and energy towards things we can control, such as how to qualitatively organize one's time during self-isolation or which recommendations to follow and to let go of things we cannot, such as other people's behavior or other external factors.

Indeed, refocusing our attention is critical to minimizing personal anxiety and interpersonal conflict. So instead of overly focusing on 'I do not want to die,' 'I do not want [somebody close to me] to die', or 'I will not be able to cope if I [or somebody close to me] get sick' (thoughts possibly at the back of most people's minds), the focus could be on 'How can I help?', 'What is and is not in my sphere of influence?', 'How can I best 'let go' of things I cannot control?', or 'What is the wisest way for me to contribute?'. Psychologists commonly recommend strengthening self-care in times of crisis. This includes both behavioral (i.e., sufficient sleep, good food, some safe exercise, relaxation, etc.) and psychological responses (i.e., being aware of one's own thinking and behavior and adjusting these patterns if needed). Spiritual and religious practices have been shown to be beneficial in crises as well (i.e., 'Let go and let God'), providing they do not cause the erroneous application of 'faith-based solutions' in the material world, where fact-based solutions are necessary. The best way forward is: 1. Choosing the thoughts and actions that minimize the possibility of violence arising now and in the future, and 2. Using existing conflicts to create something new, a better future. The guiding metaphors could be: 'The Kindness (to oneself and others) Pandemic' or 'Self-Others care'.

EMERGENCE: CREATING INNER AND OUTER BALANCE

Finally, conflict theorists also commonly mention that every conflict can become a golden opportunity to create something new. For example, perhaps we could use this time to pause and reevaluate some personal values and practices (i.e., from 'big life questions' such as: 'how should I live my life knowing that I can die unexpectedly and suddenly', to smaller questions such as: 'how should I organize my daily activities during this forced pause', or, 'how could I best be of service to others')?

We can also inquire into solutions that are needed to improve existing social structures, systems and institutions. Perhaps the coronavirus and other environmental changes could help us rethink the human-nature relationship so that this relationship is also improved? Indeed, there is an opportunity to generate a strong global response to the climate crisis, and out of the "ashes of the corona crisis [create]something new" (Watts, 2020).[20] Or, given the difficulties nations and states face to solve global problems, perhaps we could investigate what type of global and, alternatively, communal/regional/local institutions we should create or enhance?

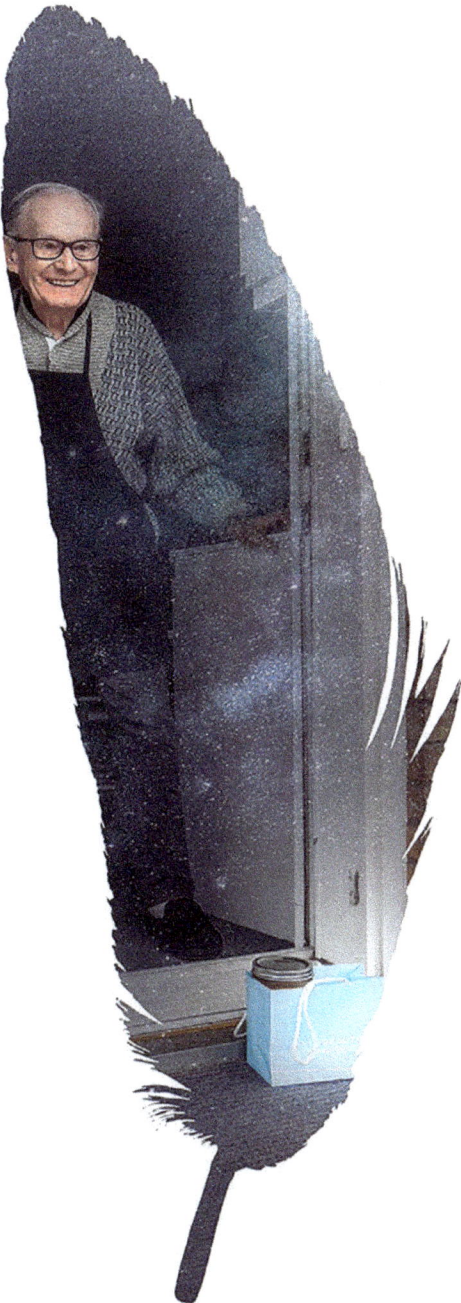

We are already seeing efforts to coordinate global health efforts, even transform existing economic and social structures as well as the worldview behind them. For example, a joint statement of the G20 leaders framed the COVID-19 pandemic as a 'powerful reminder of our inter-connectedness and vulnerabilities' (G20, 2020)[20]. Because 'the virus respects no borders' they committed to 'presenting a united front against this common threat' (ibid.). Their call for action should be replicated as a springboard for a host of other problems – from climate change to global inequality – conflicts around COVID-19 thus truly becoming an opportunity to create something substantially better for the future. In their words, what is needed is 'a transparent, robust, coordinated, large-scale and science-based global response in the spirit of solidarity' (ibid.). Beyond dealing with this pandemic, there is much work left to be done. In addition to addressing pandemics, a global campaign for 'a new just world economic system, where all nations work for the benefit of the other in a win-win fashion' is also needed – 'we need to change our outlook, or we [humans]will perish' (Askary, 2020).[22] Indeed, countless individuals and organizations have already been working on workable solutions towards such a transition for decades.

And yet, we do live in an imbalanced nation-based geopolitical system. We are in the middle of numerous conflicts, inner and outer. Some entrenched values and worldviews are behind structures and systems that reward inequity and injustice. Alternatives are all around us, though they remain marginalized. Balancing acts are never easy. Yet, depending on how skilled we are or become in the process of minimizing versus enhancing thoughts and behavior that give rise to conflict, we can influence the development of more or less peaceful futures. Indeed, with each and every action we take these days, we already do so. Hope remains that we can all use this illness as a way to make ourselves, others, and the planet healthier. The new guiding metaphor could be: 'A different, better world and the best possible selves are possible'.

Summary Table

Source and Type of Conflict	Makes it worse	Makes it better
Information	Inability to discriminate between false and real information	Relying on scientific, evidence-based and reputable sources of information
Resources	Uncertainty and unfairness of allocation	Clear and fair rules based on community needs
Relationships	Blaming, scapegoating, stereotyping	Compassion and concern towards others
Structure	Measures that help the more powerful	Measures that help the most vulnerable
Values	Insularity, rigidity	Dialogue, openness
Intrapersonal	Focusing on thoughts and actions that enhance fear, create controlling behavior and lead to being overwhelmed	Awareness, self-other care, balancing sub-personalities, gratitude, surrender to what's outside of one's control

Source and Type of Conflict	Detrimental guiding metaphor	Helpful guiding metaphor
Information	I see, I share	Accurate information, timely shared; Information hygiene
Resources	Me/We first; First come, first served	There is (will be) enough for all; Solidarity and fairness
Relationships	'They' are causing the pandemic	We are all in this together
Structure	Survival of the fittest	Flattening the inequity curve
Values	Natural immunity; We/humans are powerless	In government/our leaders/scientists/ health workers we trust; Community mobilizes
Intrapersonal	The sky is falling	Kindness pandemic

Table by: Dr Ivana Milojević, Metafuture, www.metafuture.or

AUTHOR

Dr. Ivana Milojević is a researcher, writer and educator with a trans-disciplinary professional background in sociology, education, gender, peace and futures studies and Director of Metafuture. She has held professorships at several universities and is currently focused on conducting research, delivering speeches and facilitating workshops for governmental and academic institutions, international associations, and non-governmental organizations. Dr. Milojević can be contacted at ivana@metafuture.org

The author would like to thank Charmaine Sevil for her creativity on the images in this article. Charmaine Sevil is a futures designer and her website is www.sevilco.com.au

REFERENCES

Burke, A. (2020, April 14). Peace and the Pandemic: The Impact of COVID-19 on Conflict in Asia. *Devpolicy Blog*. https://devpolicy.org/peace-and-the-pandemic-the-impact-of-covid-19-on-conflict-in-asia-20200414/.

Chotiner, I. (2020, March 3). How Pandemics Change History. *The New Yorker*. https://www.newyorker.com/news/q-and-a/how-pandemics-change-history.

Executive Intelligence Review (2020, March 27). *Xi and Trump Confer; Global Collaboration Grows Against Pandemic; New Economic Systems is the Key*. https://larouchepub.com/pr/2020/20200328_Xi&Trump_Confer.html.

G20. (N.D.). Recover Together: Recover Stronger. https://g20.org/.

Gearin, M., and Knight, B. (2020, March 29). *Family Violence Perpetrators using COVID-19 as 'a form of abuse we have not experienced before'*. https://www.abc.net.au/news/2020-03-29/coronavirus-family-violence-surge-in-victoria/12098546.

Gordon, El, and Carrot, F. (2020, April 8). Coronavirus in Conflict: The Fight Has Hardly Begun. *The Interpreter*. https://www.lowyinstitute.org/the-interpreter/coronavirus-conflict-zones-fight-has-hardly-begun.

Kelly, M. (2020, March 26). Trauma Surgeons Brace for Surge in Domestic Violence-Related Injuries. *The Canberra Times*. https://www.canberratimes.com.au/story/6698842/trauma-surgeons-brace-for-surge-in-domestic-violence-related-injuries/.

Kluth, A. (2020, April 1). How the Coronavirus Pandemic Will Lead to Social Revolutions. *Bloomberg* https://www.bloomberg.com/opinion/articles/2020-04-11/coronavirus-this-pandemic-will-lead-to-social-revolutions.

Kraybill, R. (2001). *Peace Skills: Manual for Community Mediators*. Jossey-Bass.

Milanovic, B. (2020, March 19). The Real Pandemic Danger is Social Collapse. *Foreign Affairs*. https://www.foreignaffairs.com/articles/2020-03-19/real-pandemic-danger-social-collapse.

Relationships Australia (2020, April 16). *How to Manage Relationship Tensions during COVID-19*. https://www.relationshipswa.org.au/news-events/current-news-and-events/2020/april/how-to-manage-relationship-tensions-during-covid-1.

United Nations (2020, April 21). *As Families of 'biblical proportion' look, Security Council urged to 'act fast'*. https://news.un.org/en/story/2020/04/1062272

Vatikiotis, M. (2020, April 18). COVID-19 is Fuelling Conflict: New Ways Will be Needed to Make Peace. *New Straits Times*. https://www.straitstimes.com/opinion/covid-19-is-fuelling-conflict-new-ways-will-be-needed-to-make-peace.

Watts, J. (2020, April 23). Earth Day: Great Thunberg calls for 'new path' After Pandemic. *The Guardian*. https://www.theguardian.com/environment/2020/apr/22/earth-day-greta-thunberg-calls-for-new-path-after-pandemic.

COVID-19 & PANDEMIC PREPAREDNESS:

*Foresight Narratives and
Public Sector Responses*

Ivana Milojević

The management of the COVID-19 pandemic is a novel global challenge being addressed in real time. While some countries and regions of the world have had more recent experience managing similar viruses (such as SARS), all have had to deal with the new corona virus and the novel challenges that it presents. Public policy responses are rapidly changing, sometimes daily. This article focuses on how foresight narratives have impacted policymaking as related to the COVID-19 pandemic. More specifically, it provides an overview of the use of foresight within the public sector prior to the pandemic. It also investigates the key narratives in circulation during the implementation of governments' strategic objectives and the realization of visions of a 'pandemic-free' society. The approach used here is that of narrative foresight which predominantly focuses on the stories that individuals, organizations, states and civilizations tell themselves about the future. In addition to the overarching narratives, the article also investigates more specifically the most commonly used metaphors prior to and during the COVID-19 pandemic. The goal of the article is to ascertain which lessons we can learn in terms of successes and failures of narrative 'foresight in action', so as to be able to utilise this knowledge for future global problems. Finally, the article argues that many current metaphors and narratives are linked to 'futures fallacies' – detrimental thinking patterns about the future. It then concludes by briefly investigating alternative narratives and metaphors which are more likely to facilitate the desired future of adequate pandemic preparedness.

COVID-19: WERE WE WARNED?

"'No', I said, 'nothing new has happened. Plagues are as certain as death and taxes.'" ([Krause 1982] cited in Krause, 1993, xviii)

The role of hindsight is salient if we wish to enhance foresight. The role of historical events, insights and warnings is critical for any informed foresight work. That is, we need to know what we can learn from history and we need to know how we can improve our thinking about the future both now and in the future.

Previous research on public sector foresight processes strongly indicates gaps in knowledge (e.g. Calof & Smith, 2012; Cameron, Georghiou, Keenan, Miles & Saritas, 2006; Coates, 2010; Conway & Stewart, 2004; Cook, Inayatullah, Burgman, Sutherland & Wintle, 2014; Cuhls & Georghiou, 2004; Da Costa, Warnke, Scapolo & Cagnin, 2008; Dator, 2007, 2011; Dreyer & Stang, 2013; Greenblott, O'Farrell, Olson, Buchard, 2018; Havas, Schartinger, & Weber, 2010; Jennings, 2017; Kuosa, 2012; Savio & Nikolopoulos, 2009; Schartinger, Wilhelmer, Holste & Kubeczko, 2012; Solem, 2011; UNDP, 2014). A "dramatic lack of forward thinking and planning" specifically related to pandemics (Rubin, 2011, p. 63) has also previously been identified. Moreover, "lessons learned" from previous infectious disease outbreaks and "recommendations for the future" related to pandemic preparedness were encapsulated in a number of publications over the last two decades (e.g., Brundtland, 2003; WHO, 2009; Rubin, 2011; Morse, Mazet, Woolhouse, Parrish, Carroll, Karesh, Zambrana-Torrelio, Lipkin, & Daszak, 2012; WHO, 2015; Ross, Crowe & Tyndall, 2015; UN, 2016; WHO, 2017; WHO, 2018; GPMB, 2019). This article intends to link together previous findings in the context of 'foresight in action' (Van Asselt, Van Klooster, Van Notten & Smits, 2010) – i.e., whether and how this knowledge was utilised.

The first point I make here is that, contrary to views held by some, foresight related to the forthcoming pandemic was NOT in "tragically short supply" (Davies, 2020). Certainly, the stories different actors tell about the past, present and future are vastly different and, indeed, the narratives of *"nobody knew"*, "who would have thought?", *"never before"* and *"pandemic shock"* have been abundant. However, so have the narratives of *"it is just a matter of time"*, *"we need to start preparing now"* and *"time is running out"*. This latter set of narratives is present in numerous documents published by various global and national bodies as well as in academic research papers and books anticipating the possibility of a pandemic. The majority of them repeat the 'mantra' of concern for: (1) the impending pandemic, and (2) the lack of preparedness at all levels of governance. Before I address the issue of the lack of preparedness for the current pandemic, I first provide examples of the application of foresight – anticipating risks and challenges – in the public sector.

COVID-19: FORETOLD AND FOREWARNED BUT NOT FOREARMED?

When COVID-19 was first identified in Wuhan, China, in December 2019, there were already many documents published by various global and national bodies as well as academic research papers and books that anticipated the possibility of a pandemic. Some 'highlights' include the following:

And for the next outbreak, of SARS, or, perhaps a new, more infectious and more deadly illness. We may have very little time. Let us use it wisely. [Brundtland, 2003, para. 44]

Future pandemic threats will emerge and have potentially devastating consequences. [UN, 2016, p. 8]

> ... despite ... the looming threat of a pandemic ... [n]ational health security is fundamentally weak around the world. No country is fully prepared for epidemics or pandemics, and every country has important gaps to address. [Cameron, Nuzzo, & Bell, 2019, pp. 6, 9]

In addition to the citations above, similar warnings were part of various publications emphasising the narrative of the forthcoming pandemic and lack of preparedness. For example, a discussion about "a major pandemic outbreak" including efforts to "upgrade our global preparedness to identify and isolate new diseases" features in the World Economic Forum's 2007 *Global Risk Report.* It then reappears in 2008, as follows:

> A pandemic disease jumps from the animal population to humans, with high mortality and transmission rates. [WEF, 2008, p. 22]

> [And since] global travel patterns have made the risk of a pandemic homogenous across the world [a]ll countries are equally vulnerable to a pandemic that originates in one country. [WEF, 2008, p. 29]

An academic publication from the same year [Jones, Patel, Levy, Storeygard, Balk, Gittleman & Daszak, 2008, p. 990] similarly argued that:

Emerging infectious diseases (EIDs) ... have risen significantly over time ... the majority of these (71.8%) originate in wildlife ... EID origins are significantly correlated with socio-economic, environmental and ecological factors, and provide a basis for identifying regions where new EIDs are most likely to originate (emerging disease 'hotspots').

Many decades prior, Richard Krause, the author of *The Restless Tide: The persistent Challenge of the Microbial World* (1981) warned that "...emerging viruses know no country. There are no barriers to prevent their migration across international boundaries or around the 24 time zones." (Krause, 1993, p. xvii)

In 2009, the World Health Organisation (WHO) issued a *Whole of Society Pandemic Readiness* document wherein they asked the question of "Why do pandemic planning beyond health care?" and to which they responded in the following manner:

Given that a pandemic of any severity will have consequences for the whole of society, it is essential that all organizations, both private and public, plan for the potential disruption that a pandemic will cause ... While many countries have made substantial efforts to prepare for the health consequences of pandemics, not all countries have yet given sufficient attention to preparing for the economic, humanitarian and societal consequences. (WHO, 2009, p. 5)

Warnings about the economic fallout that could arise if we were to experience a pandemic were given as well. For example:

...the world [is] highly vulnerable to massive loss of life and economic shocks from natural of human-made epidemics and pandemics. ... The inclusive costs of the next ... pandemic could be US$570 billion each year or 0.7% of global income ... Given the magnitude of the threat, we call for scaled-up financing of international collective action for epidemic and pandemic preparedness. (WHO, 2017, p. 742)

A few years prior, the President of the World Bank called for the creation of a new pandemic emergency facility:

planning must … begin for the next pandemic, which could spread much more quickly, kill even more people [than Ebola] and potentially devastate the global economy. [The World Bank, 2014, para. 3]

Concerns were also raised about "the increasing frequency of pandemics occurring over the last few decades." [Ross, Crowe & Tyndall, 2015, p. 89] Specifically, and "worryingly" [Ross et al., 2015, p. 89]:

…the frequency between pandemics seems to be disturbingly shorter as evident with Severe Acute Respiratory Syndrome [SARS] in 2003, Influenza A H1N5 [bird flu] in 2007, H1N1 [swine flu] in 2009, Middle East Respiratory Syndrome [MERS] in 2012 and Ebola in 2014. … Clearly, the window of opportunity to act is closing.

Given this context, the UN Secretary-General established the High-level Panel on the Global Response to Health Crises in April 2015 [UN, 2016]. The Panel also noted that:

…the high risk of major health crises is widely underestimated, and that the world's preparedness and capacity to respond is woefully insufficient. Future epidemics could far exceed the scale and devastation [of previous outbreaks]. [Their emergence] could rapidly result in millions of deaths and cause major social, economic and political disruption. [UN, 2016, p. 5]

Over time, the warnings became more alarmist. In May 2018 the World Bank and the WHO co-convened the Global Preparedness Monitoring Board which in their first annual report on global preparedness for health emergencies stated the following:

…there is a very real threat of a rapidly moving, highly lethal pandemic of a respiratory pathogen killing 50 to 80 million people and wiping out nearly 5% of the world's economy. A global pandemic on that scale would be catastrophic, creating widespread havoc, instability and insecurity. The world is not prepared. [GPMB, 2019, p. 6]

EXAMPLES OF PANDEMIC AWARENESS AND FORESIGHT AMONG NATIONAL AND REGIONAL GOVERNMENTS

Parallel to global bodies or globally-oriented analysis, various national governments and academics analysing specific countries' or regions' pandemic preparedness were also aware (and gave warnings) of the emerging threat of infectious diseases (EID). Here are some US-based examples:

> ...a growing concern by senior US leaders ... the growing global infectious disease threat. ... New and re-emerging infectious diseases will pose a rising global health threat and will complicate US and global security over the next 20 years. (NIC, 2000, pp. 1, 5)

> If we wait for a pandemic to appear it will be too late to prepare. And one day many lives could be needlessly lost because we failed to act today. (George Bush, 2005, cited in Mosk, 2020, para. 24)

In the UK, a series of 2006 publications were part of the foresight project entitled *Infections Diseases: Preparing for the future* which looked 10-25 years ahead in order to "consider infectious diseases in humans, animals and plants" (Brownlie, Peckham, Waage, Woolhouse, Lyall, Meagher, Tait, Baylis & Nicoll, 2006, p. 64). Whilst recognising that "predicting our disease future with precision is not possible" (Brownlie, et al., 2006, p. 63), nonetheless, amongst the "eight global disease threats" the authors identified "new pathogens or novel variants of existing pathogens" and "zoonoses" (Brownlie, et al., 2006, p. 23). They also wrote the following:

> Nearly 40 'new' human pathogens were first reported in the last 25 years, and the majority of these had zoonotic origins. The risk of zoonotic infection shows no sign of diminishing and may well increase in the future ... diseases that cross species [are] ... one of the top future risks. (Brownlie et al., 2006, p. 32)

Moreover, in the section investigating "China – future trends in human and animal infectious diseases" the authors recognised "the importance of Asia as a source of zoonotic diseases, and China as an important country in the region" (Brownlie et al., 2006, p. 64). Finally, future gaps and trends in vulnerabilities in China for human and animal infectious diseases were also identified, such as:

> Illegal practices ... Lack of interaction between policy and regulatory agencies leading to delays in detection and identification ... [and] Problems across international agencies, particularly barriers to the sharing of data. (Brownlie et al., 2006, p. 68)

Such very specific warnings are also present in academic papers, for example:

> The presence of a large reservoir of SARS-CoV-like viruses in horseshoe bats, together with the culture of eating exotic mammals in southern China, is a timebomb. The possibility of the reemergence of SARS and other novel viruses from animals or laboratories and therefore the need for preparedness should not be ignored. (Cheng, Lau, Woo & Yuen, 2007, p. 694)

Similar narratives are replicated elsewhere. For example, a thorough 2008 analysis of national preparedness plans in the African region concluded the following (Ortu, Mounier-Jack & Coker, 2008, pp. 161-169):

> With 35 countries of 53 having drafted and approved plans since November 2005, preparation efforts for an influenza pandemic in the African region have advanced considerably. ... Africa faces many challenges and the limited surveillance capacity to pandemic ...the human health care sector is ill-prepared.

More recent (Kinsman, Angrén & Elgh, 2018, p. 2) analysis of "Preparedness and Response Against Diseases with Epidemic Potential in the European Union" ascertained that:

> Infectious disease outbreaks remain as an ongoing threat. Efforts are required to ensure that core public health capacities for the full range of preparedness and response activities are sustained.

The same year, the World Bank analysed pandemic preparedness in East Asia and the Pacific and highlighted the following:

> Countries in East Asia and the Pacific made tremendous efforts to tackle emerging infectious diseases; however, many challenges remain to ensure that resilient health systems and pandemic preparedness are sustainably financed. [The World Bank, 2018, para. 2]

The MENA region as well, had previously:

> ... missed out on opportunities to advance patient research during prior infectious disease outbreaks caused by the Severe Acute Respiratory Syndrome, Ebola, and the Middle East Respiratory Syndrome, as evidenced by the lack of concerted research and clinical trials from the region. [Ibrahim, Kamour, Harhara, Gaba & Nair, 2020, p. 106106]

These examples are just the tip of the iceberg when it comes to the use of foresight prior to the COVID-19 pandemic. In summary, the current pandemic was widely anticipated and many warnings in terms of actions needed to ameliorate human suffering and economic cost were given. There is also a consensus that even the most alarming warnings did not adequately translate into the level of preparedness in the public sector which such a future pandemic would require. The next section of this article aims at suggesting that in addition to the usual 'suspects' – e.g., a lack of political will, coordination or funding – detrimental thinking patterns about the future, termed futures fallacies, [Milojević, 2020a] were also salient.

COVID-19 FUTURES FALLACIES

Futures fallacies are a broader issue which I've investigated in three previous publications [Milojević, 2020a, 2020b, 2020c]. In the following sections of this article, I further explore the futures fallacies as they relate specifically to lack of adequate preparedness for COVID-19. The purpose of this investigation is to: (1)

map some of the reasons behind the lack of pandemic preparedness related to how we often think about the future, and (2) enhance narrative foresight within the public sector at the global, national and local level. The narratives under investigation have been circulating in both public policy documents (inclusive of academic publications) and public discourse (inclusive of political discourse) – in relation to epidemics/pandemics in general and COVID-19 in particular.

It is very clear from this investigation that a number of cognitive and futures fallacies converged so as to prevent an adequate pandemic preparedness response. They ensured that the strategies needed to manifest desired longer-term futures were missing or insufficiently applied (Miojević, 2020a, 2020c). They also ensured that the best existing evidence, facts, and logic, of relevance to emerging futures, fell on deaf ears (Milojević, 2020a, 2020c).

DENIAL: JUST A FLU

To start with, one of the longest and best documented cognitive fallacies **– denial –** has been abundantly present in narratives both before and during the pandemic. One example of this fallacy is the narrative of COVID-19 being *'just a flu'*. What is problematic in this narrative is perhaps not so much comparison with the flu, but more the adverb 'just'. The yearly global toll from 'just the flu', as estimated by WHO (2019), is 1 billion cases, of which three to five million are severe cases, "resulting in 290 000 to 650 000 influenza-related respiratory deaths". Unfortunately, foresight itself may have contributed to this narrative. Since the early 1990s, many epidemiologists and governments anticipated that a new pandemic might be related to influenza (e.g. Webster, 1997; WHO, 1999; NIC, 2000; HSC, 2005; AHMPPI, 2014; Ross et al., 2015). Even though those reports warned of 'other' possible infectious diseases, and also new emerging influenza viruses to which there is no immunity, timely vaccine or adequate treatment, the 'just the flu' narrative seemed to have stuck. And perhaps "[framing a new EID as a flu] was a mistake; telling people the next pandemic would be caused by influenza didn't make it seem nightmarish at all. The flu? I get that every year. We have a vaccine for that." (Henig, 2020)

Foresight based documents also repeatedly warned that no pandemic can be accurately predicted. Still, the warnings were often about the details of the prediction rather than whether prediction discourse is in itself problematic. For example:

With such a small number of cases, it is impossible to predict future numbers of cases of the human disease... [Murphy, 1998, p. 433, italics added]

Although the timing cannot be predicted ... [HSC, 2005, p. 1, italics added]

While the source and virulence of the next emerging pathogen are difficult to predict... [UN, 2016, p. 29, italics added]

African experts concurred with the prediction that HIV/AIDS, malaria and respiratory infections including tuberculosis will remain the most important infectious diseases in Africa in coming decades. [Brownlie et al., 2006, p. 35, italics added]

PREDICTION: THE BOY WHO CRIED WOLF

Once again, the problem here is not in trying to identify early warning signals and emerging issues, but the futures fallacy of **prediction** [Milojević, 2020a, 2020c]. The main danger with this fallacy is that genuinely valid warnings about the future are not heard due to previously 'failed predictions', even though, given the sheer volume of predictions made on a daily basis, it is always possible to find predictions which have, in retrospect, been shown to be true. The metaphor of *'the boy who cried wolf'* perhaps best summarises this futures fallacy in the context of COVID-19. Krause [1993, p. xviii] for example, describes efforts to forestall a 1975 epidemic amongst a small number of soldiers at Fort Dix, NJ, USA. In order to prevent a possible repetition of the 1918 flu pandemic, "within 9 months a specially formulated vaccine was mass produced and millions of Americans were immunized" Krause in Morse, 1993, p. xviii]. However, for whatever reason, that particular flu did not go global. In fact, except for AIDS, the same was the case with many other emerging infectious diseases [EIDs], e.g., SARS in 2003 [mostly stayed in Asia], MERS in 2012 [mostly stayed in the Middle East] and Ebola in 2014 [mostly remained in west Africa]. Which may explain why – having seen so many *"This Is the Big One"* threats flaming out, we ended up "inured to the real threat of a true international crisis" [Henig, 2020] prior to and at the beginning of COVID-19 pandemic.

Given how long *'the most likely to endanger us'* lists have been getting, it's not surprising many became overwhelmed or simply gave up. The public sector in most countries is stretched and struggling to meet competing and changing demands. So on one hand, in our globalised and interconnected world, humanity is better equipped to manage pandemic risks. On the other hand, the exponential rate of social change and the cultural, demographic, environmental, technological and economic challenges of our time make such tasks increasingly difficult. COVID-19 response has been termed "the greatest global science policy failure in a generation" (Horton, 2020a). And yet, when governments did act successfully in the past, for example, during the outbreak of the 2009 swine flu pandemic, many were subsequently critiqued for their 'over-reactiveness' as well as high spending on the vaccine and other medical supplies. In 2010 the German magazine *Spiegel*, for example, asked the question of how and why the world overreacted, using terms such as *'the swine flu panic'* and *'reconstruction of a mass hysteria'*. *'Damned if you do, and damned if you do not'* may be a metaphor best summarising public sector dilemma in face of the type and intensity of a response to be chosen.

OVERINFLATED AGENCY: 'OTHERING' THE VIRUS

The futures fallacy of **overinflated agency** which commonly relegates and reaffirms responsibility (Milojević, 2020a, 2020b, 2020c) – in this case to the public sector and government leaders – only adds fuel to the fire. The fallacy of overinflated agency is also behind conspiratory thinking which proportions blame to an individual, organisation or group of people – e.g., Bill Gates, George Soros or Huawei and 5G networks, as heard during the COVID-19 pandemic. Moreover, 'mysterious' and 'unconquered' diseases, in particular, tend to unleash a "tsunami of hate and xenophobia, scapegoating and scaremongering" (Guterres, 2020). The ascent of HIV-AIDS in the 1980s, for example, engendered fear and hatred against social groups seen as combatants in the "AIDS invasion of North America" (Gilman, 1987, p. 87). Those were the "five 'H's – homosexuals, heroin addicts, Haitians, haemophiliacs and hookers" (Cohn, 2012, p. 538). The current *"China-virus"* or *"kung-flu"* metaphors similarly aim to apportion blame. What is behind it is yet another powerful metaphor of *"nation-as-organism"*, where "just as the body may be threatened by contaminating foreign elements, the social body is treated as vulnerable to corruption by invading sub-groups" (Bin Larif, 2015, p. 97). This group of people could include anybody deemed as 'the other', from foreign nationals, migrants and refugees, to recently returned travellers (UN, 2020).

OVERINFLATED AGENCY AND PREDICTION: WARNINGS VERSUS PREDICTIONS

Returning to the futures fallacy of prediction, this fallacy makes anticipation in general and distinguishing between the *'signal and the noise'* (Silver, 2012) in particular even more precarious. For example, "between 1940 and 2004 there were 335 emerging infectious diseases (EID) origins reported globally" (Ross et al., 2015, p. 90). It is "estimated that there are 354 generic infectious diseases in the world today [2017]" (BFI, 2017). Since 1980, "a new infectious disease has emerged in humans at an average of one every four months." (UNEP, 2016, p. 65). In the period between 2009 and 2019, the (now defunct) PREDICT program has "identified 1,200 different viruses that had the potential to erupt into pandemics, including more than 160 novel coronaviruses" (Baumgaertner & Rainey, 2020). Over 90 infectious disease outbreaks were identified by WHO in 2018 and nearly 120 in 2019 (WHO, 2020a). In the year 2020 "pneumonia of unknown cause – China" (5 January) and "novel coronavirus - China" (23 January) make an appearance. But so do Ebola, MERS-CoV, Measles, Lassa fever, Yellow fever, Dengue fever, Dracunculiasis (Guinea worm disease), Influenza A(H1Ns), Plague, Chikungunya and Monkeypox – all in multiple parts of the world. Most of those diseases were, once again, contained to particular regions. But so was 'novel coronavirus-China' on 11 and 12 January 2020 (WHO, 2020b):

> The evidence is highly suggestive that the outbreak is associated with exposures in one seafood market in Wuhan. ... Among the 41 confirmed cases, there has been one death. ... Currently, no case with infection of this novel coronavirus has been reported elsewhere other than Wuhan.

Fast forward to 1 October 2020 where 41 confirmed cases in one Chinese city has grown to 33,842,281 confirmed cases and 1,010,634 deaths with cases present in 235 countries, areas or territories (WHO, 2020c). Volumes will be written about 'what went wrong' and how come this particular virus/case – amongst so many – spiralled 'out of control'. Of course, all this will be done retrospectively.

The problem with the future fallacy of prediction is that it may exacerbate some government's reluctance to get on board with important projects or politicians' criticism of organisations doing 'prediction' for not getting it *'exactly right'*. Important recommendations may be seen as a *'waste of time and money'*, given that prevention rarely gives politicians *'hero status'* or *'helps them cut the ribbon'* (Inayatullah, 2018, p. 20). Spending time on getting 'the right signal amongst the noise' or deciding what should be on the top of 'the most likely to endanger us' lists is understandable. In the changing world, citizens and governments want some certainty which prediction discourse is more than happy to provide. At the same time, efforts there may mean that more important messages are 'lost in the process of translation'. For example, the messages about: (1) the importance of early warning systems, (2) addressing underlying drivers for the diseases, (3) putting generic preventative measures in place, (4) developing futures literacy in general, (5) developing a foresight-oriented agile public sector in particular, and (6) acting early and decisively while also (7) being flexible in needed responses as circumstances change. In other words, the underlying assumption is that warning signals can safely be ignored until they become a full-blown problem. The difference between warnings which are about possibilities and predictions which are about certainties may be subtle. However, this difference is critically important and it is crucial that we find a way to communicate it more clearly in future foresight projects.

THE ARRIVAL AND THE EXEMPTION: THE WEST AS AN INFECTION-FREE UTOPIA

Three other futures fallacies go hand in hand with the futures fallacy of prediction: (1) **linear projection**, (2) **ceteris paribus** and (3) **the arrival** futures fallacies (Dorr, 2017). Taken together, they presume (Dorr, 2017): (1) that future change will be a simple and steady extension of past trends (such as extrapolation of past pandemics), (2) that it is sufficient to consider only one single aspect of change (such as the spread of the pathogen) and (3) that possible futures are envisioned as static objects like a destination or goal (such as arresting the epidemic's spread, elimination of the virus/pathogen).

For example, the linear projection fallacy has been behind the long-standing belief that infectious diseases were *'conquered'* and nature *'controlled'* by science and technology. While prior to the twentieth century it was thought that infections were part of the human condition (Wilson, 1994), modern scientific and technological advances had "facilitated the control or prevention of many infectious diseases, particularly in industrialized nations." (CISET, 1994). Antibiotics and other drugs, vaccines against childhood diseases, and improved technology for sanitation (CISET, 1994), made it appear that we had arrived, or were in the process of arriving, to *'post-nature'* societies. This led both the public and many experts to expect nearly complete freedom from infectious diseases (Wilson, 1994).

Influenced by the linear projection, ceteris paribus and the arrival futures fallacies, the mainstream global discourse of the mid to late 20th century has thus been one where, at least partially, it is assumed that the western industrialized nations 'have arrived' to the stage of an *'infection-free utopia'*. It was also assumed that the rest of the world will follow, providing it adopts the same standards of hygiene, immunisation and medical care.

FUTURE PERSONAL EXEMPTION: OUT OF SIGHT, OUT OF MIND

However, yet another futures fallacy – of **future personal exemption** – made industrialized nations blind to the facts of the old and new infectious diseases elsewhere. Numerous regulatory frameworks, including those by the International Health Regulations (IHR), World Health Organisation (WHO) and World Health Assembly (WHA), were critiqued on the basis that the regulations pose an enormous obligation for all but are "primarily developed to protect the health and welfare of developed nations" (Ross et al., 2015, p. 91). COVID-19 has laid bare errors in governance committed by the "global health leaders", more than 80% of whom are nationals of high-income countries and half being nationals of the UK and the USA (Dalglish, 2020, p. 1189). Moreover, "85% of global organisations working in health have headquarters in Europe and North America; two-thirds are headquartered in Switzerland, the UK, and the USA" (Dalglish, 2020, p. 1189). And, consequently but short-sightedly, "the majority of the scientific and surveillance effort [is] focused on countries from where the next important EID is least likely to originate" (Jones et al., 2008, p. 990).

This global power imbalance has had two important implications. First, *'out of sight, out of mind'*, including questions of what constitutes an epidemic worth looking into (Henig, 2020). And, second, the myopia blinding us globally to "the strengths of the COVID-19 [and other EID] response in Africa and Asia", i.e., in some countries which have, despite limited resources, adopted measures perhaps "worth imitating" (Dalglish, 2020, p. 1189).

Dynamics similar to those which takes place globally can be observed within a single country as well. For example, the UK's government advisers are "narrowly drawn as scientists from a few institutions ... [consequently they] took narrow a view and hewed to limited assumptions (Grey & MacAskill, 2020). Policy makers all around the world tend to have similar backgrounds (educated, middle- or upper-class background, dominant ethnic or religious group) – they "often unintentionally frame policy problems from a narrow world view, and often it is their own" (Terranova, 2015, p. 372). Expertise that exists in a number of marginalised spaces – e.g., local, indigenous knowledge – may thus be neglected. But it is precisely this type of knowledge and expertise – from various globally marginalised places – that has to be included if the fallacy of future personal exemption is to be addressed.

To strengthen this latest point, it is perhaps worth mentioning that in the 2019 *Global Health Security Index*, an assessment of 195 countries' capacity to face infectious disease outbreaks – compiled largely by US-based experts – it is the USA which is ranked first in terms of overall preparedness score, followed by the UK, Netherlands, Australia and Canada (Cameron et al., 2019). In light of the devastating COVID-19 death rate and other policy failures in the US, the authors of the GHSI have since provided a further elaboration as to the "significant preparedness gaps" in the US (GHSI, 2020, para 2):

> The United States' response to the COVID-19 outbreak to date shows that capacity alone is insufficient if that capacity isn't fully leveraged. Strong health systems must be in place to serve all populations, and effective political leadership that instils confidence in the government's response is crucial.

It is beyond doubt that *'leveraging capacity'*, having a *'strong public health system'* and *'effective political leadership'* are all critical for any future pandemic preparedness and adequate response. But so is addressing the fallacy of future personal exemption which makes it less likely for wealthy and powerful nations and individuals to help address the root causes and drivers most commonly identified as being behind epidemics and pandemics outbreaks. Some of those drivers include (but are not limited to): poverty, inequity, violent conflict, inadequate public health provision, inadequate funding for prevention, the lack of an adequately integrated and well-funded 'One Health' global approach (WHO, 2017), environmental pressures and degradation, habitat destruction and human/host/reservoir interaction. Addressing the root causes and drivers behind epidemics is a monumental task but one which needs to be undertaken if we are to succeed in *"coming together"* (Brundtland, 2003) to prevent yet another global catastrophe.

TYPHOID MARY 2.0 OR ALL IN THE SAME STORM

Alternatively, we are left with metaphors and narratives that externalise both the risk and the blame. For example, the poor (and 'the other') may be blamed for their 'reckless' behaviour – such as eating wild life, exploiting animals, or going back to unsanitary wet markets. This is akin to the blaming of the poor Irish immigrant to the US Mary Mallon some hundred years ago for her 'persistence' in working as a cook despite being an asymptomatic carrier of the highly contagious typhoid fever. To this day, instead of being a symbol of the refusal of the well-off to address the underlying conditions which made Mary Mallon (and others) forced to go back to the very same conditions that influenced the spread of the disease, she continues to be remembered as 'Typhoid Mary' – a killer of the affluent. Of course, if we are to prevent Typhoid Mary 2.0, 3.0, etc. we need to discard the fallacy of future personal exemption, as it makes many of us blind to the significance of minimising the previously mentioned drivers behind the spread of infectious diseases.

Being in the *"same storm but not in the same boat"* is the metaphor that probably best summarises the current situation. It is also important to point out the differential treatment different 'boats' (real and metaphorical) receive, depending on how close they are to wealth and power. Consequently, some were blind as to the possibility of luxury cruise ships being carriers of the dangerous diseases. This in turn led to numerous outbreaks of COVID-19, most notably in Japan and Australia: because how could *Diamond Princess* or *Ruby Princess* possibly be *Typhoid Mary 2.0?*

PRESENT ATTENTION AND FATALISM: LATEST NEWSWORTHY ISSUE AND DODGING THE BULLET

Yet more futures fallacies played a role in our collective lack of preparedness for COVID-19. The futures fallacy of **present attention**, for example, while helpful in futures issues framing, is also notable for its "narrow focus on the latest newsworthy issue" [Milojević, 2020a]. Our cognitive biases influence us in a way that makes us tend to "assess the relative importance of issues by the ease with which they are retrieved from memory" [Kahneman, 2011, p. 8]. And since "few of us have experienced a pandemic [such as COVID-19] … we [were] all guilty of ignoring information that doesn't reflect our own experience of the world" [Horton, 2020a]. Even when epidemics spread in some countries or regions of our common world, the rest of 'us' *"kept on dodging a bullet* [as] it was easy to attribute everyone else's susceptibility to things that didn't exist in our … way of life" [Henig, 2020, italics added]. Those of us that "didn't ride camels … eat monkeys [or] … handle live bats and civet cats in the marketplace" [Henig, 2020] – not being 'complicit', felt safe.

Such "biases of intuitive thinking" are apparent in "assigning probabilities to events, forecasting the future, assessing hypotheses, and estimating frequencies" [Kahneman, 2011, p. 8]. As a consequence, pandemic preparedness and response in the public sector oscillate between cycles of *'panic followed by neglect'* [WHO, 2017; Cameron et al., 2019; World Bank, 2017; UN, 2016]. In other words, global panic during the latest potentially growing epidemic is usually followed by complacency and inaction when said epidemic subsides. Consequently, recommendations in relation to preparedness for future outbreaks are not implemented. As epidemic cycles wax and wane, due to the futures fallacy of present attention, over-reaction is followed by under-reaction, and much-needed consistency is found wanting. This, sadly, results in "a significant and preventable loss of life" [UN, 2016, p. 6].

The fallacy of present-attention is related to logical fallacies known as availability, attention or anchoring bias, which ignore or minimise phenomena that exist but cannot be remembered or retrieved with ease [Milojević, 2020a, 2020c]. This may explain yet another finding by psychologists, as to why our *'imaginations about the future'* are, by and large, *'not particularly imaginative'* [Gilbert, 2007]. We can see this in the frequency of risks framed in terms of the extrapolation of the present or recent situations. For example, the previously cited Global Risk Report by the World Economic Forum features pandemics as a major risk (amongst the top five) in 2007 and 2008 – in the aftermath of SARS 1 outbreaks – but not in the Global Risk Reports 2009-2019. 2013-2017 widespread Ebola outbreak is reflected in a number of "Futures Decks" during that period – decks used in workshops within the public policy sector. For example, here are concerns for the future, during the Ebola pandemic:

> Ebola mutates into a virus as contagious as the flu, creating a global pandemic. (ForesightNZ, 2016)

> What if India is hit by Ebola? India has yet to be hit really hard by a global epidemic. India's large population, inadequate health care and absence of a proper sanitation system would be hugely problematic in the face of something like Ebola. (The Takshashila Future Deck, 2014)

And, in the aftermath of MERS, there were reports which:

> ...focused on preparedness for a respiratory viral pandemic, with the Middle East respiratory syndrome (MERS) given as the specific disease of concern. (ECDC, 2015, p. 1)

As I argued in the previous futures fallacies articles (Milojević, 2020a, 2020c), all of the fallacies have some benefits as well. Arguably, the countries praised for having both a good level of preparedness as well as acting early and decisively on the warning signs were the ones with a fairly recent and similar epidemic experience with SARS 1. Despite, or perhaps more accurately, due to their proximity to where COVID-19 first originated, Taiwan, Japan, Singapore and Vietnam were all praised for successfully limiting the spread of the virus early on in the crisis. While certainly not being the only factor, *the ability to imagine the spread of the virus in the future* – either based on past experiences or the understanding that it can happen to 'us' as well – seemed to have been helpful.

FATALISM: LETTING IT RUN

Another helpful approach was to NOT succumb to the futures fallacy of **fatalism.** Fatalism in the context of pandemic preparedness refers to a "feeling that sudden disease outbreaks will emerge in capricious ways as 'acts of God'" (Morse, 1993, p. 10]. Fatalism is one of the oldest – indeed, millennia-long – discourses in relation to pandemics. It co-existed with other alternative explanations in the past, and so to this day it co-exists with the alternative discourses which provide different explanatory narratives and subsequently request different measures. The table below summarises some key pre-20th Century pandemic discourses.

Examples	Cause & death toll	Explanatory narratives	Measures
Antonine Plague, Plague of Justinian, Black Death/Bubonic Plague, Smallpox, Cocoliztli, Russian Flu, Cholera	Viruses and bacteria From 1million to 200 million	**Dominant:** The wrath of gods/evil spirits Devil's work God's punishment **Alternative:** "The Other" (foreigners, minorities) The imbalance among 'bodily fluids' known as 'humours' Miasma – pollution theory	Appeasement of gods 'Quaranta giorni'/40 days quarantine Bleeding and purges Early vaccination Sanitation

Table 1. Pre 20th C Pandemics

All of those discourses continued to play a role in relation to the general lack of preparedness and adequate responsiveness in the COVID-19 pandemic. Humours and miasma transformed into 'balance' and 'toxins' discourse within contemporary alternative and complementary medicine (Shapiro, 2008). They joined forces with some equally powerful long-standing metaphors such as 'natural selection' and 'the survival of the fittest'. During the COVID-19 pandemic, they transformed once again, this time into the narratives of 'only those with pre-existing conditions' and 'herd immunity'. The –'building up 'natural immunity' and 'letting it run' narratives are seen by some to be 'the only realistic approach' in managing COVID-19. Moreover, their proponents believe that "the price of natural selection ... [remains] ethically acceptable" (Lederberg, 1993, p. 4). Whatever the case may be, such narratives endure because they tap into our general "difficulty to accommodate to the reality that Nature is far from benign", or, at the very least it "has no special sentiment for the welfare of the human versus other species" (Lederberg, 1993, p. 3). Their endurance is also related to the horror we feel when imagining "the emergence of new infectious agents as threats to human existence", including viewing pandemic as a "recurrent, natural phenomenon" (Lederberg, 1993, p. 3).

Since looking at that reality of human existence is difficult, an alternative approach was taken during late 20th and early 21st centuries. *'Natural'* and *'supernatural'* explanations have formed an alliance which has been undermining governments' and public health sectors' epidemic/pandemic responses – previous, current and planned. Concretely, the natural/supernatural alliance is commonly behind anti-vaccine or vaccine hesitancy stances as well as anti-isolation/protection measures such as quarantines and the wearing of masks. Unfortunately, given their resilience throughout human history, we can assume that they will continue to influence the pandemic response (or the lack thereof) in the future. However, fortunately, many alternatives to these narratives also exist. A detailed exploration of these alternative discourses is beyond the scope of this paper, which aims to help us better understand the lack of pandemic preparedness and adequate response. What will suffice here is to briefly raise a couple of dilemmas which are explored in the final section of this paper.

FROM WAR TO SYNDEMICS

The main measures currently in place to contain the COVID-19 pandemic – isolation, physical distancing, and hygiene/sanitation – are the direct result of the paradigmatic victory of 'germ theory'. However, a number of researchers have raised questions regarding the usefulness of the *'man vs microbe'* (Garrett, 1996) narrative as well as its connection to military/war narratives. While perhaps useful for previous and current levels of preparedness and response, these narratives are increasingly seen as problematic for the future, for various reasons.

To start with, viewing EID challenges – by researchers, policy makers and general public – as a *"battlefield* where the final outcome may be some form of victory in the continuing battle against disease", has been problematised because such discourse "fails to take into account broader socio-economic dynamics or a holistic systems perspective" (Black, 2015, pp. 138-139, italics added). Over the last several decades, some researchers have thus argued for the abandonment of such approaches and metaphors. Many have also argued for the rethinking of solutions which predominantly arise from an anthropocentric worldview. Seeing *'humans at the centre of an environment'* that contains microbes which should be eradicated so as to assure 'infection-free' human survival is, they argue, not only short-sighted, it is also probably impossible [Wilson, 1994]. These researchers have argued for an alternative, eco-centric view instead, one which envisions the *human as one of many species* co-existing and competing with others [Wilson, 1994]. Like most other living organisms, microbes are 'opportunistic'; they *"thrive in the undercurrents of opportunity* that arise through social and economic change, changes in human behaviour, and catastrophic events such as war and famine" [Krause in Morse, 1993, p. xii, italics added]. So instead of, or in addition to, waging full-fledged wars against them, perhaps a better approach would be to minimise those undercurrents of opportunities.

The narrative and metaphor that best expresses this alternative and emerging approach is probably the one of *"syndemics"* [Merrill, 2009]. In a nutshell, the syndemics approach encourages focus "not just on disease interactions but on the fundamental importance of the social conditions that foster disease clustering and interfaces" [Merrill, 2009, p. 16]. The syndemics approach no longer construes an infectious disease purely in terms of the notion of the "organism as a closed ... self-contained, independent ... unit and of the hostile causative agents invading it" [Fleck cited in Merrill, 2009, p. 19]. It has become fairly obvious by now that COVID-19, like most other infectious diseases, has disproportionally affected those with 'underlying conditions'. Underlying conditions, or an array of non-communicable diseases, for their part, cluster "within social groups according to patterns of inequality deeply embedded in our societies" [Horton, 2020b, p. 874]. The syndemic perspective, therefore: "... does not stop with the consideration of biological connections (myriad, complex, and fascinating as they may be), because in the human world disease develops within and is significantly influenced by the social contexts of diseases sufferers" [Merrill, 2009, p. 21]. Rather, this perspective provides a conceptual framework for "understanding diseases or health conditions that arise in populations and that are exacerbated by the social, economic, environmental, and political milieu in which a population is immersed" [The Lancet, 2017, p. 881].

Perhaps COVID-19 will provide opportunities to move away from an anthropocentric worldview and the battlefield-based germ metaphors. Ideally, it may even help us address major issues such as "global warming, environmental degradation, global health disparities, human rights violations, structural violence, and wars [all of which] exacerbate syndemics with damaging impacts on global health" (Hart & Horton, 2017, p. 888). This will require integration of multidisciplinary, including social science, research "into models of infectious disease emergence and evolution" (Morse et al., 2012, p. 1959) in order to better understand pandemics. And it will require the integration of data with narratives, metaphors as well as community input (Next Strain, 2020).

CONCLUSION

> Some may say that AIDS has made us *ever vigilant for new viruses*. I wish that were true. Others have said that we could do little better than to sit back and *wait for the avalanche*. I am afraid that this point of view is much closer to the reaction of public policy and the major health establishments of the world, even to this day, to the prospects of emergent disease. (Lederberg, 1993, p. 3, italics added)

Based on the investigation in this paper, we can assume that the public sector will continue to be impacted by futures fallacies well into the post-COVID era. To what degree this will be the case will depend on the type of narratives, including metaphors, we choose. To clarify two basic choices, the following table recaps the metaphors discussed in this article.

Table 2. Key Narratives and Metaphors

Lack of Preparedness	Improved Preparedness
Nobody knew	It's just a matter of time
Never before	Pandemics as certain as death and taxes
Who would have thought?	Time is running out; Use time wisely
Panic or neglect	Ever vigilant

Sit back and wait for the avalanche	If you fail to plan, you plan to fail
Let it run	Infection-free utopia
Just the flu	New disease, new approach
Acts of God	Man vs microbe
Survival of the fittest	Germ theory
Natural selection	One Health: human, animal and environment
Herd immunity	Awaiting vaccination
The next big one	Act now
The boy who cried wolf	Responding to the signals amidst the noise
Damned if you do and damned if you don't	Governments and citizens
Out of sight, out of mind	All in this together
Dodging a bullet	Battlefield
Not me and not 'us'	All of 'us' are vulnerable
Nation as organism	Emerging viruses know no country
Typhoid Mary	Removing undercurrents of opportunity
Kung flu	Same storm, different boats
China virus	Coming together
Only those with pre-existing conditions	Syndemics

The table is based on narratives and metaphors that circulated prior to and during the first six months of COVID-19 pandemic. Those on the left tend to decrease our agency, our ability to act. Those on the right tend to enhance our preparedness. The analysis is limited to publications in English and it would be of use to analyse narratives within different linguistic and cultural settings. More narratives and metaphors will certainly emerge as the pandemic evolves. Debates about the best use of (always limited) resources, as well as what are the most effective ways to address root causes of the specific emerging infectious diseases, will continue.

Finally, key recommendations already published in numerous government documents as well as in expert/scientific papers will be critical in how we collectively respond to the consequences of COVID-19 as well as how well we start preparing for the next pandemic. In this process, the choice of overarching narratives and key metaphors will be critical. Carefully chosen narratives and metaphors can enhance the ability to prepare for future pandemics. They can help ensure that we move toward a world where doing nothing moves to a syndemics-type approach. That is, we see 'us' – humans and nature – all in this together, as we co-evolve. Alternatively, unhelpful narratives and metaphors will continue to contribute to future realities in which most of us are ill-prepared or only a few of us are ready. In that scenario we continue to commit futures fallacies. Thus, the key question for the future is whether we can create and collectively choose stories that help us not only prevent EIDs but also create a better, more equitable and all-round healthier planet.

ACKNOWLEDGEMENTS

The research reported in this article was supported by the First Futures Research Grant, awarded by the Prince Mohammad Bin Fahd Center for Futuristic Studies (PMFCFS) and World Futures Studies Federation (WFSF). Its content is solely the responsibility of the author.

REFERENCES

Australian Government, Department of Health. (2014). *Australian Health Management Plan for Pandemic Influenza.* https://www1.health.gov.au/internet/main/publishing.nsf/Content/ohp- ahmppi.htm

Baumgaertner, E. & Rainey, J. (2020, April 2). Trump Administration Ended Pandemic Early-warning Program to Detect Coronaviruses. *Los Angeles Times.* https://www.latimes.com/science/story/2020-04-02/coronavirus-trump- pandemic-program-viruses-detection

Bin Larif, S. (2015). Metaphor and Causal Layered Analysis. in S. Inayatullah & I. Milojević (Eds.), *CLA 2.0: Transformative Research in Theory and Practice.* Tamkang University.

Black, P. (2015). Causal Layered Analysis: Case study of Nipah virus emergence. in S. Inayatullah & I. Milojević (Eds.), *CLA 2.0: Transformative Research in Theory and Practice.* Tamkang University.

Brownlie, J., Peckham, C., Waage, J., Woolhouse, M., Lyall, C., Meagher, L., Tait, J., Baylis, M. and Nicoll, A. (2006). *Foresight. Infectious Diseases: Preparing for the Future.* Future

Threats. Office of Science and Innovation.

Brundtland, G.H. (2003, June 18). *New Global Challenges: Health and Security from HIV to SARS*. Geneva Centre for Security Policy. https://www. who.int/dg/brundtland/speeches/2003/genevasecuritypolicy/en/

BFI (2017). *Brunei Futures Deck*. Brunei Futures Initiative. Centre for Strategic and Policy Studies.

Calof, J.L. & Smith, J.E. (2012). Foresight Impacts from Around the World. Editorial. *Foresight*, 14(1), 5-14.

Cameron, H., Georghiou, L., Keenan, M., Miles, I., & Saritas, O. (2006). *Evaluation of the United Kingdom Foresight Programme Final Report*. PREST, Manchester Business School, University of Manchester.

Cameron E., Nuzzo J., Bell J. (2019). *Global Health Security Index: Building Collective Action and Accountability*. Nuclear Threat Initiative and Johns Hopkins Bloomberg School of Public Health.

Cheng, V.C.C., Lau, S.K.P., Woo, P.C.Y., and Yuen, K.Y. (2007). Severe Acute Respiratory Syndrome Coronavirus as an Agent of Emerging and Reemerging Infection. *Clinical Microbiology Reviews*, 20(4), 660-694.

CISET (1994). *Global Microbial Threats in the 1990s*. Report of the NSTC Committee on International Science, Engineering, and Technology (CISET) Working Group on Emerging and Re-emerging Infectious Diseases.

Coates, J. F. (2010). The Future of Foresight: A US perspective. *Technological Forecasting & Social Change*, 77,1428-1437.

Cohn, S.K. (2012). Pandemics: Waves of disease, wave of hate from the Plague of Athens to A.I.D.S. *The Historical Journal*, 85(230), 535–555.

Conway, M. & Stewart, C. (2004). *Creating and Sustaining Foresight in Australia: A Review of Government Foresight*. Swinburne University of Technology, Australian Foresight Institute.

Cook, C.N., Inayatullah, S., Burgman, M.M., Sutherland, W.J., & Wintle, B.A. (2014). Strategic Foresight: How planning for the unpredictable can improve environmental decision-making. *Trends in Ecology & Evolution*, 1-11.

Cuhls, K. and Georghiou, L. (2004). Evaluating a Participative Foresight Process: 'FUTUR – the German research dialogue. *Research Evaluation*, 13(3), 143-153.

Da Costa, O., Warnke, P., Scapolo, F., & Cagnin, C. (2008). The Impact of Foresight on Policy Making: Insights from the FORLEARN mutual learning process. *Technology Analysis and Strategic Management*, 20(3), 369-387.

Dalglish, S. (2020, April 11). COVID-19 Gives the Lie to Global Health Expertise. *The Lancet*, 395(10231), 1189.

Dator, J. (2007). Governing the Futures: Dream or survival societies? *Journal of Futures Studies*, 11(4), 1-14.

Dator, J. (2011). Futures Studies and Futures Research, in W.S. Bainbridge (ed.) *Leadership in Science and Technology*. SAGE Reference Series on Leadership, SAGE: Thousand Oaks, CA.

Davies, K. (2020, April 17). *Blinking Red: 25 Missed Pandemic Warning Signs*. GEN: Genetic Engineering & Biotechnology News. https://www.genengnews. com/a-lists/blinking-red-25-missed-pandemic-warning-signs/.

Dorr, A. (2017). Common Errors in Reasoning about the Future: Three informal fallacies. *Technological Forecasting & Social Change,* (116), 322–330.

Department of Health and Ageing (2003). *Returns on Investment in Public Health: An epidemiological and economic analysis*. Commonwealth Department of Health and Ageing, Australian Government.

Dreyer, I. & Stang, G. (2013). Foresight in Government: Practices and trends around the world. *EUISS Yearbook of European Security*. European Union, Institute for Security Studies.

ECDC (2015). Preparedness Planning for Respiratory Viruses in EU Member States: Three case studies on MERS preparedness in the EU. European Centre for Disease Prevention and Control (ECDC): Stockholm. https://www.ecdc.europa. eu/sites/portal/files/media/en/publications/Publications/Preparedness%20planning%20 against%20respiratory%20 viruses%20-%20final.pdf

Garrett, L. (1996). *Microbes Vs Mankind: The Coming Plague*. Foreign Policy Association.

GHSI (2020, April 27). *The U.S. and COVID-19: Leading the World by GHS Index Score, not by Response*. Global Health Security Index News. https://www.ghsindex.org/news/the-us-and-COVID-19-leading-the-world-by-ghs- index-score-not-by-response/.

Gilbert, D. (2007). *Stumbling on Happiness*. Vintage books.

Gilman, S.L. (1987). AIDS and Syphilis: The Iconography of Disease. *MIT Press*, (43), 87-107.

GPMB (2019). *A World at Risk. Annual Report on Global Preparedness for Health Emergencies*. Global Preparedness Monitoring Board.

Greenblott, J.M., O'Farrell, T., Olson, R., & Buchard, B. (2018). Strategic Foresight in the Federal Government: A survey of methods, resources, and institutional arrangements. *World Futures Review* 11(3): 245-266.

Grey, S. & MacAskill, A. (2020, April 8). RPT-Special Report. *Reuters*. https://www.reuters. com/article/health-coronavirus-britain-path/ rpt-special-report-johnson-listened-to-his-scientists-about-coronavirus-but-they-were- slow-to-sound-the-alarm-idUKL4N2BV54X.

Guterres, A. (2020, May 11). COVID-19: UN Counters Pandemic-related Hate and Xenophobia. *United Nations*. https://www.un.org/en/coronavirus/COVID-19-un- counters-pandemic-related-hate-and-xenophobia.

Foresight NZ (2016). *Foresight NZ Playing Cards*. McGuinness Institute.

Hart, L. & Horton, R. (2017). Syndemics: Committing to a healthier future. *The Lancet*, 389

[10072], 888-889.

Havas, A., Schartinger, D. & Weber, M. (2010). The Impact of Foresight on Innovation Policy-making: Recent experiences and future perspectives. *Research Evaluation*, 19(2), 91–104.

Henig, R.M. (2020, July 20). Why Weren't We Ready for This Virus? *National Geographic*, https://www.nationalgeographic.com/ magazine/2020/07/why-werent-we-ready-for-this-virus/.

Horton, R. (2020a,April 9). Coronavirus is the Greatest Global Science Policy Failure in a Generation. *The Guardian*. https://www.theguardian.com/ commentisfree/2020/apr/09/deadly-virus-britain-failed-prepare-mers-sars-ebola- coronavirus.

Horton, R. (2020b). COVID-19 Is Not a Pandemic. *The Lancet,* 396, 874.

HSC (2005). *National Strategy for Pandemic Influenza*. Homeland Security Council.

Ibrahim, H., Kamour, A.M., Harhara, T., Gaba, W.H., and Nair, S.C. (2020). COVID-19 Pandemic Research Opportunity: Is the Middle East & North Africa (MENA) Missing Out? *Contemporary Clinical Trials September 2020* (96): 106106.

Inayatullah, S. (2018). Foresight in Challenging Environments. *Journal of Futures Studies*, June 2018, 22(4), 15-24.

Jennings, L. (2017). Foresight in the Public Sector: 2017 update. AAI Foresight: Roadmaps to Strategic Foresight. http://www.aaiforesight.com/blog/foresight-public-sector-2017-update.

Jones, K.E., Patel, N.G., Levy, M.A., Storeygard, A., Balk, D., Gittleman, J.L., and Daszak, P. (2008). Global Trends in Emerging Infectious Diseases. *Nature*, 451, 990-994.

Kahneman, D. (2011). *Thinking, Fast and Slow*. Penguin books, Random House.

Kinsman, J., Angrén, J., Elgh, F. et al. (2018). Preparedness and Response Against Diseases with Epidemic Potential in The European Union: A Qualitative Case Study of Middle East Respiratory Syndrome (MERS) and Poliomyelitis in Five Member States. *BMC Health Services Research* (18), 528.

Krause, R.M. (1993). Foreword, in Morse, S.S. (ed.) *Emerging Viruses* (xvii-xix), Oxford University Press.

Kuosa, T. (2012). *The Evolution of Strategic Foresight: Navigating Public Policy*. Gower Publishing Limited.

Lederberg, J. (1993). Viruses and Humankind: Intracellular Symbiosis and Evolutionary Competition, in Morse, S.S. (Ed.) *Emerging Viruses* (3-9), Oxford University Press.

Merrill, S. (2009). *Introduction to Syndemics: A critical systems approach to public and community health*. Jossey-Bass.

Milojević, I. (2020a, June 18). Futures Fallacies: Our common delusions when thinking about the future. *Journal of Futures Studies*. https:// jfsdigital.org/2020/07/18/future_fallacies/.

Milojević, I. (2020b). *Mirror, Mirror on the Wall, Who Should I Trust After All? Future in the Age of Conspiracy Thinking.* UNESCO Futures of Education Ideas LAB. https://en.unesco.org/futuresofeducation/milojević-mirror-mirror-wall- who-should-i-trust-after-all

Milojević, I. (2020c). Futures Fallacies. What They Are and What We Can Do About Them. *Journal of Futures Studies.* 25(4), 1-16.

Milojević, I. & Inayatullah, S. (2015). Narrative foresight. *Futures,* 73,151- 162.

Morse, S.S., Mazet, J.A.K., Woolhouse, M., Parrish, C.R., Carroll, D., Karesh, W.B., Zambrana- Torrelio, C., Lipkin, W.I. and Daszak, P. (2012). Prediction and Prevention of the Next Pandemic Zoonosis. *The Lancet,* 2012(380): 1956–65.

Mosk, M. (2020, April 5). George W. Bush in 2005: 'If we wait for a pandemic to appear, it will be too late to prepare'. *ABC news.* https://abcnews.go.com/ Politics/george-bush-2005-wait-pandemic-late-prepare/story?id=69979013.

Morse, S.S. (1993). Examining the Origins of Emerging Viruses, in Morse, S.S. (ed.) *Emerging Viruses* (10-28), Oxford University Press.

Murphy, F. (1998). Emerging Zoonoses. *Emerging Infectious Diseases,* 4 (3), 429-435.

Next Strain (2020). *Real-time Tracking of Pathogen Evolution.* Accessed 12 October 2020 from https://nextstrain.org.

NIC (2000). The Global Infectious Disease Threat and Its Implications for the United States. *National Intelligence Council.* United States.

Ortu, G., Mounier-Jack, S. and Coker, R. (2008). Pandemic Influenza Preparedness in Africa Is a Profound Challenge for an Already Distressed Region: Analysis of National Preparedness Plans. *Health Policy Plan,* 22(3). 161-169.

Ross, A.G.P, Crowe, S.M., and Tyndall, M.W. (2015). Planning for the Next Global Pandemic. *International Journal of Infectious Diseases,* (38), 89-94.

Rubin, H. (2011). *Future Global Shocks: Pandemics.* International Futures Programme and OECD.

Savio, N. & Nikolopoulos, K. (2009). Forecasting Effectiveness of Policy Implementation Strategies: Working with semi-experts. *Foresight 11*(6). 86-93.

Schartinger, D., Wilhelmer, D., Holste, D. and Kubeczko, K. (2012). Assessing Immediate Learning Impacts of Large Foresight Processes. *Foresight 14*(1): 41-55.

Shapiro, R. (2008). *Suckers: How Alternative Medicine Makes Fools of Us All.* Harvill Secker.

Silver, N. (2012). *The Signal and the Noise: Why Most Predictions Fail – But Some Don't.* Penguin.

Solem, K.R. (2011). Integrating Foresight into Government. Is it possible? Is it likely? *Foresight 13*(2), 18-30.

The Takshashila Future Deck (2014). *Future Deck.* The Takshashila Institution. http://takshashila.org.in/the-takshashila-future-deck.

Terranova, D. (2015). Causal Layered Analysis in Action: Case studies from an HR practitioner's perspective. In Inayatullah, S. & Milojević, I. [Eds.] *CLA 2.0: Transformative Research in Theory and Practice*. Tamkang University.

The Lancet (2017, March 4). Editorial. Syndemics: Health in context. *The Lancet* (389), 881.

UN (2016). *Protecting Humanity from Future Health Crises: Report of the High-Level Panel on the Global Response to Health Crises*. United Nations. https://www. un.org/ga/search/view_doc.asp?symbol=A/70/723.

UNEP (2016). *UNEP Frontier 2016 Report: Emerging Issues of Environmental Concern*. United Nations Environment Programme, Nairobi.

UNDP Global Centre for Public Service Excellence (2014). *Foresight: The manual*. Global Centre for Public Service Excellence and UNDP.

Van Asselt, M., Van Klooster, S., Van Notten, P. & Smits, L. (Eds.). (2010). *Foresight in Action: Developing policy-oriented scenarios*. Earthscan.

Webster, R.G. (1997). Predictions for Future Human Influenza Pandemics. *The Journal of Infectious Diseases*, (176),14-19.

WHO (1999). *Influenza Pandemic Plan. The Role of WHO and Guidelines for National and Regional Planning*. WHO/CDS/CSR/EDC.

WHO (2009). *Whole-of-Society Pandemic Readiness*. World Health Organization. https://www.who.int/influenza/preparedness/pandemic/2009-0808_wos_pandemic_readiness_final.pdf?ua=1.

WHO (2015). *Anticipating Emerging Infectious Disease Epidemics, WHO Informal Consultation Meeting Report*. World Health Organization.

WHO (2017). Financing of International Collective Action for Epidemic and Pandemic Preparedness. *The Lancet*, (5), 742-744.

WHO (2018). *Memorandum of Understanding Between the United Nations Food and Agriculture Organization and The World Organization for Animal Health and The World Health Organization*. https://www.who.int/zoonoses/ MoU-Tripartite-May-2018.pdf?ua=1.

World Health Organization (2019). *WHO Launches New Global Influenza Strategy*. https://www.who.int/news-room/detail/11-03-2019-who-launches-new-global- influenza-strategy.

World Health Organization (2020a). *Emergencies Preparedness, Response. Disease Outbreaks by Year*. https://www.who.int/csr/don/archive/year/en/.

World Health Organization (2020b). *Emergencies Preparedness, Response. Disease Outbreaks by Year*. https://www.who.int/csr/don/archive/year/2020/en/.

World Health Organization (2020c).*COVID-19 Pandemic. Numbers at a Glance*. https://www.who.int/emergencies/diseases/novel-coronavirus-2019.

Wilson, M. (1994). Disease in Evolution. New York Academy of Sciences.

The World Bank (2014, October 10). *World Bank Group President Calls for New*

Global Pandemic Emergency Facility. https://www.worldbank.org/ en/news/press-release/2014/10/10/world-bank-group-president-calls-new-global- pandemic-emergency-facility.

The World Bank (2017). *From Panic and Neglect to Investing in Health Security. International Working Group on Financing Preparedness* (IWG) Report. http://documents1.worldbank.org/curated/ en/979591495652724770/pdf/115271-REVISED-FINAL-IWG-Report-3-5-18.pdf.

The World Bank (2018, February 28). *Making Pandemic Preparedness Financially Sustainable in East Asia and the Pacific*. https://www.worldbank.org/en/ news/feature/2018/02/28/making-pandemic-preparedness-financially-sustainable-in- east-asia-and-the-pacific.

World Economic Forum (2007-2020). *Global Risks*. World Economic Forum.

"SYSTEM OF LIFE"

A Metaphor For Re-Imagining
the COVID-19 Pandemic

Rafeeq Bosc

May 19th, 2020

This paper describes the deliberations of a group of nine Foresight practitioners in our consulting firm's Strategy practice. In the wake of the transition to working from home, a number of us in different cities around North America decided to come together virtually to use the four layers of the Causal Layered Analysis (CLA) method to examine the COVID-19 pandemic. The intent of the exercise was to identify some themes at each of the four layers of CLA and to surface some lessons about how to facilitate foresight work in virtual settings.

After some initial comments about how the exercise was structured, this paper is organized along the lines of the four CLA layers viz. litany, systems, worldview/discourse and myth/metaphor (see Figure 1). We also proposed an alternative myth from which to respond to the outbreak of COVID-19. Finally, we present some learnings and insights emerging from the process.

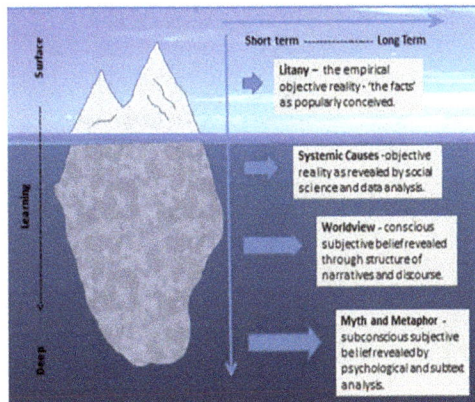

Figure 1: Four Levels of Causal Layered Analysis – taken from Martin Haigh's paper "Fostering Deeper Critical Inquiry with Causal Layered Analysis", Journal of Geography in Higher Education, vol. 40 no.2 (2016)

PROCESS

The process started with a chat thread in the company's internal Microsoft Teams site. This asynchronous round of collaboration surfaced initial observations at the four layers of the CLA method from various team members. These were then carried forward into the subsequent live collaboration sessions using the Miro virtual collaboration tool.

The discussion group also identified the set of participants for the live collaboration sessions, as everyone who had contributed to the chat was invited to the live sessions. The live collaboration participants had varying exposure to the CLA technique. One had come across CLA as part of a postgraduate Futures Studies program while four others had encountered the technique in a corporate training event on Strategic Foresight. The remainder of the participants were engaging as observers to see how the technique may be applied.

This group attempted to build a CLA model in two live sessions using the content from the Teams discussion as a starting point. A loose collaboration structure was adopted, with no-one functioning as a designated facilitator.

Observations were generated at all four layers during the two live sessions. However, none of the items identified at the Litany layer were explicitly taken down through the successive layers as prescribed in the CLA method.

A final live retrospective session was conducted to reflect on the process and the application of the four layers of CLA. The outcomes of those discussions are captured below.

LITANY LAYER

At this surface level, we noted plenty of discussion in popular media, print media, podcasts, news channels, etc. about the outbreak.

Most discussion was characterized by panic and fear. Litanies included death and disease (as seen in televised daily government ministry briefings and tracking statistics on government health websites), economic disruption (loss of value on stock markets), and varying degrees of social disruption (from voluntary social distancing to total lockdown).

The aggregation of the news stories and personal experiences led to the emergence of an overarching theme that "we are all experiencing the pandemic virtually". What this means is that while the pandemic was ostensibly about the outbreak of a disease, the effect of the pandemic was to drive a lot more of our day-to-day experience into the virtual realm (moving to work from home, contacting family members in quarantine via telephone or video conference etc.)

SYSTEMS LAYER

Two key observations were made at the Systems level. First, is the characterization of the pandemic as a "Black Swan" event by some commentators. This was viewed as an interesting proposition to advance because it implies an element of unpredictability of the pandemic.

This characterization is at odds with warnings about the inevitability of such a pandemic in the past decade since the outbreak of the Severe Acute Respiratory Syndrome (SARS) coronavirus (Hoffower, 2020). The motivation behind this characterization was called into question, and it was noted that this characterization started within the investment fund management fraternity (Sequoia Capital, 2020). It was speculated that this narrative was possibly a damage control move in advance of economic fallout and associated stress on the investment fund management fraternity.

The second observation was the holding forth of a vaccine as the countermeasure against the virus. Language about "flattening the curve" and "buying time" all seem to culminate in a "success" scenario in which a vaccine is finally available to protect humanity from the ravaging effects of the viral spread (World Health Organization, 2020a). This narrative implicitly advanced technological solutions to a biological problem.

Alternative narratives advancing social behaviors, hygiene practices, good health promotion, and resilient public health systems as enduring solutions seemed curiously absent. There seems to be little discussion (yet) about permanently increasing the capacity or improving the resilience of healthcare facilities (ventilators, beds, PPE). And a prevalent paradigm of "revenue per square foot" militates against the adoption of social distancing as a permanent new social etiquette. This paradigm is reflected in the configuration of restaurants, airplanes, schools, and other places where people gather in groups.

Although some discussion was observed about the power of (natural) human immunity mechanisms (World Health Organization, 2020b) (Altmann et al., 2020), these were not imbued with the same prominence and hope for deliverance as manufactured vaccine options.

WORLDVIEW/DISCOURSE LAYER

At the worldview layer, three themes were observed. The first is viewed through the lens of our observer group, all based in North America. The worldview discernable from the above layers was that the virus was something "out there", and making its way "over here". The notion is one of inevitable and impending disaster. At the root of this discourse was the notion of disconnect between humans in different parts of the world. What is absent from this discourse was the impulse to assist the humans suffering "out there" and rather focus on preventing the problem getting "over here".

The second discourse observed was around the existence of "wet markets", which are understood to be the source of this outbreak (Infection Prevention and Control – Canada, 2020). This discourse is somewhat related to the previous one because it separates humans on the basis of cultural practices. The group was not particularly au fait with the origins of eating exotic animals but found the characterization of certain animals as "exotic" to be interesting and invertible depending on the observer. The discourse around safe and hygienic nutrition in general is surrounded in various presuppositions about industrial capacity, cultural beliefs about eating live animals, relative aggregate health outcomes associated with outputs of industrialized food production systems e.g. the population health cost of artificial food and sugar-rich diets fostered by industrialized food production or the climate price of massive industrial-scale cattle farming.

Third, there seemed to be a worldview about preserving the status quo, especially the economic status quo. Social interventions like social distancing, work from home or full country lockdown were seen as temporary measures to be endured for a time until "normalcy" could be resumed. In the initial weeks of the pandemic, there was still very little discussion about how to entrench the benefits of a world operating in a fundamentally different mode.

Allied to this was the remarkable demonstration of government power to curtail the free movement and interaction of people. Some enforcement was required, but by and large whole countries complied to a large extent with calls to make highly inconvenient changes to their personal daily patterns (Human Sciences Research Council, 2020) (Smyth, 2020). These compromises were all made against the backdrop of daily statistics awaiting the bending of curves as indicators that we could return to the way things were before the outbreak. This return was invariably a return to economic- and consumption-based activity.

MYTH/METAPHOR LAYER

Finally, at this level, we discerned two operative myths. One was the "hostile world" myth. In this story, the world outside us is always trying to destroy us. Danger lurks at every turn. The person next to us may unwittingly be the porter of the seed of our destruction.

There was a second myth advanced which is of the "human superiority". Viruses, although devastating and always mutating, were no match for human ingenuity. Humans have claimed their place as the apex species. Viruses crossing the "barrier" from animal to human were somehow flouting a law of human primacy but will be taught a lesson when humans bring to bear their formidable technology to obliterate the threat they pose.

The two myths are lightly linked and play into a larger myth about competition between species for dominance at the expense of each other. We proffer an alternate myth to form the basis of different discourse, systems discussion, and ultimately litany. That myth is a "system of life".

In this myth, the existence of viruses, animals, and humans are all seen as co-existing components of a broader system. The system is one in which humans indeed occupy a privileged position, but that privilege arises because of, not despite, the presence of other categories of species. For the price of the odd viral infection, the human herd achieves viral immunity. Mutating viruses keep this system constantly engaged and therefore optimized. The aggregate outcome is a flexible "life space" able to accommodate all species.

With this as the myth, we believe focus will shift away from panic and anxiety, to preparation and graceful management of the expected. Society will embed a learning capacity, somewhat mimicking the body's immune response to these epidemiological events. Freed from the fear associated with myths of hostility and superiority, human society can turn its energy and attention to more productive responses. The increasing risk of pandemics brought about by the evolution of human society (globalization, air travel, longer life expectancies) demands the optimization of those attentions and energies.

Ascending the CLA layers from this metaphor, we can expect to find a worldview that sees the outbreak of viral pandemics as a natural consequence of the interplay between species in the system of life. Crucially, in this worldview, the incidence of epidemics is truly anticipated. This means that mechanisms and systems capacity exist for detecting and responding to early signals that potentially epidemic infections have occurred. A good analogy for this kind of sentinel function can be seen in the weather monitoring systems which warn of hurricanes, tornados and other large-scale weather or seismic events. Within this worldview, we anticipate much less of the recrimination we see today that result in victimization of people of certain ethnicities or the proliferation of conspiracy theories about viruses deliberate developed in shadowy bio-tech laboratories.

An additional alternative worldview-level idea is the interconnectedness of all of humanity. The notion that the occurrence of a virus in one part of the world or in one community is not likely to affect all of humanity is thoroughly broken down in the context of the new metaphor. In a world interconnected through globalized commerce, communication, and travel, the idea that something like a potentially lethal virus is not a global threat should inspire a much higher level of cooperation about epidemiological response than we have observed in the case of COVID-19.

These worldviews should give rise to health systems that are much better prepared with procedures and capacity designed to absorb the additional burden of disease and decrease the exposure of vulnerable sectors of the population. In this instance, it was the elderly and immune-compromised who were most at risk, but well-prepared systems would be versatile enough to identify and protect whoever is most at risk from a particular threat.

The other shift at the system level is to place more focus on good health practices i.e., those behaviors which boost human immunity and consequently the ability to recover from viral infection. This notion would see an expression in food production systems, placing more emphasis on good, wholesome nutrition. Work habits that postpone regenerative rest and recovery or promote excessive, continuous stress would also fall away without the systemic reward for such immuno-destructive behaviors.

PROCESS LEARNINGS

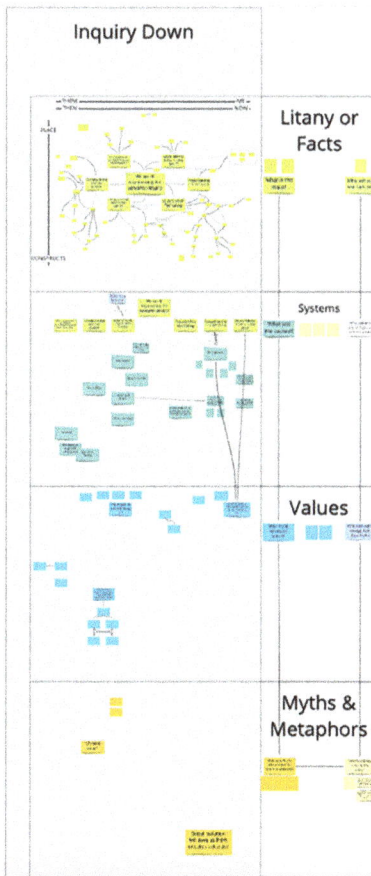

The consensus view on the CLA method was that the process of using the four layers was a good way to grasp the nuances of post-structural critical enquiry (as held forth by Inayatullah in his early writings on the technique in 2002 and 2003). We did feel that the scope of the CLA we pursued was very wide, and one thought was to keep the target of a CLA more focussed to avoid too much discussion at the Litany level.

A key learning in the group using the four layers of CLA was to allow time for the themes to emerge. These may not always be apparent during the discussion and involves some creative contemplation by participants who excel naturally at detected themes in a wide array of facts.

There was an expectation that the virtual whiteboarding tool would naturally facilitate collaboration, but the learning was that the tool does not replace the need for skilled and prepared facilitation. What the tool does solve is the challenge of co-location (or lack thereof).

We were also intrigued about how much further we may have gotten with the aid of an expert CLA facilitator. An expert facilitator would have encouraged deeper vertical enquiry and the creation of connections between items in the various levels (as prescribed by the CLA method).

CONCLUSION

In using the four layers of CLA on COVID-19, the group identified two driving myths which propelled the discussion at the litany layer. An alternative myth was proposed which was intended to refocus the response of society. It is anticipated that pandemics will be a more regularly recurring phenomenon and hence a better response is necessary to mitigate the societal fallout from such events.

This paper represents only a portion of the observations and insights that emerged during the exercise. Figure 2 is a snapshot of the very busy Miro virtual whiteboard on which we recorded our observations at the various CLA layers. This snapshot is intended to show that a large proportion of ideas generated during this process, are unrepresented in this write-up.

We recognize that even this is not an exhaustive or conclusive analysis of the pandemic. Another exercise, with perhaps a different group of participants, and applying the CLA method—rather than just using the layers—would likely generate a different set of insights, especially at the deeper levels of the analysis where the interpretation of observations occurs.

NOTE

The contributors to this article are all consultants at Slalom, a modern consulting firm focused on strategy, technology, and business transformation. Learn more at slalom.com.

CONTRIBUTORS

Alexandra Reese, Portland (alexandra.reese@slalom.com)

Boris Vishnevsky, Seattle (borisv@slalom.com)

David Ontaneda, Vancouver (david.ontaneda@slalom.com)

Jeremy Pollack, Hartford (jeremy.pollack@slalom.com)

Michelle Senkiw, Toronto (michelle.senkiw@slalom.com)

Rafeeq Bosch, Vancouver (rafeeq.bosch@slalom.com)

Rahul Shankar, Seattle (rahul.shankar@slalom.com)

Shane Mikes, Seattle (shane.mikes@slalom.com)

Tamarah Usher, St. Louis (tamarah.usher@slalom.com)

REFERENCES

Altmann, D. M., Douek, D. C., & Boyton, R. J. (2020). Comment What policy makers need to know about COVID-19 protective immunity. *The Lancet*, 6736(20), 19–21. https://doi.org/10.1016/S0140-6736(20)30985-5

Hoffower, H. (2020, December 15). Bill Gates has been warning of a global health threat for years. Here are 11 people who seemingly predicted the coronavirus pandemic. *Business Insider*. https://www.businessinsider.com/people-who-seemingly-predicted-the-coronavirus-pandemic-2020-3

Human Sciences Research Council. (2020). *HSRC Study on COVID-19 indicates overwhelming compliance with the lockdown*. South Africa Department of Science and Technology. http://www.hsrc.ac.za/en/media-briefs/general/lockdown-survey-results

Infection Prevention and Control – Canada. (2020, April 29). *Coronavirus (COVID-19)*. https://ipac-canada.org/coronavirus-resources.php

Sequoia Capital. (2020, March 5). Coronavirus: The Black Swan of 2020. *Medium* https://medium.com/sequoia-capital/coronavirus-the-black-swan-of-2020-7c72bdeb9753

Smyth, J. (2020). New Zealand and Australia open up after coronavirus success. *Financial Times*. https://www.ft.com/content/c4200db9-3eb5-484d-818a-00355a99c649

World Health Organization. (2020, April 24). *"Immunity passports" in the context of COVID-19*. https://www.who.int/news-room/commentaries/detail/immunity-passports-in-the-context-of-covid-19

World Health Organization. (2020, April 29). Update on WHO Solidarity Trial – Accelerating a safe and effective COVID-19 vaccine. https://www.who.int/emergencies/diseases/novel-coronavirus-2019/global-research-on-novel-coronavirus-2019-ncov/solidarity-trial-accelerating-a-safe-and-effective-covid-19-vaccine

CREATING A NEW RENAISSANCE:

Can Responses To COVID-19 Pivot Us a to a Transformed World?

Sohail Inayatullah

In this essay, we ask if there are any weak signals for a pivot toward a new renaissance trigged by COVID-19. Using the work of Arundhati Roy as a starting off point, we suggest that six pivots are possible: [1] the shift from GDP to Wellbeing; [2] From Roads, Rates, and Rubbish to the Anticipatory City; [3] From Central Fossil Fuel Systems to Decentralized Distributed Renewable Systems; [4] Toward a Green, Fair, and Coordinated Asian Region; [5] Toward Inclusion and Partnership; and [5] Toward the Inner. Of course, while in the long run, we may create a wiser world, equally possible is a descent into an era of pandemics, catastrophic climate change, and violent tribalism.

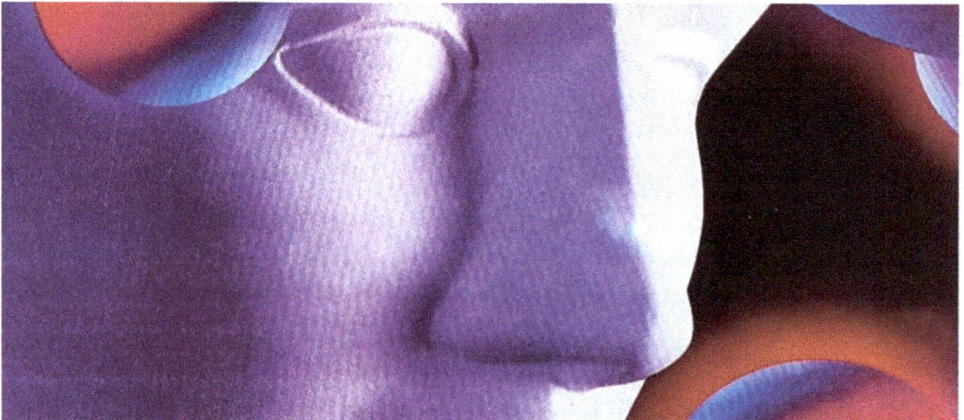

Cover of New Renaissance Magazine. Vol. 3. No. 1, 1992). Used with permission from A.V. Avadhuta.

1 THE PORTAL

While there are many reflections on the implications of COVID-19 and planetary futures, I would like to begin with the door of possibility. Writes novelist Arundhuti Roy (2020):

> Historically, pandemics have forced humans to break with the past and imagine their world anew. This one is no different. It is a portal, a gateway between one world and the next. We can choose to walk through it, dragging the carcasses of our prejudice and hatred, our avarice, our data banks and dead ideas, our dead rivers and smoky skies behind us. Or we can walk through lightly, with little luggage, ready to imagine another world. And ready to fight for it.

Thus: can COVID-19 can help us create a new Renaissance - a transformation of self and society, home, and plant. There have been two historical renaissances. The Asian Renaissance was personal: the quest for inner peace, enlightenment, the utopia of the mind. The European Renaissance challenged dogma, allowing science and art to flourish, creating the possibility of revolution after revolution against authority that does not serve the greater good. The question now is can we integrate the two for the next stage in human history.

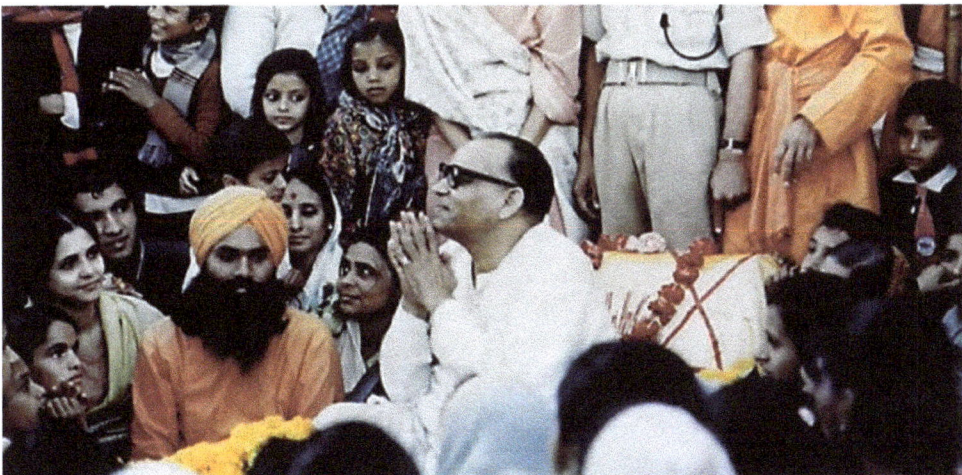

Shrii P.R Sarkar Public image from https://www.facebook.com/Ananda-MARGA-Pracaraka-Samgha-1067799116566003/

The world philosopher Shrii P.R. Sarkar (1988) suggested as much decades ago. He argued that "humanity was sleeping, and now it must wake up from the Cimmerian slumber (47) " and transform the physical (science and technology), the social (equity and inclusion) and the spiritual (inner practice and purpose) in "all strata of life (47)."

2 MAKING THE PRESENT MALLEABLE

Can we create such a novel future? If so, how do we go about it. Part of the solution comes from the study of possible and preferred futures. In this approach, theories of change are analysed and the future is used to change today. We learn from where we wish to be: we see the present as not eternal, but remarkable, merely the fragile victory of one possible trajectory over other pathways. The future thus becomes malleable, allowing agency to challenge structure. Going back many decades, I remember well the resistance to the study of the future. Indeed, one of my professors at the University of Hawaii in in 1978 called the study of the future "a can of worm," a waste of time. The future does not need to he studied as it is stable. Looking back at the last forty years, it is stunning how wrong he was. Whether the fall of the Berlin Wall, the spread of the Internet, the development of the Human Genome Project, the rise of China, depopulation and other demographic shifts in large parts of the world, the Global Financial Crisis, the impacts of Climate Change, and now COVID-19, it is clear the world has dramatically changed. Indeed, instead of a can of worms, the study of the future is now a capability one must have as the head of Strategy of INTERPOL Anita Hazenburg has often commented (Sheraz, 2019; Vettorello, 2021).

3 POSSIBILITIES OF CHANGE

Are there any weak signals for this latter future, this portal to profound change? Or will we return to the pre-COVID world? Again, this is hard to predict, however, there are weak signals, possible pivots to a different world. They may develop or may disappear, destroyed by a regression to the narrative of blame or inertia or from the outbreak of war (caused by the possibility of a hegemonic shift).

3.1 TO WELL-BEING

The first pivot is the shift from GDP to Well-being. In dozens of workshops that we have led around the world what has emerged is the search for a new model of work (hybrid), accounting (expanded), and success (wellbeing) [Inayatullah, 2017]. This is the possible shift from the economy as everything to models where there is a quadruple bottom line, that of prosperity plus social inclusion plus nature plus spirit or purpose. In a project for a national government, we focused on the futures of infrastructure, it was understood that infrastructure would need to be smarter, greener, and more participatory in design, but the meta question was what might infrastructure look like if designed from the principle of wellbeing? They concluded that infrastructure would be preventive based and aligned with creating community and social cohesion, not just roads. With wellbeing in mind, infrastructure could be used to create partnerships, enhance mental health, reduce carbon emissions, reconnect with nature, and design for personalized education and health (Inayatullah and Milojević, 2021).

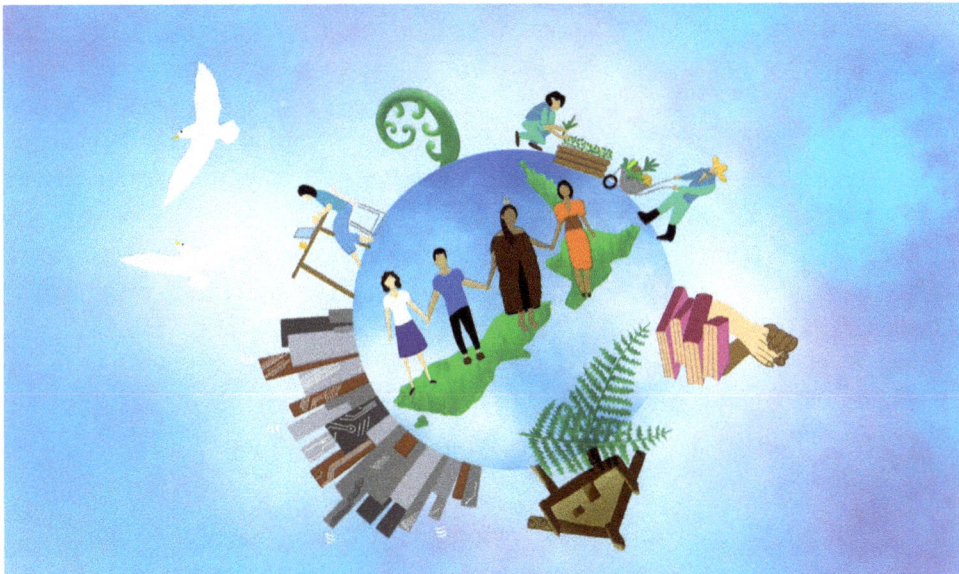

Image by Charmaine Sevil. charmaine@sevilco.com.au

3.2 TO THE ANTICIPATORY CITY

But where will the sites of change be? Cities, it seems. Traditionally cities have been focused on short-term planning, expanding roads, and collecting garbage. In several recent projects, what has emerged are discussions on the rise of the anticipatory city. In this new image of the city, using big data, cities become sites where we can anticipate tomorrow's problems: flooding, psychological depression, pandemic spread and on the positive side, areas of well-being, longevity, and indeed even bliss. With big and real time data, public policy shifts to becoming more science and foresight led (Russo, 2016). Without science-led policy, we will continue to see health disasters as with India, Brazil, and Trump's USA, for example, where religious dogma and fascist politics ensured the spread of COVID-19.

3.3 TO RENEWABLE AND DISTRIBUTED ENERGY SYSTEMS

With prices of solar energy decreasing monthly, another pivot has been the shift to renewable and distributed energy systems. Numerous energy companies we have worked with all imagine a future where their role is not the supplier of energy per se but both the connector, ensuring household solar systems are connected to the broader grid and the energy wizard, providing real time energy information systems. Thus, the new system is decentralized – household self-reliance-nested in a new decentralized but integrated system. The goal is a shift toward full renewables with each person having full data access to energy use, much as we do with mobile phone plans, knowing the daily gigabyte use and the costs entertained. More imaginative companies such as Tenaga Nasional Berhad of Malaysia envision a world with the "genie" of energy, much like telecommunications utilities, giving citizens real time energy whenever they need it. More and more, coal mines will become stranded assets and the worldviews psychic sunk costs.

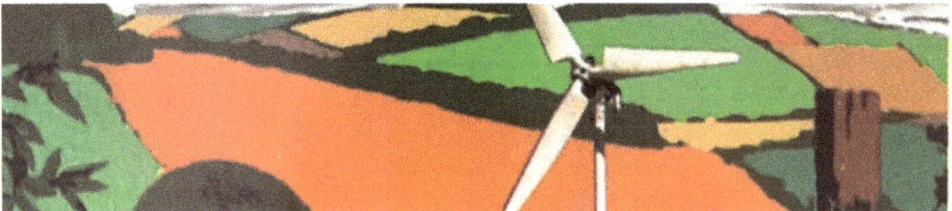

Part of the illustration cover of New Renaissance Magazine. Vol. 3. No. 3, 1992. Used with permission from A. V. Avadhuta.

3.4 TO A GREEN, CLEAN, AND FAIR COORDINATED REGION

In recent work with the United Nations Economic and Social Commission for Asia, experts and advisors explored the region in 2040 [UNESCAP, 2021]. What emerged was the focus on a shift from pollution as an individual issue or as a negotiation between states to pollution as a collective issue: form my air to our air. To create the new air commons, an Asian confederation or harmonization of laws would be required [Inayatullah and Na, 201]. The region needed to move together to create a greener and fairer region. If the region is to lead the planet, then it must become not just more prosperous but far fairer and greener. Along with pollution, eco-health systems need to be revitalized, stopping the encroachment of cities into wildlife areas. Climate change threatens to unleash more and more COVID-19 pandemics – zoonotic diseases - unless a new narrative is created for the region [Naicker, 2011; Shrestha, 2019]. However, it is not just that one region needs to become greener but that all planetary regions need to coordinate and move toward a Gaian polity [Thompson, 1985].

3.5 TOWARD INCLUSION AND PARTNERSHIP

In a series of foresight workshops with a leading medical centre in the region, while there were many novel ideas what participants were most passionate about, they key pivot was the move toward inclusion. As the head of the centre said: "we need to challenge a system that creates more white buildings with white labs run by one gender wearing white coats." His point was that diversity would enhance creativity, diversity would create new ideas, help the medical centre and knowledge centre as a whole transform. For example, more and more data asserts that gender inclusion, for example, enhances productivity, it optimizes [Turban, Wu, and Zhang, 2019]. As Sarkar has argued, "Society should have cooperative leadership, not a subordinated leadership: there should be coordinated, cooperative leadership between males and females" for a renaissance to be possible [Sarkar, 1987: 49]. Others need to be brought in who have different worldviews thus making the entire system more resilient. Science itself needs to move from the corporatist model to a non-profit open science discovery model. We are seeing early indications of this with the COVID Moonshot project (Chodera, Lee, London and Delft, 2020) but much more needs to be done to move toward a global right to vaccination regime, a global right to preventive health. Science, again as Sarkar has written, must like art exist for "service and beatitude [Sarkar, 1988 p. 47]. As we have seen with COVID-19, exclusion enhances the spread of the virus i.e., an integrated inclusive system protects all, while a system that excludes minorities can enhance vulnerability. In a workshop for the Government of Egypt on the futures of manufacturing, participants suggested that the most important and radical scenario was one in which the informal sector was integrated through platform cooperatives and artificial intelligence [Inayatullah, Jacob, and Rizk, 2020]. Up to date data on pricing, climate, pollution, and pricing could help those on the street enhance their wealth, make rapid decisions, and contribute to the national economy. Instead of seeing the informal sector as the problem, it could become the solution, what Sarkar has called the people's economy [Sarkar, 1992 p. 40].

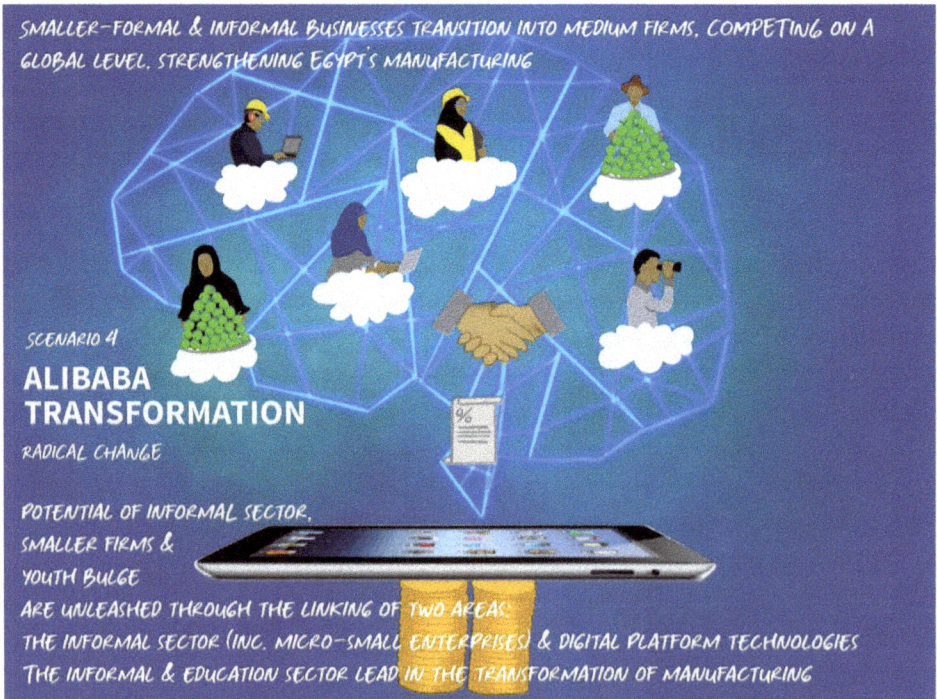

SMALLER-FORMAL & INFORMAL BUSINESSES TRANSITION INTO MEDIUM FIRMS. COMPETING ON A GLOBAL LEVEL. STRENGTHENING EGYPT'S MANUFACTURING

SCENARIO 4
ALIBABA TRANSFORMATION
RADICAL CHANGE

POTENTIAL OF INFORMAL SECTOR,
SMALLER FIRMS &
YOUTH BULGE
ARE UNLEASHED THROUGH THE LINKING OF TWO AREAS:
THE INFORMAL SECTOR (INC. MICRO-SMALL ENTERPRISES) & DIGITAL PLATFORM TECHNOLOGIES
THE INFORMAL & EDUCATION SECTOR LEAD IN THE TRANSFORMATION OF MANUFACTURING

Image by Charmaine Sevil. charmaine@sevilco.com.au

3.6 TOWARD THE INNER

The final pivot as the continued shift toward the inner. This is the great pause – using restriction as a way to become more mindful, enhance quiet time, to go deeper into one's life, moving away from the litany of noise, and toward silence (Katyal et al, 2020). The data is conclusive. Meditation works by first enhancing efficacy, second by increasing efficiency (Rathi, 2015), and third by increasing compassion. and its spread has become easier through new apps that increase accessibility. Indeed, research as well suggests that through meditation we can train ourselves to be more compassionate toward others. It appears that cultivating compassion and kindness through meditation affects brain regions that can make a person more empathetic to other peoples' mental states, say researchers at the University of Wisconsin-Madison (Land, 2008).

4 CHANGING IMAGE

In this reading, COVID-19 becomes a leverage point toward possible transformation. It is a potential move toward a wiser world where wellbeing leads the way. Health is wealth, as the saying going. To move through the portal to a different future, we need to imagine complex and guided evolution: humans cooperating and co-evolving with nature, technology, and spirit. If we don't then instead of a new Renaissance, we can easily see a descent into an era of pandemics, catastrophic climate change, and violent tribalism. All three are equally dangerous.

They all reinforce national politics and power instead of regional and global governance, the necessary new inclusive global commons. However, successful and failed responses to COVID-19 have clearly taught us that society progresses when all are included, when everyone moves together (Guterres, 2020; Milojević and Inayatullah, 2021).

REFERENCES

Chodera, J., Lee, A., London, N., Delft, F. (2020). Crowdsourcing Drug Discovery for Pandemics. *Nature Chemistry*. https://www.nature.com/articles/s41557- 020-0496-2.

Guterres, A. (2020, April 23). *We are all in this Together: Human Rights and COVID-19 Response and Recovery.* United Nations. https://www.un.org/en/un-coronavirus-communications-team/we-are-all-together-human-rights-and-COVID-19- response-and

Inayatullah, S., and Milojević, I. (2021). *Visions of Wellbeing for Aotearoa New Zealand: 2050-2070.* Government of New Zealand, Ministry of Transport.

Inayatullah, S., Jacob, A., and Rizk, R. (2020, November 3). Alibaba and the Golden Key. *Journal of Futures Studies*. https://jfsdigital.org/2020/11/03/alibaba-and- the-golden-key/.

Inayatullah, S. (2017). *Prout in Power*. Proutist Bloc of India.

Inayatullah, S., and Na, L. (2018). *Asia 2038*. Tamkang University.

Land, D. (2008, March 25). *Study Shows Compassion Meditation Changes the Brain.* https://news.wisc.edu/study-shows-compassion-meditation-changes-the-brain/.

Milojević, I., and Inayatullah, S. (2021). Narrative Foresight and COVID-19: Successes and Failures in Managing the Pandemic. *Journal of Futures Studies*. 24(3), 79-84.

Naicker, P. (2011). The Impact of Climate Change and other Factors on Zoonotic Diseases. *Archives of Clinical Microbiology*. 2(24), 1-6.

Rathi, A. (2015, October 22). Meditation and Yoga Dramatically Cut our Need for Health care services. *Quartz*. https://qz.com/529654/meditation-and-yoga-could-dramatically-cut-our-need-for-health-care-services/.

Roy, A. (2020, April 4). The Pandemic is a Portal. *Financial Times*. https://www.ft.com/content/10d8f5e8-74eb-11ea-95fe-fcd274e920ca

Russo, C. (2016). Mapping Planning and Engagement Systems Applied by Four Queensland City Futures Initiatives. *Journal of Futures Studies*. 21(2), 1-20.

Sarkar, P.R. (1988). *Renaissance in all the Strata of Life. A Few Problems Solved.* Ananda Marga Publications.

Sarkar, P.R. (1992). *Proutist Economics*. Ananda Marga Publications.

Sheraz, U. (2019, 25 October). Exploring the future of INTERPOL and Policing: an interview with Anita Hazenburg. *Journal of Futures Studies*. https://

jfsdigital. org/2019/10/25/exploring-the-future-of-interpol-and-policing-an-interview-with-anita- hazenberg/

Shrestha, S. [2019, August 30]. What Asia can do to Protect against Animal-borne diseases. *Development Asia*. https://development.asia/explainer/what- asia-can-do-protect-against-animal-borne-diseases.

Katyal, S.,Hajcak, G., Flora, T.,Bartlett, A. Goldin, P., [2020]. Event-related Potential and Behavioural Differences in Affective Self-Referential Processing in Long-term Meditators Versus Controls. *Cognitive, Affective, and Behavioural Neuroscience*. 20, 326-339.

Thompson, W. [1985]. *Pacific Shift*. Sierra Club Books.

Truban, S., Wu, D., and Zhang, L., [2019, 11 February]. Research: When Gender Diversity Makes Firms More Productive. *Harvard Business Review*. https://hbr. org/2019/02/research-when-gender-diversity-makes-firms-more-productive

UNESCAP [2021]. *Raising Ambitions: Asia and the Pacific in 2040*. United Nations.

Vettorello, M. [2021, June 15]. Anita Hazenburg: Police Futures. *Journal of Futures Studies*. *The Briefing Today*. https://jfsdigital.org/2021/06/21/thebriefingtoday/.

FUTURES STUDIES RESPONDS TO THE PANDEMIC

PANDEMIC-3.0 – FROM CRISIS TO TRANSFORMATION

Exploring the COVID-19 challenge and opportunity with synergistic pathways and visual foresight

Joe Ravet

While the COVID-19 global pandemic has caused death and disruption around the world, it has also exposed underlying tensions, traumas and conflicts. There are many hard lessons in disaster management, public health, economic recovery and so on – and also many inspirational examples of mutual aid and reciprocity. In this Perspective I would like to look more deeply and widely, to sketch-map some of the systemic transformations now in motion, both negative and positive – and then explore what kind of systemic pathways could help steer from one kind of outcome to another. Drawing on the synergistic methods set out in Deeper-City (Ravetz 2020), this argument is in four sections: –

- Exploring the scope of collective intelligence in many pandemic-related systems, social, bio-medical, economic, political or cultural;
- Mapping or designing Pathways towards societal transformation; methods, tools, outcomes;
- Exploring the scope and nature of relevant knowledge, both scientific, policy and practical;
- One example of the scope of a 'Pandemonics-3.0' is the 'Visual foresight' method: the graphics below show work in progress on the 'Corona games', with an alternative view on pathways based on the archetypal game-plays of actors and interactions.

SCOPING THE 'COLLECTIVE PANDEMIC INTELLIGENCE'

A **Pandemonics-3.0** is basically a frame for a 'system of systems', working both in public health and more broadly, with the capacity to turn crisis towards transformation. A Pandemonics-3.0 follows the principles of collective intelligence, in bio-medical, government, technology, urban design, social policy and many other areas. Such collective pandemic intelligence can be seen by its absence, when organizations are disconnected and rigid: and also by the aspiration and potential for organizations and social networks to learn, think ahead, co-create and co-produce. It also seems the vital qualities of collective intelligence can be mapped onto three main levels or 'Modes' of system organization, ranging from the functional to the co-evolutionary. In summary,

- **Mode-I systems** are framed as technical problems, to be fixed by functional solutions: so the Pandemonics-1.0 looks for solutions in positivist epidemiological modelling, with linear type applications in public health and medical care systems;
- **Mode-II systems** are framed with evolutionary 'winner takes all' competition. For the Pandemonics-2.0, we look to markets, incentives and smart innovations, which generally come with the typical side-effects of myopia, waste and inequality.
- **Mode-III systems** are framed as co-evolutionary 'winners are all', with synergies between many layers of social, technical, economic, ecological, political, cultural logic and value. A Pandemonics 3.0 system mobilizes deeper forms of collective intelligence, across wider communities, for a further scope of cause-effects, to bring all these together. Synergistic and intangible qualities, such as trust in governance, mutual aid and reciprocity across social groups, then come to the fore as the keys to turn crisis towards opportunity.

In practice all three Modes are needed to work in parallel, as shown in the examples at the end. While Mode-I does the basic material-functional problems, Mode-II works with incentives, competitions and psychology: and then Mode-III brings all layers together for a Pandemonic-3.0 level of transformation. Such inter-dependency also shows up in gaps and failures. For instance the UK experience in 2020 showed some Mode-I competence, but lacked much of the Mode-II incentives: and after a brief start the Mode-III qualities in connecting citizens, enterprise, government and science seemed to fall back [Calvert & Arbuthnott 2021].

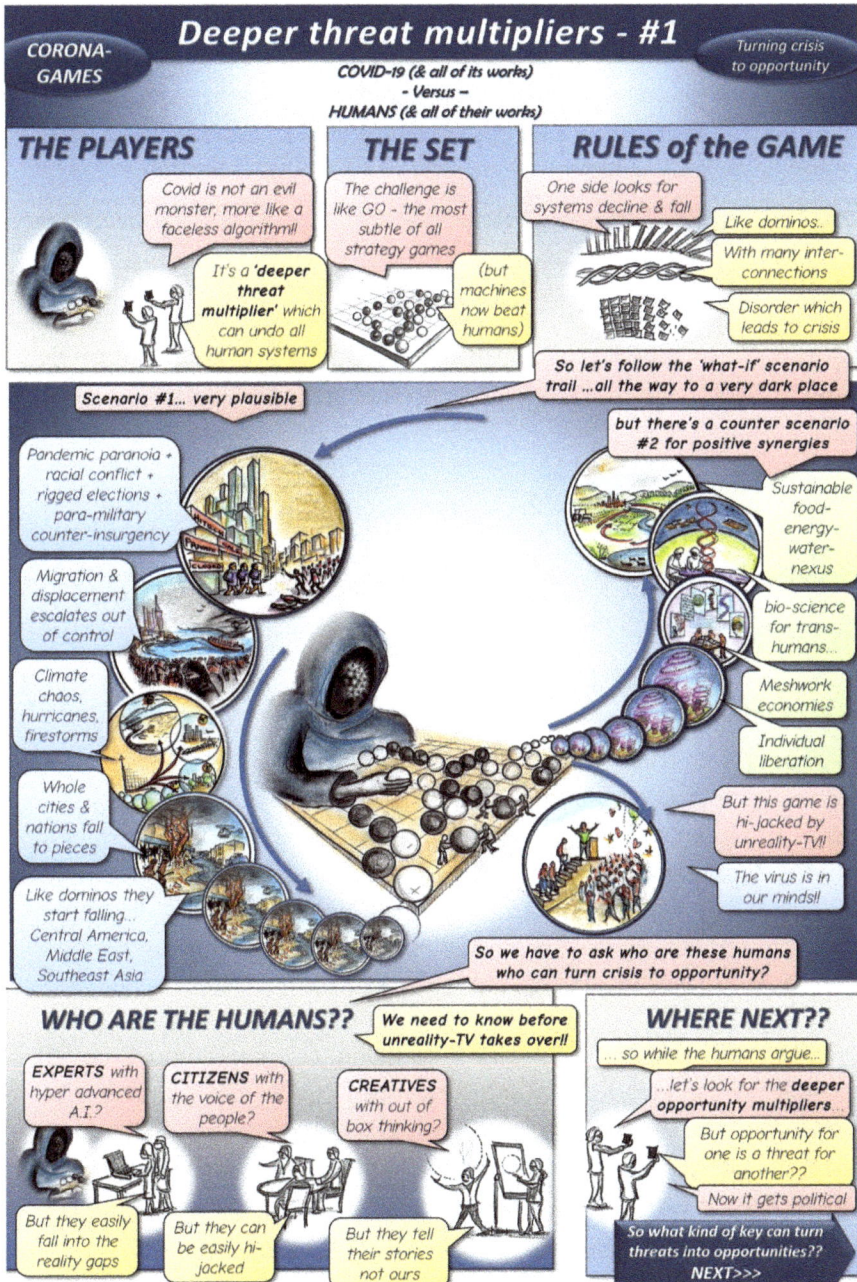

Figure: 1

A GAME OF DEEPER THREAT MULTIPLIERS

In such global crisis, challenges such climate change or rampant inequality are not likely to disappear overnight: they seem more likely to magnify up, as new forms of power and wealth and hierarchy emerge. If this COVID-19 pandemic can be contained or resolved, then we can get back to work on these challenges and others: but if it continues (which after 15 months seems likely) to be messy and divisive, or indeed as the next wave or the next variant arrives, then we face new challenges alongside the old. We can use the notion of Deeper Threat Multipliers (as in the USA security / defence industry), visualized as a scenario game-play, to illustrate the challenge and opportunity when multiple challenges of deeper complexity all interact. The graphic in Figure 1 is one of a series of so-called Corona Games, which use the visual game-play format to explore both challenges and opportunities (from work in progress on www.urban3.net/mind-games):

FORESIGHT 3.0 AS COLLECTIVE ANTICIPATORY INTELLIGENCE

It seems for these situations of high urgency, uncertainty, conflict and controversy, the **Foresight-III** approach from the Synergistic Toolkit is very useful (Ravetz and Miles 2016). The methods and tools of Foresight Mode-III or 3.0 extend from standard practice, to explore the scope of collective anticipatory intelligence, the learning and creative potential of whole communities and societies. With simple visual thinking tools, we can begin to explore and map pathways, directions for forward change, not only in crisis management, but of transformation in all systems 'social-technical-economic-ecological-political'.

The sketches below shows three angles on this global crisis of critical danger and opportunity. They start with the saying 'never let a good crisis go to waste' – and then ask, if new systems of Mode-III social-political-economic cooperation can emerge from this crisis, how to enable these to grow and flourish? And how to counter or bypass the forces of 'winner takes all' populism, of exclusion and intolerance, hijack of truth and expropriation of livelihoods? This is a brief sketch of a planet-sized challenge: and if this can help to contain or resolve this crisis, then we may be better prepared for the next....

SCENARIOS – UNKNOWNS OR UNKNOWABLES?

As of mid 2021, it's an unknown whether COVID-19 can be contained, or continues to multiply or re-emerge: but it's a deeper kind of unknown as to how social and economic and political systems might interact with the direct effects of the COVID-19. It's an even deeper unknown (perhaps 'unknowable'), whether or not social-economic-political systems could return to the old normal, or transform towards some kind of 'new normal'. So it's interesting to map out the combinations, as possible 'what-if' scenarios, each with a mix of danger and opportunity, and each with a mix of external forces and internal dynamics. Here in Figure 2 is a basic map of alternative futures:

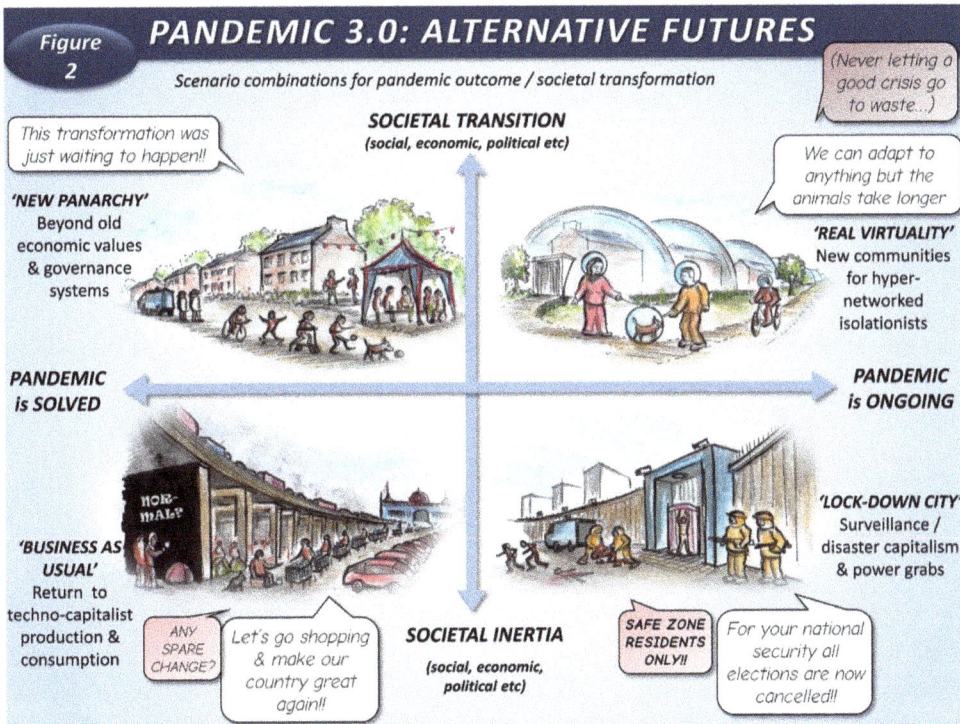

Figure: 2

- **'new panarchy':** we ask, what-if progress is resumed and the pandemic solved, while staying vigilant for the next one? Meanwhile there is deeper and wider learning from the 2020 episode, and a serious agenda to look beyond old-style hierarchies and extractive systems.
- **'business as usual':** as the general direction of most official or corporate prospectives (OECD, MGI etc), this simply looks to the other side of the pandemic, and aims to reconstruct the familiar game of capitalist-materialist production and consumption.
- **'real virtuality':** here everything has changed, with technology as the enabler for hyper-networked- isolationists, a new normal of video-holograms, decontamination suits and sterile pods. While humans are endlessly adaptable, this future brings huge challenges for individuals and communities, and maybe opportunities.
- **'lock-down':** a familiar techno-dystopia of 'Blade-runner' surveillance / disaster capitalism. Here the ongoing pandemic and its effects of disruption and trauma, is an open door for power-mongers and warlords who merge with the tech corporates. The graphic shows how 'safe zones' can easily turn into zones of exclusion and oppression.

It gets more interesting, as it emerges these scenarios are not only neutral visions of a possible alternative futures – they are more like active and contested grabbing of the present and very near future (a week or month at the time of writing). We can also explore such scenarios, not as distinct and separate, more like different angles on a chaotic bundle of deeper realities.

SOCIETAL TRANSFORMATIONS – BY ACCIDENT OR DESIGN?

To unpack such a bundle, we can follow the domains of social, technology, economic, ecological, political ('STEEP' for short), around the material facts of the pandemic, in the centre of a nexus of inter-connections. As sketched on the left of Figure 3, each of these involves not only material facts such as economic growth, but also the underlying layers of discourse and myth between all involved (Inayatullah and Black 2020). This could be the beginning of a long project, to explore and map the many cross-connections between each of the circles or domains, many of which are again 'unknowable' in any rational sense. And for each part of such a nexus there's also a potential counter-case, shown in the connexus on the right, where we explore and map the synergies. With both sides in view, with the synergistic methods we could begin to design and map potential pathways from one to the other, and cultivate the seeds and catalysts of potential transformation.

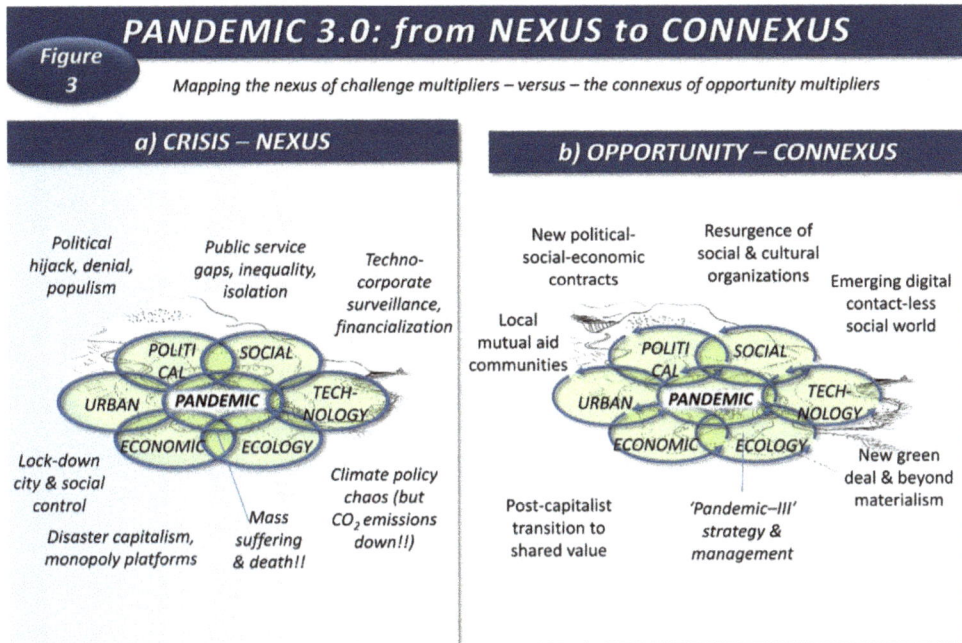

PANDEMIC 3.0: from NEXUS to CONNEXUS

Figure 3

Mapping the nexus of challenge multipliers – versus – the connexus of opportunity multipliers

a) CRISIS – NEXUS

Political hijack, denial, populism

Public service gaps, inequality, isolation

Techno-corporate surveillance, financialization

POLITICAL   SOCIAL
URBAN   PANDEMIC   TECH-NOLOGY
ECONOMIC   ECOLOGY

Lock-down city & social control

Disaster capitalism, monopoly platforms

Mass suffering & death!!

Climate policy chaos (but CO_2 emissions down!!)

b) OPPORTUNITY – CONNEXUS

New political-social-economic contracts

Resurgence of social & cultural organizations

Emerging digital contact-less social world

Local mutual aid communities

POLITICAL   SOCIAL
URBAN   PANDEMIC   TECH-NOLOGY
ECONOMIC   ECOLOGY

Post-capitalist transition to shared value

'Pandemic–III' strategy & management

New green deal & beyond materialism

In the social domain, the pandemic response in lock-down has shut most forms of direct social interaction, along with one third of economic activity in service consumption: it also exposes the gaps and shortfalls in public services, and the underlying inequality and exclusion. However there's a resurgence of social and cultural values, organizations and systems in different countries, from singing on balconies to a mass volunteering in the health service.

For technology, the door is open ever wider for techno-corporate surveillance and financial-ization: while local businesses go down, and while community apps and 3D printing emerge, the global 'GAFA' platforms are expanding without limit. Meanwhile in a possible future world of distancing and 'contactless community', the same digital platforms and networks will also be indispensable keys to interaction and collective action.

Production in the global economic system has been through possibly its greatest shock and growth reduction for a century, with untold suffering from the newly sick, unemployed, uninsured and homeless. However, there are new patterns of part-time and home-working, along with a deeper questioning of materialist debt-fuelled production and consumption, in an emerging collective economic intelligence.

For the ecological and climate agenda, the pandemic slowdown has brought clear skies for the first time in generations, even while climate change, species extinction and toxic overload continues. While international cooperation will be more difficult, it seems possible that in a post-pandemic era, new forms of the green deal will emerge along with non-material lifestyles.

Political implications spread in all directions – the most obvious being the extraordinary acts of the state (in some countries) in underwriting businesses and workers – and the most extreme, where large (tax-avoiding) corporates carve up the multi-billion bailouts. Again in a post-pandemic era we look for pathways for transformation, with new political-social-economic games in play, and a potential emerging collective political intelligence.

EMERGING KNOWLEDGE FOR THE PANDEMONICS-3.0

It seems these emerging transformations – social, economic, political, and all their inter-connections – call for new forms of knowledge, with deeper layers of value and wider constituencies.

Most scientific activity rests on underlying assumptions which are mainly hidden. These can work well for some 'problem frames', but less so for others, and the emerging science of the COVID-19 – here titled as a new 'Pandemonics' – is a classic example of multiple layers:

a. For **mode-I** problem frames – generally tangible, tractable, uncontested (general consensus on facts & values) – the 'normal' scientific model can work well; epidemiological models can provide robust forecasts and policy options.

b. For **mode-II** situations where scientific expertise is in competition with other forms of cognitive order (cultural, political, mythological etc), there may be huge pressure on the institutions of science. Systems of research methods, publication, peer-review, training etc, may be easily undermined and/or expropriated by other institutions – those of power, money, or ideology. In practical terms the science has to rapidly make many new connections – to understand the interactions of social psychology, community networks, organization change, complex system modelling, emergency project management, to name a few.

c. This suggests a co-evolutionary path towards a **mode-III 'collective scientific intelligence'.** The cognitive multiplicity and inchoate deeper complexity of real-world human phenonema, is not only a competition between rational science and other kinds of reality: it can be the source of deeper and wider understandings of cognitive multiplicity. It seems post-normal science is one way to approach this, if it can link 'science' with other forms of knowledge (Waltner-Toews et al 2020): but we should talk about not only 'post' but 'pre'-something, in this case a synergistic Science 3.0 [Ravetz and Ravetz 2016].

Some likely implications of this co-evolutionary mapping are summarized in Table 1: *Table 1: the science of Pandemonics: a co-evolutionary mapping Source: the author*

	Mode-I Linear	Mode-II Evolutionary	Mode-III Co-evolutionary
	'CLEVER': complex	'SMART': emergent complexity	'WISE': deeper complexity
SCIENCE GENERAL			
Scientific paradigm	Universalist, materialist	Dynamic, evolutionary	Reflexive co-evolutionary multi-versities

Science education	Assimilation of 'facts'	Competition & innovation	Mature creative minds
Archetypes & myths	Science for problem solving	Science for evolutionary innovation / competition	Science for co-evolutionary transformation
PANDEMONICS			
Empirical evidence	Data on cases, impacts	Social speculation & gaming of data & causal links	Reflexive deliberation on cases, impacts, causal links
Cognitive causality	Covid cases cause illness & death	Covid cases lead to synergistic effects with accelerated mortality	Covid is a symptom of a systemic disorder in the socio-bio-technical multiplicity
Policy guidance & recommendations from 'the science'	Socio-economic broad lockdown, pending vaccine and/or herd immunity	Socio-economic segregation for risk & vulnerability	Socio-economic engagement & open deliberation, for systemic risk & vulnerability:

COLLABORATORIUM – FROM EVOLUTION TO COEVOLUTION

The trillion dollar question is then, how to shift from crisis to opportunity, and what kind of pathways might enable this. In reality consensus is lacking on the goals of such transformation: and meanwhile many players are not 'letting their crisis go to waste' – rather they are pushing their interests by whatever means, as shown in Figure 4. Another time we would map in this way, the whole disaster cycle, from anticipation to preparation, initial response and recovery, and then to resilience and/ or transformation. For now, we just sketch a typical process of learning, thinking, co-creation and co-production – asking the question, how would different kinds of actors adapt and evolve with these challenges and opportunities, with very different goals, strategies, myths and archetypes? Again it's useful to frame this with different levels of system organization and learning, from the linear (Mode-I), to evolutionary (Mode-II), to the co-evolutionary (Mode-III).

With a **linear** Mode-I response, seen on the left of *Figure 4,* we plan ahead with best available evidence, with enforcement on transmission paths, with supplies of medical equipment, and with functional social communications (seen in one or two countries so far). This is the implicit framing of epidemiological analysis, such as the modelling study which informed the initial UK response (Imperial College 2020).

When the shortcomings of the linear emerge, then *Mode-II* **evolutionary** thinking then comes into play, with advanced risk management, socio-psycho 'nudges' or incentives, and smart urban micro-engineering (also on the left of *Figure 4*). But

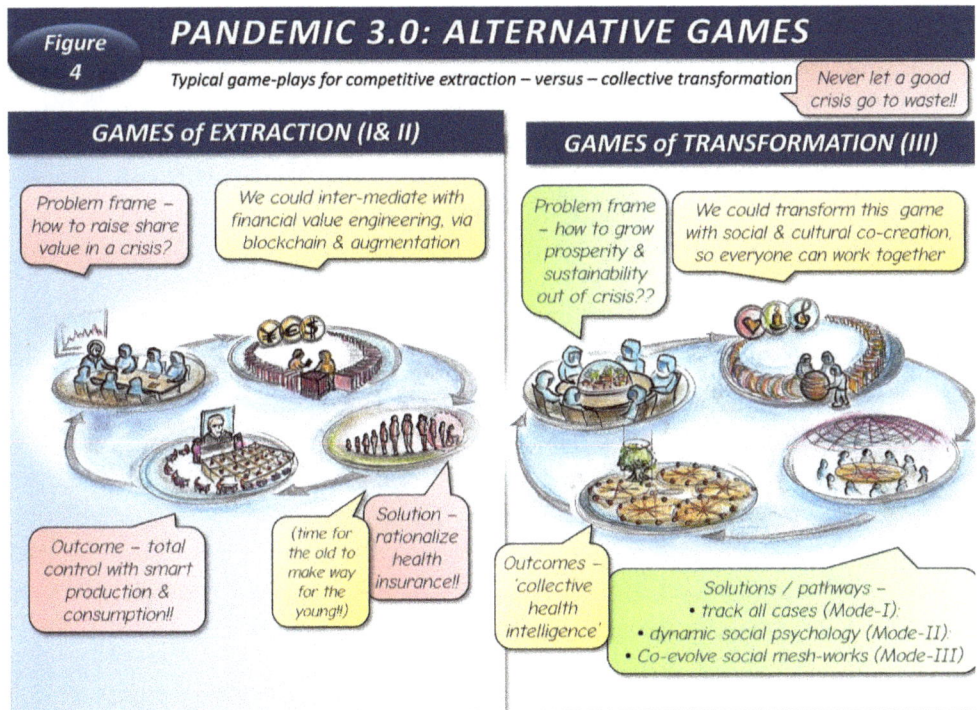

Figure 4

PANDEMIC 3.0: ALTERNATIVE GAMES

Typical game-plays for competitive extraction – versus – collective transformation   Never let a good crisis go to waste!!

GAMES of EXTRACTION (I& II)

Problem frame – how to raise share value in a crisis?

We could inter-mediate with financial value engineering, via blockchain & augmentation

Outcome – total control with smart production & consumption!!

(time for the old to make way for the young!!)

Solution – rationalize health insurance!!

GAMES of TRANSFORMATION (III)

Problem frame – how to grow prosperity & sustainability out of crisis??

We could transform this game with social & cultural co-creation, so everyone can work together

Outcomes – 'collective health intelligence'

Solutions / pathways –
• track all cases (Mode-I);
• dynamic social psychology (Mode-II);
• Co-evolve social mesh-works (Mode-III)

if the overall problem 'frame' is how to maintain business or power structures, the crisis is also an opportunity to accelerate the power game of 'control'. The sketch on the left of Figure 4 shows the result, a dystopian logic of digitally-enabled social engineering solutions.

In contrast the **co-evolutionary** Mode-III, on the right side of *Figure 4*, shows a possible results of many deeper aspirations – where the problem 'frame' is about how to use such a crisis for transformation of social-economic-political systems. Here we are talking not only 'solutions' but extended pathways, which combine all three Modes. We look for advanced systems of integrated tracking of cases and transmissions *[Mode-I]:* and for the best dynamic social psychology, with incentives and communications for hearts and minds *[Mode-II]*. And most of all we look for a co-evolutionary mesh-work structure *[Mode-III]*, a collective social intelligence, in the learning and thinking capacity of communities / organizations / networks.

Some countries such as New Zealand, Taiwan and many of the Nordics, have demonstrated the basic societal qualities, of trusted leadership, social reciprocity, and a functioning public health system (and is it coincidence that many such countries have female leaders?) (Fukuyama 2020). Beyond that, there's a call for a next generation of social systems: regenerative finance, positive health systems, inclusive social mesh-works, socio-eco-business models, deliberative-associative multi-level governance, to name a few. Each of these can be explored and designed with the principles of *collective intelligence*, as pieces of the *Pandemonic 3.0* jigsaw.

Again the implications can be tracked here as very practical guidance for pandemic management: with the material facts of hands, face, space and so on. The pandemic has (at the time of writing) has seen rapid learning in every walk of life: the distancing and masking policies which started in 2020 as unwelcome bureaucracy, have now largely adapted towards a new way of socio-spatial order. However such adaptation may take place at a local level, while leaving unchanged other social structures, so that the more deprived groups still live at higher risk with less resources or protection (Calvert & Arbuthnott 2021).

Table 2: Practical Pandemonics: a co-evolutionary mapping Source: the author

	Mode-I Linear: 1.0	Mode-II Evolutionary: 2.0	Mode-III Co-evolutionary: 3.0
Hands	Enforced sanitizing: contact-less & hands-free	Sanitizing incentives, games, activities	Integration of sanitizing into workplaces, communities etc
Face	Regulation of mask use	Mask incentives, fashions, brands etc	Integration with workplaces, social communities etc
Space & distance	Surface level observation of rules	Adaptive design & behaviour interactions	Rethinking collective space use for new normal
Track & Trace	Digital solutions lacking social linkages	Partial social acceptance, take-up & responses	T&T is new normal with built in civil liberties
[PROBLEMS]	Digital divide, top down system, low takeup	Partial success with many side-effects	
Test	Basic service provision in right time & place	Data access, analysis, interpretation, feedback	Integration of results to social & economic life
Isolation / shielding	Basic rules for isolation	Adaptive behaviour with gaps & barriers	Full social, economic, material support
Support	Minimum functional support	Active connections with family, friends	Integrated mutual aid groups & networks
[PROBLEMS]	fragmentation, distrust, avoidance, low takeup	Many gaps barriers & side-impacts	
Treat	Bio-medical treatment	Lifestyle feedback & incentives	Integrated well-health in the community
Vaccine	Basic functional vaccine	Targetted vaccines for social groups & activities	Active vaccination, integral to economy & society
[PROBLEMS]	Social fragmentation, distrust, low takeup	Some adaptive action but with gaps & barriers	

CONCLUSION AND NEXT STEPS

Whether the future is one of hazmat suits and holograms, or communities partying in the street, this is all to emerge. The main question here is how the world can best respond to fundamental choices, between a 'bounce back' to inequality and alienation, or some kind of 'bounce-forward'. For this it will need to explore many of the 'pathways from smart to wise' which are beginning to emerge. And more than any one pathway, this crisis / opportunity calls for a collective pandemonic intelligence to realize the potential future now in front of us.

AUTHOR

Joe Ravetz, Manchester Urban Institute, Leader 'Future-Proof Cities'

Manchester University, Oxford Rd, M13 9PL, UK

joe.ravetz@manchester.ac.uk – joe.ravetz@gmail.com

www.urban3.net – www.manchester.ac.uk/synergistics

www.mui.manchester.ac.uk/research/groups/cure/

ACKNOWLEDGMENT

Some material here is supported by the UK Natural Environment Research Council, via the project 'Peri-cene'. The argument is based on ideas from the book Deeper City (Ravetz 2020), and its Post-script.

Graphics © Joe Ravetz under Creative Commons License (CC BY-NC-SA 4.0).

REFERENCES

Calvert, J, Arbuthnott, G. (2021). *Failures of State: The Inside Story of Britain's Battle with Coronavirus.* Harper Collins.

Fukuyama, F, (2020). The Pandemic and Political Order: It Takes a State. *Foreign Affairs,* 99(4), 26.

Imperial College COVID-19 Response Team, (2020). Impact of non-pharmaceutical interventions (NPIs) to reduce COVID-19 mortality and healthcare demand. *Imperial College.* https://www.imperial.ac.uk/media/imperial-college/medicine/sph/ide/gida-fellowships/Imperial-College-COVID19-NPI-modelling-16-03-2020.pdf

Inayatullah, S. and Black, P. (2020). Neither A Black Swan Nor A Zombie Apocalypse: The Futures Of A World With The COVID-19 Coronavirus. *Journal of Futures Studies.* https://jfsdigital.org/2020/03/18/neither-a-black-swan-nor-a-zombie-apocalypse-the-futures-of-a-world-with-the-COVID-19-coronavirus/

Ravetz, J, & Miles, I.D, (2016). Foresight in cities: on the possibility of a "strategic urban intelligence", *Foresight,* 18(5), 469-490. http://dx.doi.org/10.1108/FS-06-2015-0037

Ravetz, J. & Ravetz, A. (2016). Seeing the wood for the trees: Social Science 3.0 and the role of visual thinking. *European Journal of Social Science Research,* 30(1), 104 - 120. http://dx.doi.org/10.1080/13511610.2016.1224155

Ravetz, J. (2020), Deeper City: collective intelligence and the synergistic pathways from smart to wise. *Routledge.* https://doi.org/10.4324/9781315765860

Waltner-Toews, D., Biggeri, A., De Marchi, B., Funtowicz, S., Giampietro, M., O'Connor, M., Ravetz, J.R., Saltelli, A. and van der Sluijs, J.P. (2020) PostNormal Pandemics: Why COVID-19 Requires A New Approach To Science. *Discover Society*: https://discoversociety. org/2020/03/27/post-normal-pandemics-why-COVID-19-requires-a-new-approach-to-science/

POST-PANDEMIC WORLDS FOR SOCIETY, GOVERNMENT AND ECONOMY

Aftermath and Opportunities

Otto C. Frommelt

The Coronavirus (COVID-19) disease caused a pandemic that has changed our lives and future to come beyond recognition. It is still altering society, governmental policies, and economy as well as disrupting the way we work and live together. Two key drivers identified are: The evolution of business conduct in the ecosystem and the developments of health technology. Digitalization will further drive a Shut-In Economy. I advocate that we need to have a Circular Economy that makes sustainability inclusive. Not one's passport, but ones new Global Health-ID will provide access. In order to protect oneself from contagion, artificial intelligence (AI) will become the health police through an authoritarian Digital Leninism approach. I envisage that further digitalization and blockchain technology could act as an enabler to drive these changes.

INTRODUCTION

The Coronavirus disease brought about a pandemic that has changed our lives and the way we conduct business beyond recognition. Right now, we are just at the beginning of a long journey into the future in a post-pandemic world. The objective of this article is to present an outlook of possible futures with regards to the impact on society, government and our business community. It includes practical and possible new business models focusing on a circular economy business environment. In the following, I will outline key drivers and sketch plausible scenarios.

POST-PANDEMIC SCENARIOS

Considering two key drivers of change, I identified four scenarios for the future that run as follows: Shut-In Economy, Global Health-ID, Circular Economy and Digital Leninism. Figure 1 outlines the two key drivers that are the ecosystem and health technology (or in short, HealthTech) developments.

Figure 1:
In the next months and coming years, disruptive and innovative developments will require different responses to the global outbreak. In order to be prepared for a

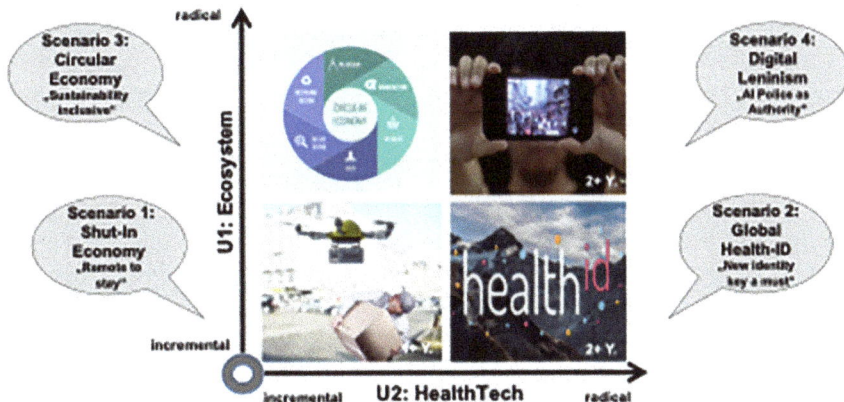

Post-pandemic scenarios for society, government and economy

Note: Ux means Uncertainty (key drivers of change)

range of possible outcomes, the following scenarios are presented, and I believe that their consideration can serve as an outlet in supporting the process of finding flexible and resilient responses:

SHUT-IN ECONOMY "REMOTE TO STAY" (SCENARIO 1)

The answer to the pandemic so far was the lock-down of people and shut down of operations to limit the contagion. Home-office and home-schooling has become the new norm. As long as there is widespread vaccination, staying at home and limiting personal contact are some of the few protections against the pandemic. Hence, online business services will continue to grow and more business will go digital where feasible. Remote access and working is going to stay. The development will transition from "shut-in-home" to "shut-in economy"[1] (Smiley, 2020). Digitalization and AI will further drive the development of on-line products and (public) services.

GLOBAL HEALTH-ID "NEW IDENTITY KEY A MUST" (SCENARIO 2)

Not one's passport, but one's new global health-ID will provide clearance to enter a country or access facilities (Mozur et al., 2020). New services can also lead to decentralized identity (DID) management that simplifies the process of issuing legal personal documents. It is, however, crucial to enforce all data protection rights according to the General Data Protection Regulation (GDPR) for the ecosystem participants, e.g. the individual that enters data should also controls it. GDPR for privacy and security was put into effect by the European Union (EU) and is currently "the toughest privacy and security law in the world and it ensures a robust business environment with clearly defined rules and responsibilities" (GDPR, 2020).

CIRCULAR ECONOMY "SUSTAINABILITY INCLUSIVE" (SCENARIO 3)

It is advocated that there is a need for a circular economy which would make sustainability inclusive. Having the necessary prerequisites, governmental policies and regulations (including CO2 tax and pricing models), new business models where sustainability is in focus will emerge. Digitalization can pave the way from „internet of things (IoT) to an economy of things (EoT)" (IBM, 2020) where an integral and holistic ecosystem is constituting the heart. The ecosystem could be managed like a digital dossier (e.g. distributed ledger technology (DLT)) where all relevant information about the entire lifecycle of products and services are stored, for example in a blockchain (Oxford, 2019). The single point of contact could be the new global health-ID for the consumer and the digital business-ID for the seller. Figure 2 outlines the notion of a circular economy with blockchain technology.

Figure 2:

Ecosystem of circular economy with blockchain technology

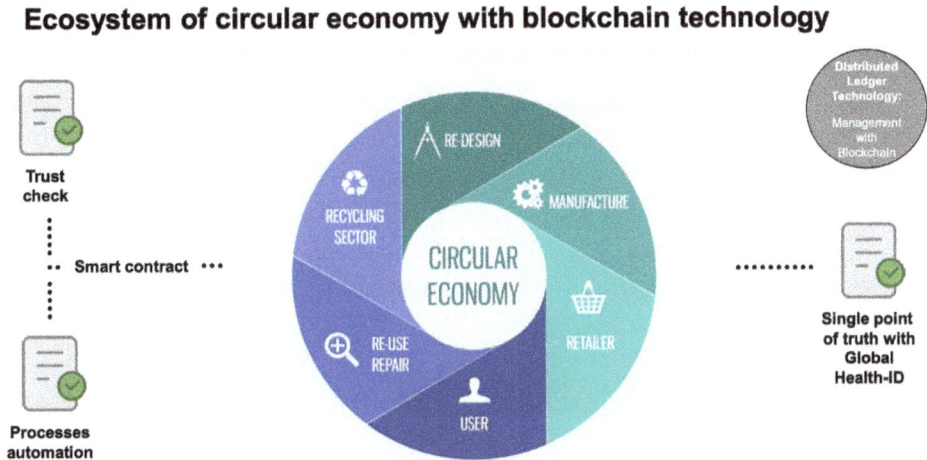

DIGITAL LENINISM "AI POLICE AS AUTHORITY" (SCENARIO 4)

In order to protect oneself from contagion, AI will become the health police and a digital leninism[2] approach is paving the way (Nass, 2019). This means that government, regional, and local authorities will know much more about a person than today. We can see this development in China or Singapore as the digital control has contributed to containing the spread of the virus (Lichfield, 2020). In Israel, the gathering and movement of persons has been controlled effectively by tracking citizens' cellphone data. Further surveillance and access technology will become the new standard, allowing one to enter a facility, cinema, restaurant, or country. This is clearly the "big brother is watching you" world where everything is noted. Suspected or prospected activities will be considered by an algorithm utilizing machine learning and AI to the maximum. Depending on the political system and laws, the development will take place at different speeds.

BLOCKCHAIN TECHNOLOGY AS OPPORTUNITY

Considering the four scenarios, I suggest that blockchain technology can act as an enabler in ushering in these changes. Blockchain is characterized by decentralization, transparency and its tamper-resistant nature. Blockchain with its DLT allows individuals to work in a decentralized and democratized manner (Frommelt, 2020). Blockchain technology could be applied in the scenarios outlined, as a means to the (four possible) ends. In Scenario 1, blockchain could be utilized to trace and track the supply chain. In Scenario 2, blockchain would bring transparency to the global health-ID. Through the tokenization of data, overview and ownership to data for the individual materializes, while allowing the government to verify this data. In Scenario 3, blockchain would bring legal certainty, since the data is mutually agreed upon and verified. Blockchain would amplify the policing enabled by AI technologies, such as tracking, in Scenario 4, by time-stamping movements.

BLOCKCHAIN DISTRIBUTED APPLICATIONS (DAPPS)

Many DApps that connect users and providers are currently emerging. Some examples and use cases for future DApps in the post-pandemic world that I identified, are: Digital business-ID, global health-ID, digital passport, bio access control, contact process mapping, health-to-go code, peer-to-peer transactions, and CO_2 circular pricing and tax modules. Process tokens and smart contracts might be an integral part. Figure 3 illustrates future DApps in a post-pandemic environment.

Figure 3

Blockchain distributed applications (DApps) platform

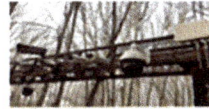

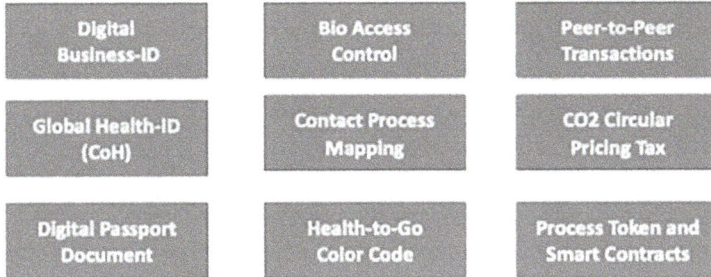

Digital Business-ID	Bio Access Control	Peer-to-Peer Transactions
Global Health-ID (CoH)	Contact Process Mapping	CO2 Circular Pricing Tax
Digital Passport Document	Health-to-Go Color Code	Process Token and Smart Contracts

Note: CoH means Certificate of Health

CHALLENGES AHEAD

In the transition to the post-pandemic future, there are also new challenges ahead. In addition to the new scenarios, a new governance model with a more circular culture and mindset needs to emerge (Figure 4). I purport that a post-pandemic future will require a new governance framework. Figure 4 presents a corporate governance matrix (CGM) where: i) HealthTech Governance is needed to manage new technology and ii) Ecosystem Governance is needed to manage new (circular) ecosystem business models.

Figure 4

Corporate governance with a circular culture and mindset

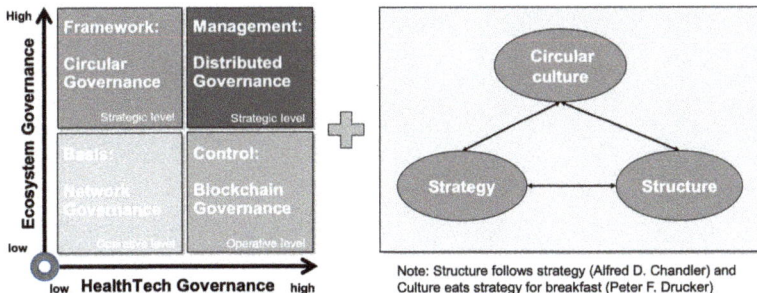

Note: Structure follows strategy (Alfred D. Chandler) and Culture eats strategy for breakfast (Peter F. Drucker)

CONCLUSION

In summary, blockchain technology is an enabler of change, constituting a bridge for a new circular ecosystem, business models and AI technology applications to emerge. In this vein, a radical transition for society, government and economy is underway to manage the post-pandemic environment and its challenges. A new way of living and working is becoming reality step-by-step.

AUTHOR

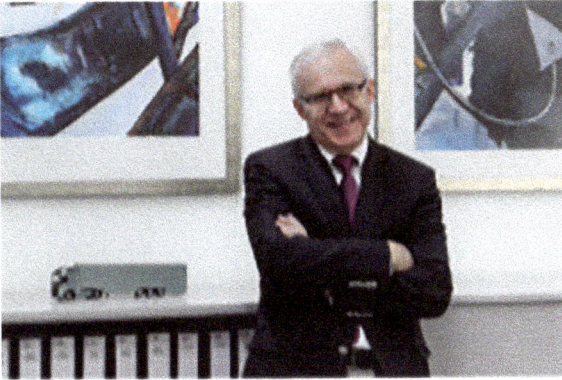

Dr. Otto C. Frommelt, MBA is Director of the National Road Office at the Principality of Liechtenstein. He has top management expertise and significant international experience within the automotive industry, governmental administration, non-profit organizations and innovative start-up companies. He is a qualified Expert in strategy development, scenario planning and foresight studies. Most recently, he published several articles about Digitalization to Touch, Autonomous Vehicles and Mobility in the Blockchain. In addition, he contributed to an European Union (EU) foresight project, conducted scenario planning workshops, hold scenario-based strategic conversations and also co-chaired the Platform Future group to develop scenarios for the future of mobility.

Linkedin: https://www.linkedin.com/in/ottocfrommelt/

Twitter: @DOFTWEET

Contact: otto.frommelt@llv.li

NOTES

1 The term "Shut-in Economy" was dubbed by Lauren Smiley (2020) in her article.

2 Example of the term is given by Matthias Nass (2019) in his article about "Digital Leninism".

REFERENCES

Frommelt O. C. (2020). 360 Vehicle Life Cycle Management with Blockchain Technology. *IfM-Impulse*, Institut für Management, 18, 14-21.

GDPR.eu. (2020). GDPR Archives - GDPR.eu. https://gdpr.eu/tag/gdpr/

IBM. (2020). The Economy of Things. https://www.ibm.com/thoughtleadership/institute-business-value/report/economyofthings

Lichfield, G. (2020). We're Not Going Back To Normal. *MIT Technology Review*. https://www.technologyreview.com/2020/03/17/905264/pandemic-socialdistancing-18-months/

Mozur, P., Zhong R. and Krolik A. (2020). In Coronavirus Fight, China Gives Citizens A Color Code, With Red Flags. *New York Times*. https://www.nytimes.com/2020/03/01/business/china- coronavirus-surveillance.html

Nass, M. (2019). Digital-Leninismus. Zeit.de. https://www.zeit.de/2019/48/china-hongkong-ueberwachung-unterdrueckung-digitalleninismus

Oxford. (2019). Oxford Blockchain Strategy Programme. Course outline. Said Business School, University of Oxford.

Smiley, L. (2020). The Shut-In Economy. *Medium*. https://medium.com/matter/the-shut-in-economy-ec3ec1294816

APPLYING THE FUTURES WHEEL AND MACROHISTORY TO THE COVID-19 GLOBAL PANDEMIC

Phillip Daffara

This paper investigates the systemic impacts of the COVID-19 pandemic and experiments with using two foresight methods with different time horizons to broaden the exploration. The Futures Wheel of consequences is applied to the global shock and pandemic of COVID-19 to firstly analyse systemic impacts of the virus within a short to medium timeframe. Then, four macrohistorical models are applied, to time two probable future trajectories resulting from the bifurcation point of the pandemic. The conclusion provides: [1] insights on the methodology of integrating the Futures Wheel and Macrohistory and proposes that they are indeed complimentary if a common spatial scale is used to link them, and [2] that the city is a practical and effective spatial scale to integrate the methods and their systemic impacts, and [3] real world actions in response to the pandemic, at the scale of the city, that may require further research.

INTRODUCTION

The Futures Wheel of Consequences [FW] is an old tool in the strategic foresight toolbox. As an architect I first learnt the Futures Wheel in 2001 in a local government leadership workshop conducted by Sohail Inayatullah. The method was first conceived by Jerome C Glenn in 1971 to visualise the direct and indirect future consequences of a change or event. [Futures Wheel, 2020]. I concede that in the suite of futures studies tools, the FW is not a method I practice often with stakeholders and I have often overlooked for other methods such as creative visualisation, scenario development and casual layered analysis.

Might this be the same within the futures studies field in general? A search of the Journal of Futures Studies database created one citation for an article that used the FW, compared to twenty-eight citations for macrohistory. Macrohistory, I believe is a more difficult method to grasp and use with participants compared to the FW.

The reason for the apparent downturn in the application of the FW, may be found within the inherent bias of timescales in each tool. The FW focusses on direct and indirect impacts in the short to medium term, handy for strategic planning. The general understanding within the Futures Studies field is that the FW is a tool that fits within the second pillar of futures thinking – anticipation (Inayatullah, 2008, p. 8). As such it may not challenge or generate alternative futures which are needed to transition out of the Anthropocene. Macrohistory (Galtung & Inayatullah, 1997) in contrast focusses on vast, intergenerational timescales to glean socio-cultural patterns and their diverse implications to anticipate long futures (Daffara, 2004a, p. 22). Within the Futures Studies field it is a method within the third pillar of futures thinking – timing the future (Inayatullah, 2008, p. 10).

So, is it possible to use both futures methods and integrate the systemic implications of the COVID-19 pandemic to encompass both short- and long-term time scales or horizons? The Futures Wheel of consequences is applied to the global shock and pandemic of COVID-19 to firstly analyse systemic impacts of the virus and identify risks and opportunities from the arising future possibilities. The benefits of the FW wheel process draw on a recent Australian case study. Secondly, the weak signals from the Futures Wheel are contextualised using macrohistorical models to time two probable future trajectories resulting from the bifurcation point of the pandemic. Causal Layered Analysis (CLA) then synthesises the multi-dimensional implications of COVID-19 gathered from the FW and Macrohistorical analyses to illustrate the different systemic focus of each method and the significance of this hinge period in human and planetary history.

FW CASE STUDY – TASMANIAN LEADERS INC

In a time of shock and crisis, such as the current global pandemic, decision makers need to respond quickly to impacts in a rapidly changing multifactorial environment. The FW tool comes into its strength during a time of global shock when quick responses are required within short time frames to anticipate possibilities. So why the FW in a time of shock? It is very quick to learn and simple to use by participants. The FW provides clarity on possible courses of action for the short to medium term with future consequences. In a time of shock where decision makers may be overwhelmed the FW provides a brief pause to suspend the biological flight or fight response that may lead to reactionary and poor decisions and allow instead considered responses.

On 26th March 2020, FutureSense hosted a 90min webinar with 25 cross-sector leaders as part of the Tasmanian Leaders Inc program, teaching them how to use the Futures Wheel of Consequences to anticipate the impacts of the COVID-19 pandemic virus on their businesses, sector or organisation. The leaders came from various sections including emergency services, cultural, not-for-profit, tertiary education, transport and energy. Angela Driver, General Manager of Tasmanian Leaders Inc., summed up the group feedback: "participants left the session feeling more connected, resilient and resourced. Three things that they are going to need to draw on over the coming months." (personal correspondence, March 27, 2020).

In preparing the FW workshop, I found that the most recent innovations to the FW methodology had occurred in the design thinking field. The methodology had been enhanced by overlaying the STEEP [1] categories to the wheel of consequences to ensure a multiplicity of contexts are explored (Behboudi, 2019). Embedding the FW within different stages of the design process is another more recent development (Figure 1). It can help in the initial stages when scanning for opportunities or later in the design process exploring how a solution may unfold. "It [FW embedded in a design process] is most useful when done with all stakeholders in the room, as it can also serve as a highly effective decision-making tool" (Behboudi, 2019).

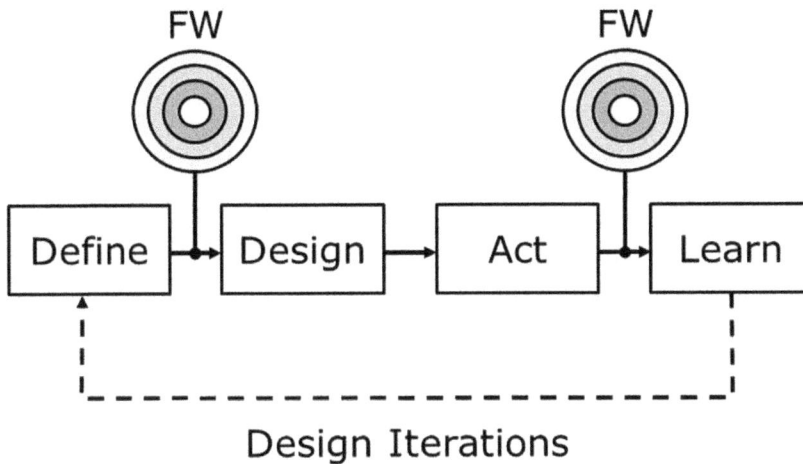

Figure 1

MAIN ARGUMENTS

From the Tasmanian Leaders case study three main arguments are evident and are presented next.

CONTEXT SPECIFIC FUTURES WHEEL APPLICATIONS

The FW workshop presented a generic global FW of possible consequences due to the COVID-19 pandemic, to demonstrate how to generate first, second and third order impacts through "what if" questioning. The adaptive capacity to climate change research, recognises generic and context specific determinants to adaptive capacity (Smith, Carter, Daffara, & Keys, 2010). Applying this to the FW methodology, the consequences generated by the FW can also be characterised as being generic or context specific. To leverage the benefits of the FW process and to build the adaptive capacity to change within participants, it is critical that participants apply the tool to their specific context. This raises their awareness of the systemic implications to their organisation, business or locality, rippling out from the initial shock of a global pandemic.

In the workshop, participants applied the FW individually to their specific context and then shared consequences within breakout groups to see if patterns emerged. Written feedback gathered from participants when asked what they learned when using the FW included:

> "Exploring some of the aspects of STEEP that may have been de-prioritized in the face of economic impacts".
> "Complexity and interrelation rather than linear cause-consequence relationship"
> "Process for systematically breaking down a complex problem".
> "Cool new tool and method to think through a complex situation and extract some useful observations regarding risks and opportunities which can be used to take action against".
> "Using the [STEEP] categories to break down a problem".

The written feedback shows how the FW with the STEEP framework facilitates multi-factorial consequences to be mapped which leads to systemic critical thinking of possible futures. That is, the search for interrelations between impacts, across social, technological, environmental, economic and political dimensions, not just casual linkages within a dimension.

GENERIC FUTURES WHEEL COVID-19 RISKS AND OPPORTUNITIES

The generic implications of a global pandemic relevant to most contexts and jurisdictions are presented in the COVID-19 Pandemic FW [Figure 2]. Three rings radiating from the core event represent the first order, second order and third order consequences. The outer field contains fourth order impacts and more. In addition to the five STEEP categories, a sixth segment allows "open space" for the mapping of other implications and in this case psychological implications emerged as a significant dimension related to a global pandemic. I stress that the mapped impacts are generic and far from complete. However, it illustrates the complexity and the critical systems thinking required to respond holistically to a pandemic. More important is the need for stakeholders (in this case everyone on the planet) to apply futures thinking using the futures wheel to their own context-specific circumstances and life conditions.

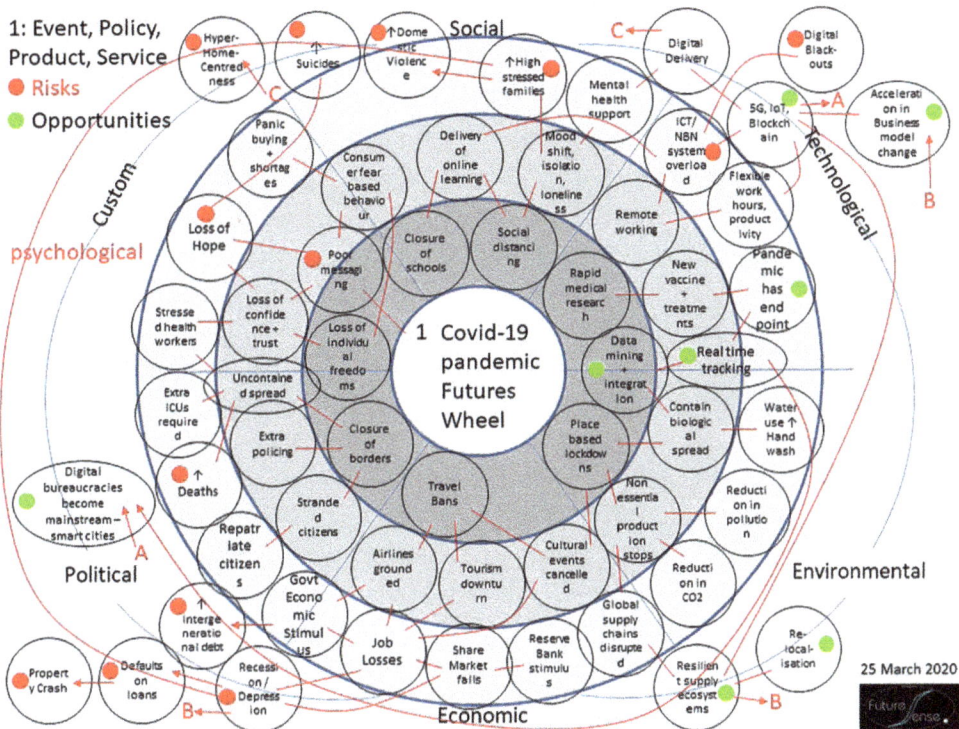

Figure 2
After the consequences are mapped, stakeholders can identify impacts that pose risks or opportunities to their specific context (place, organisation, business etc). Next, I discuss a handful of causal lines of consequence that contain significant risks and opportunities.

OPPORTUNITIES

Smart Cities: To contain the pandemic, certain countries have employed digital technologies to manage the crisis. Taiwan is using big data by integrating "national health insurance, immigration and customs databases, generating data to trace people's travel history and clinical symptoms." (The Straits Times, 2020). South Korea has employed similar digital technologies to enable real time spatial mapping of COVID-19 cases (Coronamap.site) based on extensive testing and tracking of visitors and citizens and to trace sources of the virus. (Nature, 2020). The Australian government intends to rollout Singapore's TraceTogether digital application to help trace COVID-19 contacts within communities to refine local lockdowns if required (The Guardian, April 19, 2020). No doubt, proponents for increased surveillance of the public health of populations, referred to as bio-surveillance, see the relationship between smart city innovation techno-systems and public health emergency responses. Innovations include the mining and analysis of urban sewers to monitor pathogens, virus loads and other indicators of health (e.g. drug use, alcohol consumption) to trace viral outbreaks (Senseable City Lab, 2019; The Guardian, 2016). Smart City advocates argue that "Innovative smart city technologies such as the Internet of Things (IoT), artificial intelligence (AI), 5G, open data, and analytics, offer the potential for cities to respond to the pandemic more effectively." (Chan & Paramel, 2020).

Smart Cities acting as place-based digital bureaucracies are well positioned to integrate datasets and resources to maintain public health and contain future viruses where poverty and digital divides are not major obstacles within the jurisdiction. Smart cities are not a panacea for poverty, inequality, urban apartheid, social polarisation, digital divides and urban fragmentation caused by capitalism and the informational, networked society. (Castells, 1999).

Relocalisation: Place-based lockdowns to contain the spread of the COVID-19 virus (e.g. Wuhan) effectively shut down non-essential production, which resulted in the disruption of global supply chains, particularly for medical equipment. The opportunity for the world, post COVID-19 is to design and create resilient supply ecosystems (Entrepreneur, 2020), going beyond the application of technologies within the current ecosystem, to drive a relocalisation of production and distribution. If Australia can use 3D printing technology to produce ventilators or surgical visors in a crisis when supply is constrained, why not always?

The relocalisation movement seeks to disrupt the globalisation of capital and production of food, materials and services, reducing the ecological footprint of human activities and building community resilience to future shocks (Hines, 2000).

Ecological regeneration. The great pause to the economies of the world to contain the COVID-19 pandemic through the lockdowns and home isolation of half the world's population have yielded beneficial environmental impacts. A reduction in CO_2 and pollution has been observed due to the drastic drop in road and air transportation; and manufacturing.

> "First China, then Italy, now the UK, Germany and dozens of other countries are experiencing temporary falls in carbon dioxide and nitrogen dioxide of as much as 40%, greatly improving air quality and reducing the risks of asthma, heart attacks and lung disease." (The Guardian, April 10, 2020).

The unexpected shock of the virus and the speed with which governments reigned in their respective economies, with resultant ecological benefits, provides an opportunity for perception change within communities. A glimpse of what a zero-carbon world may yield in terms of collective wellbeing and resurgent, resilient ecosystems. "The unthinkable has become thinkable" (Ibid). Rather than a return to business-as-usual:

> "UN leaders, scientists and activists are pushing for an urgent public debate so that recovery can focus on green jobs and clean energy, building efficiency, natural infrastructure and a strengthening of the global commons." (Ibid).

RISKS

The opportunities presented through a scaling up of digital capability for smart cities were previously discussed in respect to public health. The leap in the digital delivery of other services due to the pandemic such as work from home, online learning for schools, mental health support, telehealth, entertainment and creative arts and online shopping are evident in post-industrial, "informational networked societies" (Castells, 1989, 1996). Two risks emerge from the FW analysis.

Homecentredness. Firstly, the phenomenon of 'homecentredness" anticipated by Castells (1996, p. 398) has the potential to escalate during physical and social distancing measures and drastically impact daily home life and ultimately the urban-social contract. A pandemic forces people to retreat to their homes and rely on digital technologies to maintain many aspects of their work-life habits. What I call hyper-homecentredness leads to chronic social isolation and loneliness, poor socialisation within communities and poor mental health outcomes. The health impacts of loneliness are manifold and well researched:

> "The risk of premature death associated with social isolation and loneliness is similar to the risk of premature death associated with well-known risk factors such as obesity, based on a meta-analysis of research in Europe, North American, Asia and Australia (Holt-Lunstad, Smith, Baker, Harris, & Stephenson, 2015 cited in Australian Institute of Health and Welfare, 2019).

How many indirect deaths will occur due to the health impacts of social isolation and loneliness compared to the direct deaths of the virus?

The risk or prolonged forms of social isolation until a vaccine is available for the COVID-19 virus is that the enforced banning of and cessation of cultural events, festivals, sports, public gatherings and even protests may erode the public life, identity and spirit of cities, towns and communities. The conveniences of (1) home-based consumption; (2) the digital interconnectedness of devices; and (3) the delivery of products and services to the home enabled by the smart city; may also increase individualism, further straining the sense of belonging to a larger community.

Digital blackouts. Secondly, the ICT risks of digital platforms not having the system capacity to cope with the surge in demand are significant. Take for example the failure of the Australian Government's Centrelink online Jobseeker registration site within their MyGov platform to deal with the possibly, one million newly unemployed citizens caused by the pandemic's lockdown laws (The Guardian, March 24, 2020).

A worse scenario to contemplate is the internet going dark whilst the pandemic is still forcing geographic lockdowns, thereby not only physically distancing people but also socially disconnecting them from work based and personal networks. Cyber-attacks against critical platforms are a possibility during this pandemic's health crisis and economic deep freeze, adding a new dimension to the chaos that would unfold. Are we prepared for this risk, either from state-based cyber terrorists or anarchistic hackers?

Mental health risks. The FW clearly plots the causal line of consequences that ultimately impact a communities' mental health and wellbeing. Starting with lockdowns and social distancing measures, to mood shifts, increased isolation and loneliness, increased stress within families, the loss of hope and the likely increase in domestic violence and suicides. These probable impacts are well documented in a recent mental health study conducted in the countries that experienced the early outbreak of the COVID-19 virus, before a global pandemic was declared by the WHO. (Brooks, Webster, Smith, Woodland, Wessely, Greenberg, & Rubin, 2020). Related to mental health issues are the psychological factors that underpin the wellbeing of a community. Mainly poor messaging by governments on what to do and why, with a resultant loss of hope. The implications of loss of hope will be discussed in more detail next, in the context of macrohistory.

THE LITANY LEVEL· SUMMING UP OF THE FUTURES WHEEL ANALYSIS

The application of the FW of consequences to the COVID-19 pandemic, at the litany level of discourse, challenges the political messaging of governments and chief medical officers, that this virus is mainly a public health and economic emergency. Rather, the COVID-19 pandemic is a whole of systems crisis, as it impacts or disrupts multidimensional qualities of life as shown in the STEEP categories. At the system's level, I am reminded of Ian Lowe's model of transition from the pig-face systems model of sustainability to the nested systems model (Lowe, 2016, p. 230) (Figure 3). The dominant systems worldview today is the pig face, where the economy remains the dominant concern. Leaders responding to this pandemic need to be reminded that the environment and society are not here to serve the economy (like two little ears on a pigs face), but rather that the economy is to be designed to care for our society, cultures and environment (like nested spheres).

Bluntly, responding to the COVID-19 pandemic is an opportunity to redesign our economies to better serve our socio-ecological systems. But this opportunity is too daunting for most global leaders who seek a return to economic normalcy and its dominance as soon as possible.

Figure 3

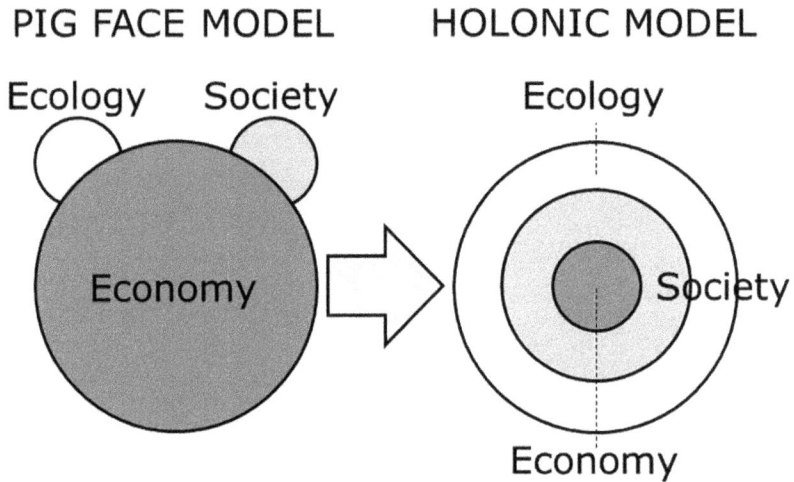

PIG FACE MODEL   HOLONIC MODEL

Transitioning between
Worldviews of Systems

WEAK SIGNALS IN THE CONTEXT OF MACROHISTORY

This part, seeks to contextualise the weak signals that emerge from the FW of a global pandemic using macrohistory and cycles of cultural change. I call the future possibilities, weak signals, because they emerge as 4th or 5th order consequences in the FW from the initial shock. As such, they normally would be beyond the awareness of participants and stakeholders. These weak signals are then contextualised using macrohistory to make some sense of the epochal shifts triggered by a pandemic. I will refer to the macrohistorical models of Sorokin, Toynbee, Teilhard de Chardin and Khaldun *(Figure 4)*.

A POST-COVID-19 WORLDVIEW – CREATIVE DESTRUCTION?

From Sorokin's macrohistorical perspective, the COVID-19 pandemic is both precursor to and trigger for a global depression and ecological chaos that exposes the weaknesses of the materialistic (sensate) cultural paradigm, holding up the mirror to the limits of growth, consumption, wealth and comfort. "If everyone is out to satisfy material needs there may not be enough to go around, and particularly if nature's needs are to be respected" [Galtung & Inayatullah, 1997, p. 117]. A grab-what-you-can mentality emerges – like people rushing into supermarkets worldwide to horde toilet paper and food – to bunker down in self isolation.

This sets the scene for a renewal phase from chaos to a new spiritual (ideational) cultural paradigm, motivated by the push forces of self-disgust "and with how the human condition has degenerated into nonhuman and even antihuman absurdities. There are also the pull forces, longing for steering and guidance" [ibid, p. 117]. Including the observed environmental spinoffs caused by the pandemic's great pause on production and human activity, such as cleaner air, water and return of wildlife to cities [The Guardian, March 23, 2020, April 10, 2020]. This possible ideational renewal may be underwritten on green and humane values, but we need to look to other macrohistorians to understand the cultural dynamics needed to motivate the creative leap from chaos to a shared universal spirituality.

Let us look to Toynbee, Teilhard de Chardin and Khaldun with a touch of Pink [3] to speculate the importance of a creative culture to respond to the global pandemic. Toynbee's macrohistory makes the point that a civilisation grows and reproduces itself through the challenge - response – mimesis (CRM cycle) by the efforts and capability of a creative minority [Galtung & Inayatullah, 1997, p. 122]. Sorokin's quantum leap back to an ideational-spiritual worldview requires Toynbee's cultural creatives to tell a unified transformative narrative to inspire the masses to contemplate a different type of planetary civilisation. Likewise, Pink's 'conceptual age' [2005, p. 48] that focusses on human empathy, story and design is relevant to provide push and pull factors for a post COVID-19 worldview that resets our sense making and memetic reproduction of meaning.

Teilhard de Chardin's "research for a synthesis overcoming the dualism of matter and spirit" (Daniela Rocco Minerbi in Galtung & Inayatullah, 1997, p. 105) is at the centre of his macrohistory. This synthesis and unity of knowledge mirrors Sorokin's idealistic cultural mentality, that integrates material concerns with those of ideas and metaphysics. Teilhard's process of personalisation and complexification towards 'noogenesis' and the 'noosphere', is an evolutionary stage of planetary culture and collective consciousness and reflection reliant on the transpersonal growth of the individual. This evolution is driven by a cosmic tendency, "towards the spirit – towards pure radial energy (love). He recognises the continual tension of the universe towards increasing entropy (disorder) within his model, and that at times the socialisation process (noogenesis) is counter-evolutionary. When this happens, society succumbs to entropy, individualism and depersonalisation, and falls away from the spiritual." (Daffara, 2004a, p. 15).

As illustrated in the FW analysis, the risk here is that the worldwide government responses to socially isolate communities to contain the global pandemic, fuels individualism and depersonalisation. Conversely, it could be argued that this decline and psychological challenge is necessary for Sorokin's and Toynbee's regeneration process.

Khaldun's macrohistory and the concept of asibiya provides key ingredients to Teilhard's emergence of the noosphere through noogenesis. Put simply without the philosophical jargon: "For Khaldun, what is important in transformational leadership is asibiya - the collective purpose, unity and memory that binds a group." (Daffara, 2004a, p. 25). The implication here, is that a post COVID-19 world and cultural paradigm or zeitgeist, requires the bottom-up co-design of a collective purpose and vision to enrol the peoples of this planet into a resilient social-ecological system.

All the above macrohistorians point to the importance of using this great global pause to reset what it means to be human, why we do what we do on this fragile planet, and how we might do better. In short, how might we design alternative futures, not so vulnerable to the cascading shocks and consequences of a global pandemic mapped by the FW.

Figure 4

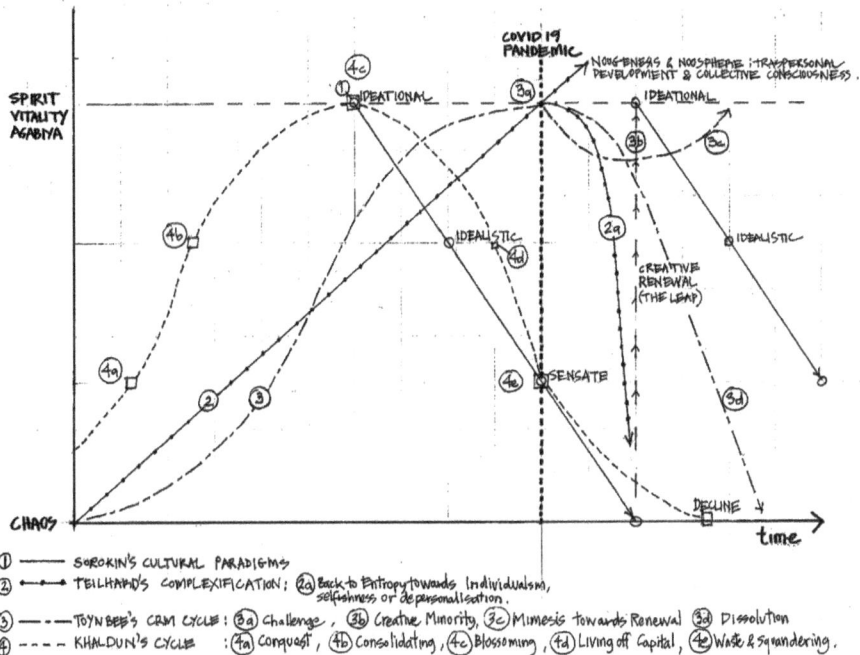

① ——— SOROKIN'S CULTURAL PARADIGMS
② —•—•— TEILHARD'S COMPLEXIFICATION; ②a) Back to Entropy towards Individualism, selfishness or depersonalisation.
③ — • • — TOYNBEE'S CRM CYCLE : ③a) Challenge , ③b) Creative Minority, ③c) Mimesis towards Renewal ③d) Dissolution
④ – – – – KHALDUN'S CYCLE : ④a) Conquest , ④b) Consolidating , ④c) Blossoming , ④d) Living off Capital, ④e) Waste & squandering .

CAUSAL LAYERED ANALYSIS: SUMMING UP THE MACROHISTORY ANALYSIS

I use Causal Layered Analysis (CLA) (Inayatullah & Milojević, 2015) as a method to summarise the FW and macrohistorical analysis so far. Previously, I have discussed the litany and systems level implications of the FW of consequences to the COVID-19 pandemic. What follows next are the worldview and myth/metaphor levels of reality. Table 1 illustrates all levels related to only two perspectives - the bifurcated choice in this hinge period in human history triggered by COVID-19.

The application of macrohistorical models to the COVID-19 pandemic, reinforces the critical importance of Western societies to respond to the systemic emergency with an awareness of cultural change dynamics. At the worldview level, we need to transition from a 'growth is good" cultural paradigm to 'positive development with zero growth' (Daffara, 2004b). The pandemic reminds us of the urgent need to avoid ecological collapse and regenerate our built and natural environments.

In terms of 'timing the future', macrohistory shows that COVID-19 comes at a critical time with other converging stressors – social, environmental, economic and political. COVID-19 may be the final systemic shock or tipping point, defining a 'hinge period in human history' (Inayatullah, 2008, p. 11). A period of bifurcation between contrasting probable futures. Either humanity will respond creatively to reset our values and design and build more resilient Lifeworlds in harmony with the planet, or we risk further ecological, social and political decline and disintegration. At the myth/metaphor level of reality, each contrasting future may be aptly described by Khaldun's macrohistory (Galtung & Inayatullah, 1997. p. 28-29): 'unification with kindness' for and by team humanity verses 'fragmentation with loss of hope' with the masses monitored and controlled by powerful and wealthy plutocrats of the informational, networked society.

TABLE 1: CLA of the hinge point in human history from COVID-19		
	Decline and Disintegration	**Creative Renewal**
Litany:	COVID-19 is a public health and economic emergency. We will make decisions to return to economic normalcy as soon as possible.	COVID-19 is a whole of systems emergency. We will take this opportunity to make decisions to remake a just, caring society.
Systems:	Pig face sustainability model: The economy is dominant and is served by our natural resources and social capital.	Holonic, nested model of sustainability. The economy cares for our cultures and societies and natural global commons.
Worldview:	'Growth is Good" cultural paradigm	'Positive Development [4] with Zero Growth'[5]
Myth using Khaldun's macrohistory: Author's Metaphor: From Nature	'Fragmentation with loss of hope' Teams of Plutocrats Muddy ponds	'Unification with Kindness' Team Humanity Blossoming lotus

The above CLA of only two probable trajectories at the bifurcation point of COVID-19 is intentional to focus the attention of decision makers and stakeholders. To use Toynbee's macrohistory, either civilisations commit to slow 'suicide' or creative renewal (Galtung & Inayatullah, 1997, p. 122). The system and worldview levels draw from Lowe's perspective (2016) and Atkisson's work (1999) respectively. The myth level uses Khaldun's macrohistory to contrast the story of fragmentation versus unification. At the metaphor level, Toynbee's macrohistory provides the disintegration narrative where "the Creative Minority becomes a Dominant Minority trying to control the Internal and External Proletariat [wage-earners]" (Galtung & Inayatullah, 1997, p. 122). What I have labelled as "Teams of Plutocrats" exerting power and influence over governments and peoples, for example, through their internet based informational networks. In contrast, the metaphor of "Team Humanity" speaks for itself in the unification trajectory.

I have sought to synthesise the CLA of each trajectory and present an underpinning metaphor from nature to evoke an emotional response within readers. I propose that the futures are like muddy disparate ponds versus a riparian system that supports blossoming lotus. If we make the collective choice towards transformation and creative renewal, then diverse alternative futures within that overarching trajectory ought to be explored using the full suite of foresight technologies.

Figure 5

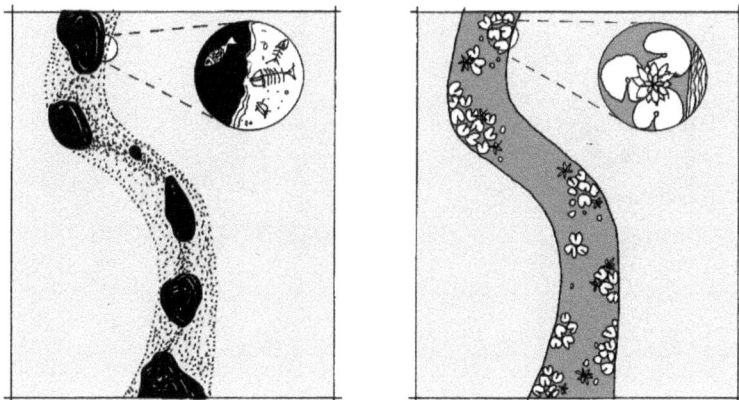

Muddy Ponds:
'Fragmentation with loss of hope'

Blossoming Lotus:
'Unification with Kindness'

CONCLUSION & FURTHER RESEARCH

The following findings are offered from the FW and Macrohistorical analyses of the systemic impacts of the COVID-19 pandemic (Figure 6). Designing a foresight process using two foresight methods with different time horizons, does broaden the exploration of impacts. The integration of the FW and Macrohistory, becomes more meaningful if a common spatial scale of analysis is used to link them. In this study, a spatial scale of analysis was not predetermined. However, during the process, the city emerged as the relevant spatial scale of study, able to link the different time scales of each method in a complimentary way and their arising systemic impacts.

Figure 6

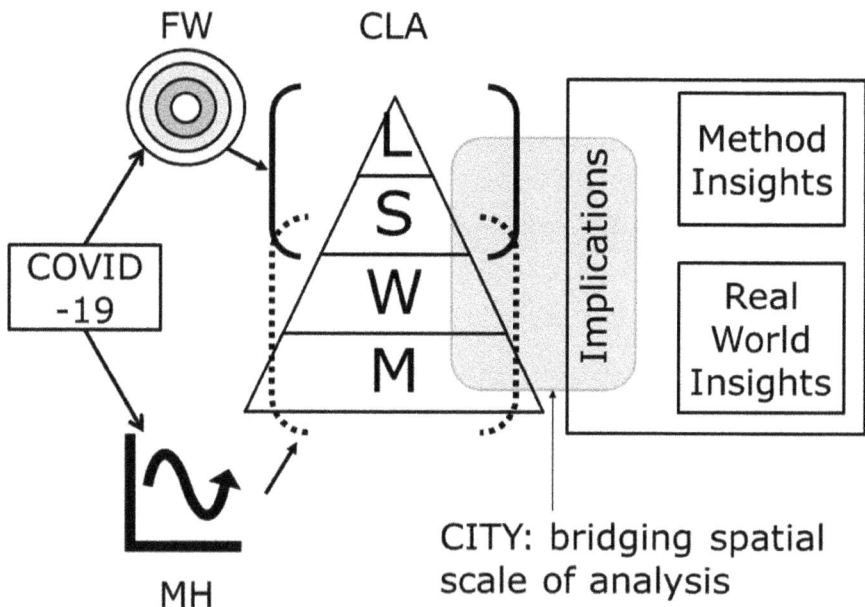

METHODOLOGICAL INSIGHTS

FW is a quick tool to grasp, giving leaders the agility to respond rapidly in the COVID-19 global pandemic as well as anticipate consequences down the causal line and their possible risks and opportunities. During the FW analysis, at the systems level, several 4th and 5th order impacts emerged, that highlighted the importance of the city in responding to the pandemic. For example: [1] relocalisation of supply chains, [2] the capacity of smart cities to trace and isolate cases and facilitate digital social connectivity, and [3] ecological renewal due to the lockdown of cities. It was found that the city could be used as a common spatial scale to provide the means of integrating the FW and Macrohistorical analyses – assisting in sense making – across CLA's different levels of reality.

As a result, the second part of the conclusion also provides real world actions in response to the pandemic at the scale of the city, and proposes areas of further research.

CLA helped to synthesise the multi-dimensional implications of COVID-19 gathered from the previous analyses and illustrates the significance of this hinge period in human and planetary history.

CLA also illustrates how the technique of the FW focusses the attention of stakeholders and participants on the litany and systems levels of reality in response to COVID-19. Whilst the comparative analysis of macrohistories draws out worldviews, cultural paradigms and myth/metaphors that influence civilisational change in response to the pandemic. The application of CLA provided a means of synthesis for making sense of the levels of reality for the two probable futures post COVID-19.

REAL WORLD INSIGHTS

Firstly, how do we allow a planet of 7.8 billion people to collectively grieve the losses caused by the global pandemic? How do we as a creative minority [futurists/ foresight practitioners] initiate the co-design of planetary asibiya – collective purposes and visions to transition towards a more ideational, integrated culture that values wisdom over technical knowledge?

Secondly, sources of hope are critical during this crisis to motivate the inner growth and personalisation of individuals as described by Teilhard and drive Toynbee's socialisation or mimesis between cultural creatives and the masses to counter Khaldun's loss of asibiya (collective purpose and vision).

Thirdly, I offer a practical path forward to respond to the second and third points mentioned previously, to be implemented at the spatial scale of the city or town. This links back to the FW impacts affecting smart cities and the relocalisation of communities and their economies. Cities are agents of change (Daffara, 2011) each a specific socio-ecological system responsible at a territorial scale for providing pluralistic, diverse futures. I propose that cities are best positioned to engage their citizens to grieve the losses caused by the COVID-19 pandemic, through truth telling fora and to facilitate personal and collective healing. Rather than erect monuments to memorialise the crisis overcome, it would be better to initiate city foresight projects to create shared values and visions for the alternative ways forward. The purpose is to create post COVID-19 "City Noospheres" – creative, learning and diverse city cultures (Daffara, 2011. p. 685) with greater adaptive capacity and resilience to respond to the next epidemic and other wicked challenges that persist such as the climate emergency and ecological destruction caused by human activity (The Guardian, March 25, 2020).

Summing up the application of the FW of consequences to the COVID-19 pandemic at the litany level of discourse, challenges the political messaging of governments that this virus is mainly a public health and economic emergency. Rather, the COVID-19 pandemic is a whole of systems crisis that presents an opportunity to redesign our economies to better serve our socio-ecological systems and the human values that underpin them.

Summing up the application of macrohistorical models to the COVID-19 pandemic, we find that we are at a hinge period in human history, critically important for Western societies to respond to the systemic emergency with an awareness of cultural change dynamics. Will the human species reset during this great pause and unite with kindness or fragment with loss of hope?

AUTHOR

Dr Phillip Daffara PhD Principal, FutureSense

PO Box 1489, Mooloolaba, Queensland 4557, Australia

p.daffara@futuresense.com.au

ENDNOTES

[1] STEEP: social, technological, environmental, economic and political categories used to describe multi-factorial issues within a system.

[2] Each quote listed from the written participant feedback represents a comment from a different workshop participant.

[3] Daniel Pink is not recognised as a macrohistorian, but his model of world change provides a useful evolution of ages. He does not provide references or sources for his synthesis, so I continue to cite Pink as the author of the "Conceptual Age" in which we currently operate in.

[4] Positive Development, developed by Janis Birkeland (2008) requires that our development must be positive, adding back to the planet's ecosystem services in every project. It demands more than nett zero carbon.

[5] Zero Growth, as discussed by Alan Atkisson (1999, p. 24–26) in this systems' view, civilization must transform itself toward "Development without Growth", away from the current course of "Growth equals Development". This is, in his view (which I share), the greatest challenge of our generation and must become humanity's fundamental project for the 21st century (Daffara, 2004b).

REFERENCES

Atkisson, A. (1999). *Believing Cassandra*. Scribe Publications.

Australian Institute of Health and Welfare. (2019, September 11). *Social isolation and loneliness*. https://www.aihw.gov.au/reports/australias-welfare/social-isolation-and-loneliness

Behboudi, M. (2019). *Futures Wheel, Practical Frameworks for Ethical Design*. https://medium.com/klickux/futures-wheel-practical-frameworks-for-ethical-design-e40e323b838a

Birkeland, J. (2008). *Positive Development*. Earthscan Press.

Brooks, S.K., Webster. R.K., Smith. L.E., Woodland. L., Wessely. S., Greenberg. N., & Rubin. G.J. (2020) The psychological impact of quarantine and how to reduce it: rapid review of the evidence. *The Lancet*, 395(10227), 912–20.

DOI: https://doi.org/10.1016/S0140-6736(20)30460-8

Chan, B., & Paramel, R. (2020). *Smart Cities & Public Health Emergency Collaboration Framework. Meeting of the Minds*. https://meetingoftheminds.org/smart-cities-public-health-emergency-collaboration-framework-33446?mc_cid=e1c88de2b3&mc_eid=a902b5de1b

Castells, M. (1989). *The Informational City: Information Technology, Economic Re-structuring and the Urban-Regional Process*. Blackwell.

Castells, M. ([1996], 1999). *The Rise of the Network Society, The Information Age: Economy, Society and Culture, Vol 1*. Blackwell.

Daffara, P. (2004). Sustainable City Futures. In S. Inayatullah (Ed.), *The Causal Layered Analysis (CLA) Reader Theory and case studies of an Integrative and Transformative Methodology* (pp. 424-438). Tamkang University Press.

Daffara, P. (2011) Rethinking tomorrow's cities: Emerging issues on city foresight. *Futures*, 43, 680–689.

Entrepreneur. (2020). *COVID-19 Will Fuel the Next Wave of Innovation*. https://www-entrepreneur-com.cdn.ampproject.org/c/s/www.entrepreneur.com/amphtml/347669

Wikipedia. (2020). *Futures Wheel*. https://en.wikipedia.org/wiki/Futures_wheel

Hines, C. (2000). *Localization: A Global Manifesto*. Earthscan.

Inayatullah, S. (2008) Six pillars: futures thinking for transforming. *Foresight*, 10(1), 4-21. DOI 10.1108/14636680810855991

Inayatullah, S. & Milojević, I. (2015). *CLA 2.0: Transformative Research in Theory and Practice*. Tamkang University Press.

Lowe, I. (2016). *The Lucky Country? Reinventing Australia*. University of Queensland Press.

MIT Senseable City Lab. (2019). *The Underworlds Book*. http://underworlds.mit.edu/

Nature. (2020). *South Korea is reporting intimate details of COVID-19 cases: has it helped?*. https://www.nature.com/articles/d41586-020-00740-y

Smith, T.F., Carter, R.W., Daffara, P., & Keys, N. (2010). *The Nature and Utility of Adaptive Capacity Research*. Report for the National Climate Change Adaptation Research Facility. https://bit.ly/3mbMkD9

Davis, N. (2016, March 27). The MIT lab flushing out a city's secrets. *The Guardian*. https://www.theguardian.com/science/2016/mar/27/lab-that-flushes-out-city-secrets-massachusetts-mit-senseable-lab-sewage

Henriques-Gome, L. (2020, March 24). Newly unemployed Australians queue at Centrelink offices as MyGov website crashes again. *The Guardian*. https://www.theguardian.com/australia-news/2020/mar/24/newly-unemployed-australians-queue-at-centrelink-offices-as-mygov-website-crashes-again#maincontent

Murray, J. & Sherwood, H. (2020, March 13). Anxiety on rise due to coronavirus, say mental health charities. *The Guardian*. https://www.theguardian.com/world/2020/mar/13/anxiety-on-rise-due-to-coronavirus-say-mental-health-charities

Watts, J. & Kommenda, N. (2020, March 23). Coronavirus pandemic leading to huge drop in air pollution. *The Guardian* https://www.theguardian.com/environment/2020/mar/23/coronavirus-pandemic-leading-to-huge-drop-in-air-pollution

Carrington, D. (2020, March 25). Coronavirus: 'Nature is sending us a message', says UN environment chief. *The Guardian*. https://www.theguardian.com/world/2020/mar/25/coronavirus-nature-is-sending-us-a-message-says-un-environment-chief

Watts, J. (2020, April 10). Climate crisis: in coronavirus lockdown, nature bounces back – but for how long? *The Guardian*. https://www.theguardian.com/world/2020/apr/09/climate-crisis-amid-coronavirus-lockdown-nature-bounces-back-but-for-how-long

Taylor, J. (2020, April 19). Australia's coronavirus contact tracing app: what we know so far. *The Guardian*. https://www.theguardian.com/world/2020/apr/17/australias-coronavirus-contact-tracing-app-what-we-know-so-far

The Straits Times. (2020, March 13). *Coronavirus lessons for the world from ground zero of Asia*. https://www.straitstimes.com/asia/east-asia/coronavirus-lessons-for-the-world-from-ground-zero-of-asia

ANCESTORS OF THE FUTURE:

The Poetry and Potency of Language

Marguerite Coetzee

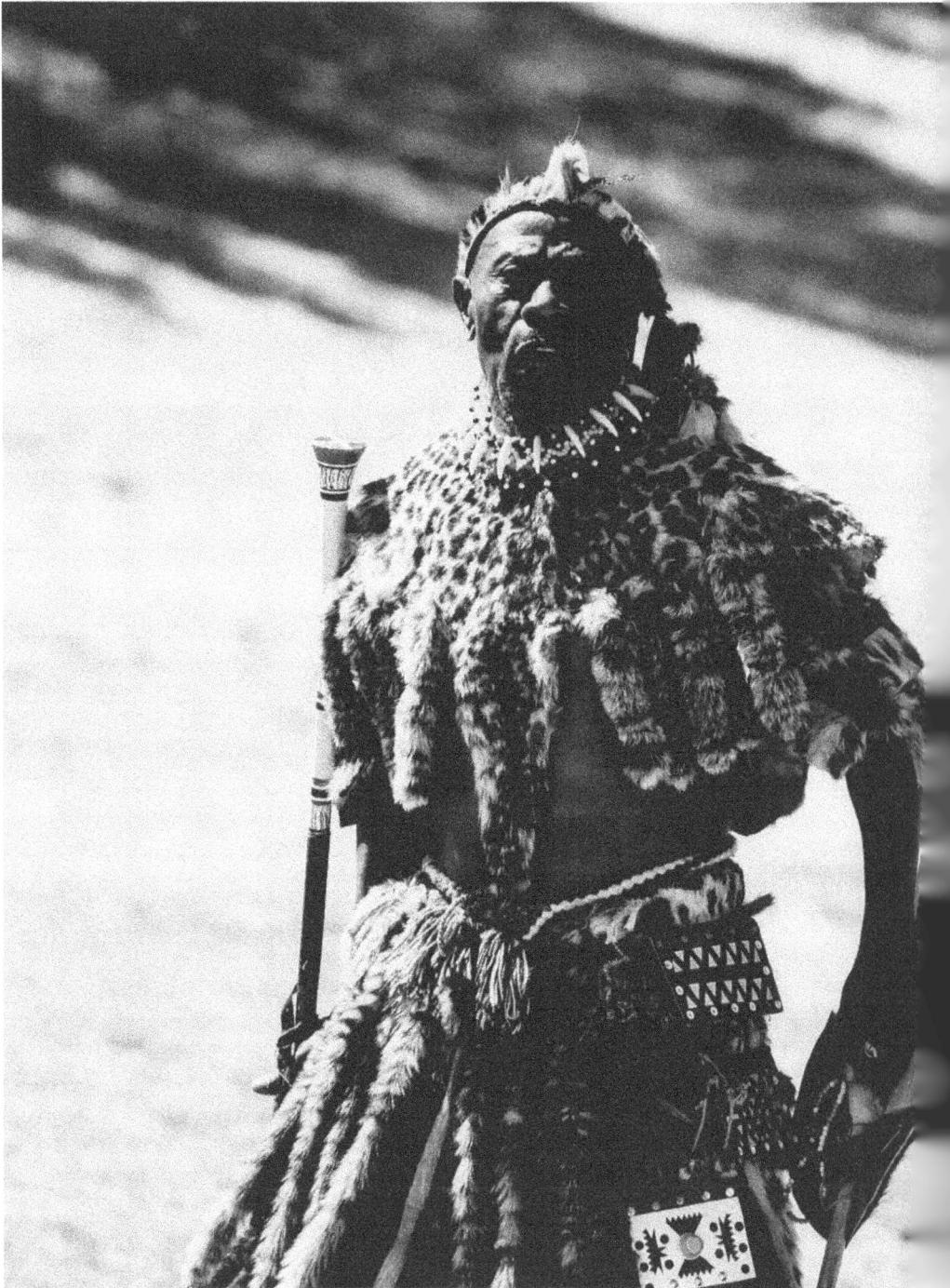

IsiZulu memorial in Johannesburg South Africa, 2019 photo by Marguerite Coetzee

In Hindu mythology, it is believed that the Earth is balanced on the backs of elephants, which are themselves supported by a World Turtle. Below that turtle? Another turtle. It is turtles all the way down. In complexity and systems thinking, it could be argued that a proposition requires justification, and the justification itself needs to be supported. No idea exists in isolation, no truth in a vacuum, no experience untethered from others. It is turtles all the way down.

By identifying layers of analysis, Causal Layered Analysis is a sense-making tool that explores the narratives used to make sense of the world. The very first layer, the litany, is the observed or obvious problem and resulting official future, second is the systemic causes or driving forces that create the conditions in which the problem or future exist, third the discourses and ideological assumptions that legitimise and support a worldview, and fourth is the layer of myth and metaphor that is linked to long-term history and emotive dimensions. In addition to developing an understanding of the world, it is used to "shape the future more effectively" and to "[create]coherent futures" (Inayatullah, 2017, p1). The intention is to map the present, unpack an issue critically, and create a preferred future reconstructed from alternative worldviews and from multiple perspectives. This leads to transformed futures that integrate difference. It is a combination of the pull of the future, push of the present, and weight of history (Inayatullah, 2017, p6).

Just as in the past, we currently find ourselves in a pandemic. How do we begin to make sense of the world we are in? "Epidemics are a category of disease that seem to hold up a mirror to human beings as to who we really are"; It reflects the relationship between people and their environment, raising questions about our ways of life (Chotiner, 2020). Metaphors are a way in which we can make concrete our imaginings, memories, and realities; they are devices with which we can play with concepts of time, blurring past, present, and future (Capo). Metaphors are meaning-making tools used in cognition and culture, shaping the way we act individually and collectively (Nerlich, 2020). In this essay I explore several dominant and emerging metaphors relating to the current pandemic, in the realms of society, technology, economics, environment, and politics. Each metaphor creates different realities, challenges, and opportunities.

SOCIAL REALM: APOCALYPSE REVOLUTION

COVID-19 has been labelled a plague. Both in religious terms – the uncontrollable mass spread of an unhealable disease – and in biological terms – a zoonotic transmission of disease from rodent to person. What results from this narrative is mass hysteria from those who fear the worst, an aura of shame around those infected, and the rise of body politics to control the contaminated and to contain the contagion. People become zombies trying to survive an apocalypse; it is the end of days. Like previous plagues, this pandemic is explained as either being a punishment for those who have wronged – morally, if from a religious perspective, or ethically, if from a biological perspective. Either society has transgressed to the point of no return (from a religious perspective), or particular populations are blamed and reprimanded and old prejudices are perpetuated (such as judging China for consuming particular animal products). The symbolism of the plague is used "to convey the suffering of the suffocation and atmosphere of terror and exile" (Zaretsky, 2020).

If we were, instead, to view the pandemic as an opportunity for revolution or renaissance – to revive or renew our world – we could see the virus as triggering a turning point in history. This narrative establishes an element of empowerment, freedom, and consent. People become agents of change, contributing to the speed and depth of the transformation. The crisis becomes a catalyst for change, enabling us to dismantle old systems of superiors and subordinates. We are in this together. In viewing ourselves as global citizens in a shared process of being and becoming – with access to communal knowledge, collective consciousness, and an evolving social commons – we are presented with an invitation to transform wicked problems into wicked opportunities (Eggers & Muoio, 2015).

An example of this is the call for an African Health Organisation that embraces – rather than undermines – traditional medicine from the continent (SABC News, 2020). It is not to say that WHO should be replaced or dominated by THO (Traditional Healers' Organisation), but rather that a collaborative relationship be formed to develop new approaches to crises. It is about leveraging Africa's strengths, not straining its weak points in favour of a homogenised, westernised method (Senbanjo, 2020).

TECHNOLOGICAL REALM· PAUSE PORTAL

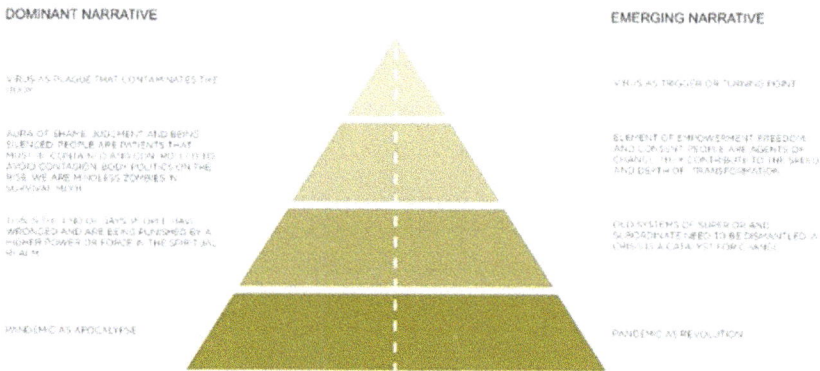

DOMINANT NARRATIVE

EMERGING NARRATIVE

PANDEMIC AS APOCALYPSE

PANDEMIC AS REVOLUTION

If all the world's a stage, as Shakespeare proclaimed, then we must be on The Truman Show. It is as if someone has hit the pause button; everything has slowed down. "Collectively we are witnessing a global phenomenon that has people everywhere staying home, slowing down, and witnessing a global pause during this pandemic" (Devaney, 2020). While we seek to digitalise everything – the way we work, socialise, learn – prospects of compromised privacy and enhanced monitoring of our online lives becomes a growing concern: "the rise and spread of digital surveillance enabled by artificial intelligence" (Wright, 2020). This brings into question the agency of the individual and the authority of the state. We have long observed the growing power of media in swaying or formulating opinion, as well as gathering data and information for commercial or political benefit (Confessore, 2018). Viewing the virus as a glitch or technical error seems to justify 'rebooting' the system. In this narrative, AI will save us, even if it is at a cost.

"Historically, pandemics have forced humans to break with the past and imagine their world anew. This one is no different. It is a portal, a gateway between one world and the next one" [Roy, 2020]. This suspended moment, from this angle, becomes a time of transition; a liminal space between reality and a dream-state. It becomes an opportunity to take a breath, put future scenarios on hold, experiment with possibilities, consider the legacy we want to leave behind, and take in the present moment, before we are transported into the new world. Doing so requires decentralised and autonomous control, as well as open source products and collaborative platforms as we co-create futures.

An example of this is the vast number of online conferences and symposiums – often made freely available to all with internet access – that have erupted from all parts of the globe. While we may have put our personal lives on pause, we are far more globally connected than we ever were before. Just look at the global foresight summit hosted by FFWD titled 'The Great Pause'. There were attendees from over 100 countries and speakers each with a one-hour timeslot over a 72-hour period.

ECONOMIC REALM· STORM DANCE

When a severe storm approaches, with little time to think or react, an instinctual response it to act quickly; to take shelter from the rain, and consider the cost of destruction after you have secured your safety. Every moment counts. Similarly, in a ship rescue, there are often those who want to contribute, but are unable to and can create confusion. Pandemic shock brings about collective trauma, crisis capitalism, and imagination paralysis (Klein, 2007). It is easy to decline into a bleak state of despair and dysfunction when in a disaster. Some are more vulnerable than others – we are not all in the same boat or equipped with the same tools to navigate Lightning bolts of disruption and tidal waves of change. Some make it to shore while others are rendered invisible amidst the throws of vicious and virtuous cycles that deepen inequality.

In a state of emergency, a utilitarian approach is often taken to ensure the immediate survival of many, even if extreme measures need to be taken. However, "once the Hammer is in place and the outbreak is controlled, the second phase begins: the Dance" (Pueyo, 2020). If we view the pandemic as a dance and the future as our dance partner, it becomes a give and take relationship of synchronisation, harmony, and collaboration. People are no longer captives to the captains of their fate, but rather dance to their own tune and choreograph their own routine.

An example of this is South Africa's declaring of the pandemic as a national disaster and focusing on providing food parcels for the hungry, shelter for the homeless, and relief funds for the financially-strained businesses. However, in its efforts to contain the spread of fear, to perform damage control, and to 'flatten the curve', its extended lockdown has come across as Draconian, or unnecessarily harsh. Many citizens argue that instead of moving to the dance phase of its strategy, leadership is repeatedly hammering the same nail. Or so it seems. While the spread of the virus is relentless – particularly across the nation's informal settlements and informal economy – leadership has put out fires elsewhere. In banning the purchase of alcohol during lockdown, the country has seen a significant decline in alcohol-related casualties (including car accidents and domestic violence). The pandemic does not operate in isolation, nor is it linear in its movements. It requires a hammer and dance approach to respond, adapt, and anticipate shadow crises, chain reactions, and satellite events.

DOMINANT NARRATIVE

EMERGING NARRATIVE

VIRUS AS LIGHTNING BOLT, TSUNAMI, OR HURRICANE - OBVIOUS, UNPREDICTABLE DESTRUCTION AND CHANGE

FUTURE AS DANCE PARTNER

THERE IS LITTLE TIME TO THINK OR REACT. A CIVILIAN RESPONSE IS RAMPED TO TAKE SHELTER FROM THE RAIN, SECURE SAFETY, AND ENSURE IMMEDIATE SURVIVAL

OPEN DIALOGUE, MUTUAL CONVERSATION, MULTIPLE INTERPRETATIONS, LIMITED EXPERIENCES SHIFTING ROLES ON-HAND, TAKING RELATIONSHIPS

IN DAILY AND DAMAGED CONTROL, TEAM OF SPARE AND DYSFUNCTION, LEADERS ARE CAPTAINS WHO ACT QUICKLY AND AGGRESSIVELY, SOME ARE MORE VULNERABLE THAN OTHERS

PEOPLE ARE DANCERS SYNCHRONISING IN HARMONY AND COLLABORATION, DANCING TO THEIR OWN MUSIC AND CHOREOGRAPHING THEIR OWN ROUTINE

PANDEMIC AS STORM

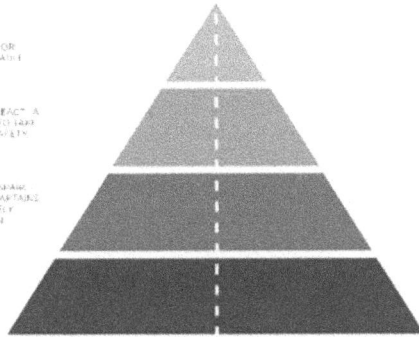

PANDEMIC AS DANCE

ENVIRONMENTAL REALM: DISASTER RIVER

Countries declaring the pandemic a national disaster are putting into place regulations and measures of control – such as providing tax relief, setting up temporary housing, responding to distress signals, and offering financial aid – to minimise damage. The virus in this narrative is perceived to be a disruption caused by natural processes beyond human control, but owing to destructive human influence. Thousands of years ago, communities the world over acknowledged the interconnected relationship between nature and culture. If there was turmoil or conflict in society, it would appear in nature – drought, fire, disease. Nature was seen to be this self-reproducing entity, not to be disturbed or exploited. It is only more recently that the western world made this 'discovery' – the Anthropocene. The disaster metaphor paints a picture of humanity as victims or survivors, volunteers or philanthropists.

While disaster management is a necessary temporary measure in extreme circumstances, there needs to be a journey of healing following the experience of loss, pain, and grief. It requires consideration for both movements on the surface and the undercurrents below; how deep do these problems run? Life in pandemic – like a river – has moments of slow calm and quick turbulence, clear shallows and murky deepness, free-flowing paths and diverging streams. Developing a dynamic map with which we can navigate uncertain terrain, anticipate obstacles, and plot strategic directions would make us explorers – not survivors – of a new world, connecting with others along the way.

An example of this is how "New Zealand has offered a model response of empathy, clarity and trust in science" (BBC News, 2020). Instead of identifying an enemy and establishing a plan of attack, New Zealand encouraged unity and working together. Prime Minister Jacinda Ardern's message stayed consistent and clear: "Be Strong. Be Kind", and so the country was a given a map with which it could navigate the course of the river it found itself on.

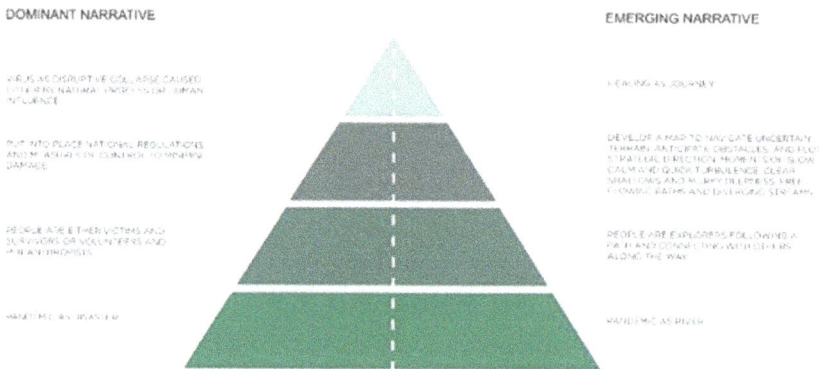

DOMINANT NARRATIVE

EMERGING NARRATIVE

VIRUS AS DISRUPTIVE OR COLLAPSE CAUSED EITHER BY NATURAL UNDER SOCIAL HUMAN INFLUENCE

HEALING AS JOURNEY

PUT INTO PLACE NATIONAL REGULATIONS AND MEASURES IN CONTROL TO MINIMISE DAMAGE

DEVELOP A MAP TO NAVIGATE UNCERTAIN TERRAIN, ANTICIPATE OBSTACLES, AND PLOT STRATEGIC DIRECTION MOMENTUM SLOW CALM AND QUICK TURBULENCE CLEAR SHALLOWS AND MURKY DEEPNESS TAKE FORMING PATHS AND DIVERGING STREAMS

PEOPLE ARE EITHER VICTIMS AND SURVIVORS OR VOLUNTEERS AND HEROES OR ENEMIES

PEOPLE ARE EXPLORERS FOLLOWING A PATH AND CONNECTING WITH OTHERS ALONG THE WAY

PANDEMIC AS DISASTER

PANDEMIC AS RIVER

POLITICAL REALM: WAR CHESS

Many the world over seem to be at war. They are united against a common enemy, fighting for a common goal: eliminate the threat to human life and national security, even if it is by violent or aggressive means. In this narrative, citizens become soldiers. It is their duty to fight for their country, protect its borders, and obey orders from power-wielding leaders. Often these power dynamics go unchecked, restrictions are enforced unquestioned, and harm in inflicted unnoticed. As many nations go into what has been termed 'lockdown', one cannot help but feel criminalised. Curfews, restrictions, bans – it starts to feel a lot like imprisonment. If we were to rather invoke the idea of a game of chess, we start to see the virus as a challenge, rather than a cage. In applying logic and strategy to develop a game plan, people enhance their mental mastery and are better prepared for future scenarios that may emerge. As players, people alternate between seemingly unassuming moves, taking risks, and making strategic decisions for the endgame – before taking on the next challenge.

An example of the war metaphor is US President Trump's naming the 'China virus' a public enemy which must be defeated. Increased border protection, rising nationalism, and enforced hero-narratives make it difficult for people to fight back and remain autonomous. When it comes to thinking things through in the form of a game of chess, we can apply Inayatullah and Black's (2020) definition of foresight as "the capacity to anticipate tomorrow's problems and [to]act today". They argue that COVID-19 is neither a black swan nor a zombie apocalypse; it was neither unpredictable nor a total surprise. Instead of focusing on what was missed or unseen, we should, they urge, prepare for the next pandemic.

CONCLUSION

"The main point is that narrative, how we describe the world structures our possibilities, what options we can see, what is possible for us to create" (Inayatullah, 2020). Many of the dominant pandemic metaphors encourage destructive discourses and promote ideas of separation or superiority. The emerging metaphors in this essay are proposed as transformational alternatives that promote interconnectedness and a process of change. There are different ways of seeing, framing, and being in the world. The language we use and the metaphors we apply, shape the way we experience reality, imagine possibility, and take on responsibility.

AUTHOR

Marguerite Coetzee | Omniology, South Africa

NOTES

The title of the paper (Ancestors of the Future) comes from a 2020 online panel in which Pupul Bisht made mention of the term in relation to decolonising the future)

REFERENCES

Chotiner, I. (2020). How Pandemics Change History. *The New Yorker.* https://www.newyorker.com/news/q-and-a/how-pandemics-change-history

Confessore, N. (2018). Cambridge Analytica and Facebook: The Scandal and the Fallout So Far. *New York Times.* https://www.nytimes.com/2018/04/04/us/politics/cambridge-analytica-scandal-fallout.html

BBC News (2020). Coronavirus: How New Zealand relied on science and empathy. *BBC News.* https://www.bbc.com/news/world-asia-52344299

Deshpande, A. (2020). Protecting women is missing from pandemic management measures in India. *Quartz India.* https://qz.com/india/1826683/indias-approach-to-fighting-coronavirus-lacks-a-gender-lens/

Devaney, J. (2020). A Global Pause as Earth Day Turns 50. *Medium.* https://medium.com/@jacobdevaney/a-global-pause-as-earth-day-turns-50-549b573ba00

Eggers, W. & Muoio, A. (2015). Wicked opportunities Part of the Business Trends series. *Deloitte.* https://www2.deloitte.com/us/en/insights/focus/business-trends/2015/wicked-problems-wicked-opportunities-business-trends.html

Inayatullah, S. (2017). Causal Layered Analysis: A Four-Level Approach to Alternative Futures [White paper]. *Prospective and Strategic Foresight Toolbox.* http://www.metafuture.org/library1/2019/CLATOOLBOX2017FUTURIBLES.pdf

Inayatullah, S. & Black, P. (2020, March 18). Neither A Black Swan Nor A Zombie Apocalypse: The Futures Of A World With The Covid-19 Coronavirus. *Journal of Futures Studies.* https://jfsdigital.org/2020/03/18/neither-a-black-swan-nor-a-zombie-apocalypse-the-futures-of-a-world-with-the-covid-19-coronavirus/

Jimenez, M. (2020). The Great Pause. *FFWD.* https://www.globalforesightsummit.com/

Klein, N. (2007). *The Shock Doctrine: The Rise of Disaster Capitalism.* Metropolitan Books.

Nerlich, B. (2020). *Metaphors in the time of coronavirus.* University of Nottingham. https://blogs.nottingham.ac.uk/makingsciencepublic/2020/03/17/metaphors-in-the-time-of-coronavirus/

Pueyo, T. (2020). Coronavirus: The Hammer and the Dance. *Medium.* https://medium.com/@tomaspueyo/coronavirus-the-hammer-and-the-dance-be9337092b56

Roy, A. (2020). The pandemic is a portal. *Financial Times*. https://www.ft.com/content/10d8f5e8-74eb-11ea-95fe-fcd274e920ca

Senbanjo, L. (2020). African countries need to challenge the idea of a homogenous approach to Covid-19. *Quartz Africa*. https://qz.com/africa/1858008/africa-needs-to-challenge-the-homogenous-approach-to-covid-19/

Traditional healers call for an African health organisation. (2020, May 16). *SABC News*. https://www.sabcnews.com/sabcnews/traditional-healers-call-for-an-african-health-organisation/

Wright, N. (2020). Coronavirus and the Future of Surveillance. *Foreign Affairs*. https://www.foreignaffairs.com/articles/2020-04-06/coronavirus-and-future-surveillance

Zaretsky, R. (2020). Out of a clear blue sky: Camus's The Plague and coronavirus. *TLS*. https://www.the-tls.co.uk/articles/albert-camus-the-plague-coronavirus-essay-robert-zaretsky/

WHAT WILL A POST VIRUS WORLD LOOK LIKE?

Garry Hone

At the time of writing Europe is the epicenter of the Coronavirus pandemic with daily death rate climbing in Italy, Spain, and the UK. Based on the news from China, the death rate should start to fall within a few weeks, and policies of social distancing and lockdown begin to be relaxed. There is still a long time before a vaccine will be made available, and there are forecasts of a resurgence and second wave to come. Much is still unknown about the virus that causes COVID-19, but the economic impact of isolation and quarantine will be severe. The world will be different on the other side.

Disruption will herald big changes in the way we live, work and interact. As someone who works in the field of risk and uncertainty, I am used to helping organizations separate their 'known unknowns' from their 'unknown knowns' to reduce uncertainty and ultimately better understand risks they face. The coronavirus throws up enormous uncertainty – political, economic, social and technical – so it seems the best way to look at future scenarios is to examine where each of these determinants might lead. The four scenarios set out below using the political-social and economic-technical axes.

Out of the four scenarios, two are optimistic, and two are pessimistic. The optimistic ones show us where humanity can benefit from this upheaval and become more resilient for future shocks. A more evolved species if you wish. The pessimistic ones show us a more regressive world where we fall back on bad habits and behaviors that have got us to where we are. These will not equip us for future shocks but will be attractive to states and institutions currently enjoying wealth and power. I have chosen to set out the pessimistic ones first:

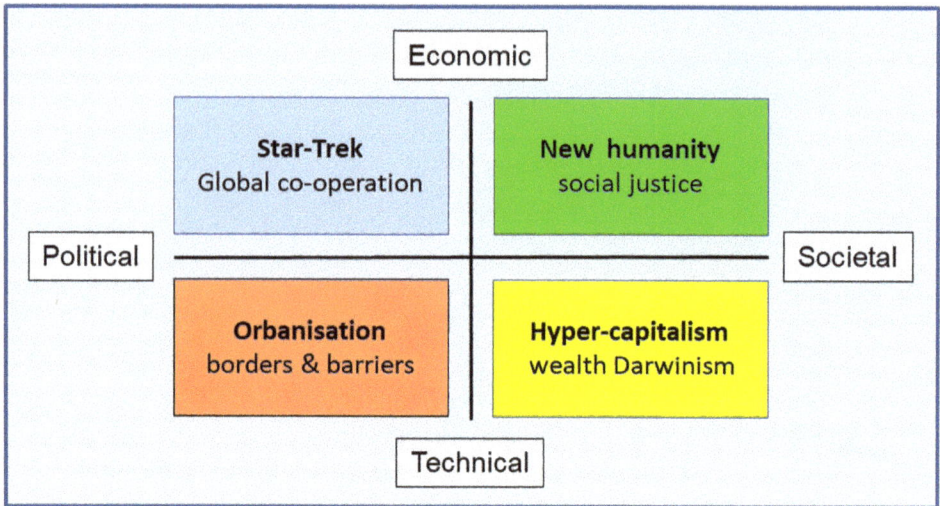

A 2x2 matrix with axes labelled Economic (top), Technical (bottom), Political (left), Societal (right):
- Star-Trek — Global co-operation
- New humanity — social justice
- Orbanisation — borders & barriers
- Hyper-capitalism — wealth Darwinism

ORBANIZATION

Named after the Hungarian leader Viktor Orban, who has suspended parliament, and intends to rule by decree indefinitely. His name serves as a label for any drift towards draconian powers seized to enforce social distancing, whether by a totalitarian or democratic government. Human rights groups fear that governments who suspend democracy or remove citizen's rights in the time of crisis are often reluctant to restore them when normality returns. Whistle-blowers are not thanked but imprisoned, authorities are intolerant of criticism and will find ways to censure or restrict voices of dissent.

Within this envisioned future we can expect a retrenched nationalism with more border controls and a surge in xenophobia. Trading blocs like the EU will retreat from the Schengen agreement of open borders and tariffs will be used as barriers for protectionism. We have already seen this between the US and China, where trade becomes a weapon of power. There will be health checks at the border and points of entry with strict quarantine at airports and ports. The virus will be portrayed as foreign and foreigners unwelcome.

Hyper-capitalism –
Under this scenario, the wealth disparity between rich and poor is exacerbated post virus. Many businesses will be forced to close by the global recession, and

many people will never work again. The world of work will be much more polarised between the 'Haves' and the 'Have-nots'. Those who have wealth will invest it for-profit and will find opportunities to gain from adversity. Those who have no wealth will find it hard to secure state support as jobs disappear to be replaced by AI or other new technology.

This could be seen as a form of wealth Darwinism where the fittest survive. In a sense, this is a continuation of a system that is exploitative and uncaring; a small few do very well through harnessing technology and adapting to a new world of work. There is very little incentive to share the wealth unless one chooses to live in a high tax culture like Denmark, where the state redistributes the wealth to create an equal society.

NEW HUMANITY

This is an optimistic scenario where the future is brighter because humanity has recognized that exploitation is unsustainable. The epidemic reminds us that the people who are paid least are actually valued by the society the most: the vast army of nurses, carers, cleaners and delivery drivers and an army of workers who keep society working and grease the wheels to keep in on the road. These people are finally recognized for the work they do in terms of societal value, what the investment firm Blackrock would call TSI – Total Societal Impact.
The virus lockdown prompts a rebalancing of values and questioning of obscene salaries paid to football players, TV celebrities and ineffective corporate leaders. This doesn't have to be a new form of socialism, but there are examples of countries like Finland experimenting with a standard basic wage so that the absence of work doesn't cause people to starve. The world of work will be different, and states will need to find a new way of providing economic support that is constructive, educational and humane.

STAR-TREK

This scenario envisions a future with an international community, not unlike that found on the fictional USS Enterprise. Full global co-operation to deal with global problems: resource management and environmental protection, never mind extra-terrestrial threats and aliens. Before we can 'boldly go' into space, we need to heal the planet and ensure that it is fit for future generations. For the past fifty years, scientists have warned that we cannot go on at the current rate and the Extinction Rebellion movement today shows how urgent this has become.

The fragmented way in which to world has responded to the virus shows not only how ineffective the World Health Organisation is, but also how badly we need a species-level response and global leaders capable of marshaling effort. The upheaval of the Second World War prompted the creation of the United Nations and World Bank; the coronavirus prompts a similar leap in co-operation for planetary stewardship. Climate change needs more than conferences; it needs action.

From these four alternative futures, the more optimistic ones, New Humanity and Star Trek, both offer hope for mankind in that they envision constructive change. The challenge for politicians and world leaders is to find ways to make these achievable against a mindset that all too easily slip back into the pessimistic and regressive alternative futures of Orbanization and Hyper- capitalism.

AUTHOR

Garry Honey is a risk consultant and founder of Chiron-risk

TRIPLE-A GOVERNANCE: ANTICIPATORY, AGILE AND ADAPTIVE

Jose Ramos, Ida Uusikyla
and Nguyen Tuan Luong

The Corona-virus pandemic has highlighted how a weak signal (the evolution of corona-viruses) can generate a wildcard event, massive disruption with huge implications. It also highlights the value of social foresight, long term thinking geared toward the public good. Unfortunately, as we are seeing with the pandemic, it is a little too late. Under-investment by governments in identifying, understanding and mitigating emerging risks has meant that most countries were not prepared. We are now experiencing the deadly consequences.

But pandemics are only one of a number of issues that as societies we need to apply foresight to. Over the past several decades we have seen an increased complexity of change: in speed, interconnectedness, and uncertainty. This new socio-ecological context brings with it new strategic risks and "wicked" systemic challenges — challenges that are like "knots" and difficult to address. These can include disruptive emerging issues such as climate change, automation, artificial intelligence, emerging diseases, social pathologies and a range of new disruptive technologies. The government has traditionally been good at dealing with social issues and problems which are static and in "silos". But the type of change we see today is overwhelming traditional planning approaches.

Many of these changes can also be seen as opportunities if we are able to identify them early and find ways of anticipating and acting on them — indeed use them to our advantage. But without anticipation and action, small problems lead to big wicked messes. New approaches to governance are needed which can help institutions express what the United Nations Development Program (UNDP) has termed "Triple-A" governance: Anticipatory, Agile and Adaptive[1]

The UNDP is leading an effort to reimagine governance in this context. To better address and respond to such challenges and help countries find faster, more durable solutions to achieve their Sustainable Development Goals, the UNDP established 60 Accelerator Labs around the world. The Accelerator Labs are a new initiative from the UNDP, which aim to drive experimentation and learning to tackle entrenched development problems. In their words: "the initiative [is]about making space for creativity in the face of problems that need new methods & new energy."[2]

"Anticipatory Governance and Experimentation" form a core capability needed in this context. The UNDP #NextGenGov initiative, which was introduced at the Istanbul Innovation Days 2018, aims to bring together partners to create the space for a new range of deliberate experiments and learning trajectories to accelerate the next generation of governance mechanisms.

ANTICIPATORY GOVERNANCE

Anticipatory Governance denotes collaborative and participatory processes and systems for exploring, envisioning, direction setting, developing strategy and experimentation for a region. Anticipatory Governance allows a region, whether city or state, to harness the collective intelligence and wisdom of collaborating organizations and citizens, to deal with strategic risks and leverage emerging opportunities for meeting development goals. It is an approach for "social navigation" — the ability of a society to navigate the complex terrain of social change.

Throughout history and even pre-history, we have seen the rise and fall of civilizations and cultures. The Mon of Southeast Asia, The Hohokam of Arizona, the Maya of Central America, and Easter Island — changed, declined or vanished. Others: Chinese, Indic, European, Bantu, and many that have become the nations of today, have changed and evolved to the present. At the most fundamental level, Anticipatory Governance is about our capacity to adapt to change, preserve what is most dear, and thrive and prosper into the future.

To do this a number of new capabilities are required.

- **First,** the ability to identify the landscape of change (foresight) and use this in organisationally useful ways;
- **Secondly,** systemic thinking and inter-organizational cooperation are needed so that the whole ecosystem can be mobilized to address wicked and complex interdependencies in the development challenges faced;
- **Thirdly,** a cultural and institutional shift that supports experimentation which can be scaled for impact and which can use experiments to drive learning.

Anticipatory Governance has different outcomes and value propositions attached to them.

This table provides an overview:

Value Proposition / Outcome	Summary
Identify weak signals and disruptors before they become problems / reduce surprise	Seeing the horizons
Cross-departmental / agency learning and collaboration	Left and right-hand talking
Avenues for citizen engagement in exploring and shaping the future	Partnership with people
Develop innovations that have a "strategic fit" with a changing and future environment	Future relevant innovation
Prioritize investment areas in research, education, industry development, markets, science, and tech changes	Strategic investments
Build systemic understandings around wicked problems that lead to more nuance "pressure point" interventions	Know the acupuncture points
Capacity to adapt quickly to changing conditions, by using experiments that can scale for impact	Adapt to change
Mobilize an ecosystem to tackle systemic level challenges	Collaborative Action
Bringing together resources that enhance all when shared	Mutualizing commons

There are different types of Anticipatory Governance, some of which are more recent and others that go back to the 1960s. As well, Anticipatory Governance approaches have been applied in different ways across a variety of contexts:

- In Finland to support ministerial and parliamentary knowledge and decision making as well as a trade mission

- In Singapore to support all-of-government future readiness for early identification of strategic risks
- In northern Europe to mobilize action to address sustainable development challenges
- In South Korea to understand citizens changing images of a preferred future and align priorities, drawing on work by the National Assembly Futures Institute (NAFI)
- In the USA dozens of states have applied participatory futures as part of anticipatory democracy processes
- In New Zealand to help rebuild the city of Christchurch after devastating earthquakes using participatory futures
- In Australia to do horizon scanning across partners organizations
- In the UK foresight has been embedded across a number of governmental systems

These are just some of the many examples.

THREE RESOURCES FOR ANTICIPATORY GOVERNANCE

Looking forward, who wants to have to go through another pandemic like the one we are experiencing now? Loss of loved ones and broken hearts, shattered businesses and lost jobs, days and days of quarantine, an economic mess, worry about the futures. The cost of short-termism is great. Yet there are other strategic risks and weak signals that can create equal or even greater pain, and so it is incumbent on our societies to invest in an Anticipatory Governance for Experimentation approach that can effectively deal with the volatile nature of our world.

Three resources for Anticipatory Governance are key: institutional futures, participatory futures, and adaptive organizational capacity.

Resource 1 — Inter-organizational Futures

Much institutional knowledge already exists in various organizations in government and in NGOs / CSOs. Many organizations already do and have research and knowledge about the future for specific areas. However, it is too common for these organizations to NOT share what they know about the future with each other. So one of the first "low hanging fruit" to pick is to bring organizations together that have a stake in an issue, and which have some tacit or explicit knowledge of the futures of that issues. Creating an inter-organizational system for sharing knowledge on a topic of shared concern leverages existing strengths and can produce quick wins. This can be done with a variety of strategies: web platforms, workshops, webinars, etc. This cooperation can then be scaled up to other aspects: shared analysis shared communication / media / public engagement, and shared experimentation.

Resource 2 — Participatory Futures

Citizens hold a wide variety of knowledge and some are "future-sensing" types while others are "future-making" types. Tapping into citizen knowledge can create the requisite awareness of change that provides agility and new pathways for regional policy, strategy and change efforts.

One potential pitfall in envisioning the future of a region is when a future vision or direction is framed by narrow interests or what Sohail Inayatullah calls 'used futures' — images created somewhere else but superimposed uncritically or serving special or hidden economic interests (Inayatullah 2008). Getting past the "used future" and having an authentic goal or vision that is particular to a region's needs and aspirations is essential. We need to include all the people in a region that have a stake in that future — not just a future framed based on narrow commercial interest, a policy clique or lobby group.

Participatory futures leverage citizens' strengths and collective intelligence and can help with mapping horizons (identifying weak signals), creating vision and purpose, charting strategic pathways, testing ideas and mobilizing change. A recent report by Nesta provides a useful overview. (Ramos, Sweeney, Peach, Smith, 2019)

Resource 3 — Organizational Capacity to Adapt

The organizational capacity to adapt is also needed. We need to create a bridge between anticipation and experimentation. This is a big challenge, especially in government where experiments can be seen as unacceptable risks. Even with government support and well resourced CityLabs, working across the messy spaces of society to generate change is challenging. There are a whole number of good strategies and frameworks for doing this, and people should just do what works. One framework that may be useful is the Anticipatory Experimentation Method (Ramos 2017).

Practically the method entails five stages:

1. Challenging the used future (questioning outdated assumptions and images of the futures)

2. Developing a preferred future or a new set of assumptions

3. Ideating a number of prototype ideas from the vision or new assumptions

4. Choosing which ideas to experiment with and running real-world

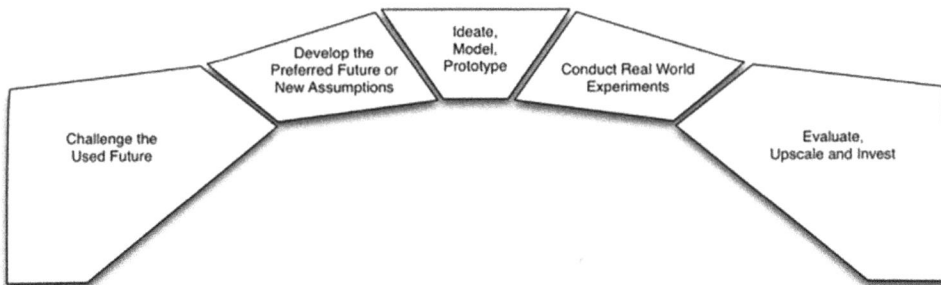

Anticipatory Experimentation "Bridge" Method, Source: Jose Ramos (2017)

experiments (e.g. action research / co-design)

5. Scaling and investing in the experiments with the best promise

Whatever approach we use, the main takeaway that we'd like to offer is that societal navigation and adaptive capacity are possible and desirable. Yes, for the most part, we have collectively "dropped the ball" with COVID-19, and now it will be painful, we will need to clean up the mess and pick up the pieces. But we can be ready for the next "surprise". This experience can be our inoculation for the challenges the future will invariably bring.

As seen from many examples around the world we can and we are building Anticipatory, Agile, and Adaptive (Triple-A) governance. Given the variety of emerging challenges we collectively face, how we each do this for ourselves, in our own regional contexts, and together, is the next big question.

AUTHORS

Dr. José Ramos is Co-Editor of the Journal of Futures Studies, Director of Action Foresight, Adjunct Senior Lecturer at the University of Sunshine Coast.

Nguyen Tuan Luong is the Head of Solutions Mapping at UNDP Accelerator Lab Vietnam, where he brings his whole heart, hands, and head to be in service to the great ambition of reimagining how development work is done.

Ida Uusikyla is a cross-unit innovator in many projects at UNDP Viet Nam focusing on inclusive and governance innovation. Ida has experience in e-governance, emerging technologies, institutional reforms, complexity science and innovation policy.

NOTES

[1] This triple A governance concept was developed by the UNDP team in Vietnam in 2019 and applied in work programs in 2020.

[2] For more information on UNDP accelerator labs see here: https://acceleratorlabs.undp.org/blog1.html

REFERENCES

Inayatullah, S. (2008). Six pillars: futures thinking for transforming. *Foresight*. 10(1), 4-21. https://doi.org/10.1108/14636680810855991

Ramos, J. (2014). Anticipatory governance: Traditions and trajectories for strategic design. *Journal of Futures Studies*, 19(1), 35-52.

Ramos, J. (2017). Futureslab: Anticipatory experimentation, social emergence, and evolutionary change. *Journal of Futures Studies*, 22(2), 107-118.

Ramos, J., Sweeney, J. A., Peach, K., & Smith, L. (2019). Our futures: by the people, for the people. *Nesta*. https://media.nesta.org.uk/documents/Our_futures_by_the_people_for_the_people_WEB_v5.pdf

CHRYSALIS

*What Emerges from
the COVID-19 Pandemic*

Jose Ramo

How do we make sense of the dramatic changes happening during the coronavirus pandemic? How do we get on an empowered footing rather than reaction and confusion? So many have simply been struck by "future shock", i.e., the future has arrived but it has arrived in a daunting pathological guise. People are not prepared, indeed many are just dumbfounded as taken for granted aspects of life are thrown asunder. Many search for meaning amid the intellectual centrifuge which is social media today, lost in the bramble of conspiracy theories, xenophobic blame and a 24 hour news cycle. Futures Studies researchers and practitioners know that psychological orientation is critical. However, we are in an ongoing process of re-orientation during these times of change.

Understanding some of the broader changes afoot can help us to re-orient, and metaphors can provide the deep structure for such re-orientation (Inayatullah 1998). The result can be a sense of empowerment, even in the face of the dramatic challenges we face. This chapter uses a simple metaphor, that of the Chrysalis, to review ten shifts we are experiencing. The intention here is not scholarship but personal-to-political reflections and sensemaking, to explore a metaphor that helps to orient, to better navigate this new landscape of change. As such it is a combination of personal viewpoints, values, hopes, weak signals and imagination.

On top of dramatic lockdowns and the physical distancing that has been mandated to stop the spread of the virus, other economic and social activities have also been partially or even fully stopped. This has put both people, our economies and society into a strange period of inwardness. We have been forced into our homes, and nations have been forced back into themselves. It has also forced each one of us into our own inner worlds. We can see this as a personal to collective and globally extensive turning inwards.

A Chrysalis is a biological formation that allows a caterpillar to fundamentally alter its physical composition and appearance. It is part of a lifecycle. A caterpillar when ready forms a Chrysalis, but from the chrysalis comes a completely different looking creature, a butterfly or moth of striking beauty and capability, able to do things on an order completely different from the caterpillar. Inside the chrysalis, the caterpillar's body breaks down into a kind of soup and is reorganized into the adult structures of the new creature!

We are living in Epic Times, historic times imbued with personal and collective meaning and logic. For each of us this story will be different, however we all have a part to play in the drama we see unfolding. Who we are, how we act, what we do, makes a difference. The era is calling forth new selves and new patterns from us. What does our world, its challenges and transition, want from us? What thinking, innovations, methods, feelings, movements? What could emerge from the Chrysalis?

1 - END OF AN ERA

It looks like the old world will never die. We need dramatic action on climate change, while the mineral industry has hampered this through lobbying (Hamilton, 2007). We need smart and decisive approaches to deal with COVID-19, but we see in too many countries (e.g. USA, Russia, Brazil) a failure of leadership that is marked by gender.[1]

Johan Galtung had forecast the end of the US "empire" several decades ago, based on 8+ structural contradictions, systemic problems that over time make the US less and less viable (Galtung, 2009). His original date for this fall was 2024, but when President George Bush Jr. invaded Iraq, he revised this to 2020. The Republican Party or the Grand Old Party (GOP) is today the champion of these contradictions: inaction on climate change, patriarchal / misogynistic attitudes, corporate privilege, anti-democratic policies, a constant stream of disinformation, race baiting.

It feels like it will never end. Yet the GOP are desperate. They know that the archaic world they represent is under serious threat. Climate change challenges US exceptionalism and their fossil fuel donors. Afro-americans and the millenial alliance through Black Lives Matter (BLM) challenges racial injustice. Obama won two terms with a rainbow coalition (women, some "white", Afro-americans, Latinos, LGBTQ, etc). Hillary Clinton won the popular vote. Republicans know they are hanging on by just a thread, due to gerrymandered voting districts. But when we're in the hurricane it is hard to see beyond it.

We see similar dynamics elsewhere, such as in Brazil, India and other countries where the historical privilege of certain groups is being ruthlessly defended. What the Chrysalis means here is that... yes we are indeed in the midst of a kind of breakdown, but on the other side of this there is the potential for transformation whereby we break through the chokehold on power of the historically privileged. A new pattern can emerge which expresses inclusive leadership that affirms the value of all people, with strengthened democracies, respect for women and disadvantaged minorities, and a planetary ethos through action on climate change.

2 - RETURN OF THE STATE

One of the lessons of COVID-19 is that we need a well oiled and disciplined state which can respond in a coordinated way to this crisis and future crises. We've seen in stark terms the difference between countries with poor, indecisive or dithering political and state responses (USA, Brazil, Mexico, UK) and those with decisive and well resourced responses (Taiwan, S. Korea, New Zealand, China, Vietnam).[2] In general terms, the states that best combined available resources with preparation, coordination and discipline are the ones that have responded to the pandemic the best.

What emerges is a greater appreciation for the role of the state in spear-heading responses to crises. This is in fact what we need with the climate crisis- i.e., decisive leadership to rapidly draw down carbon emissions. However this has been hamstrung because the climate crisis is not immediate—it is a crisis of future generations—and the fossil fuel industry has worked hard to muddy the message.[3]

From this Chrysalis, I can imagine new approaches for a "partner state" - where the state is empowered to create an ambitious "framework" for change, but where communities are in control of the "where, what and how". In governance terms this is the principle of "subsidiarity" (Ramos, 2015). And while we need the state we also see how statism is being abused in many places during the pandemic. China opportunistically re-writing the laws in Hong Kong, Trump opportunistically using BLM to argue for military lockdown/repression. So we need deeper and more sophisticated democratic controls and systems (not less) as state's powers expand to deal with emerging crises. From the Chrysalis emerges innovations of new governance systems that are on one hand more inclusive, while increasing the power and resources of the state to act in the public interest.[4]

3 – SCIENCE AND AN ECOLOGY OF KNOWLEDGES

Every time Trump uses magical thinking and says COVID-19 is going away this is in stark contrast to Dr. Fauci and others saying, sorry it isn't. Trump is one of the best advertisements for science the world has ever seen. Anti-science can be put into a broader context now. Anti-science means poor understanding of COVID-19 and an inept response costing the lives of millions. Anti-science means no action on climate change.[5] Anti-science means anti-vaxxers spreading misleading information on disease and vaccines, with greater spread of diseases society wide (Benecke & DeYoung, 2019).

What emerges from this Chrysalis is a greater appreciation for science and the domain expert, and a greater wariness and precaution against conspiracies, magical thinking, disinformation and armchair facebook 'experts'. The pattern that may emerge is a new humility about what one knows and does not know, and an understanding that humility and critical subjectivity saves lives. A smart or a dumb facebook share has real consequences.

We need many knowledges to navigate through the pandemic, not just bio-medical science. Meditation, computer science, community mental health and wellness, new economic thinking, deep sustainability, and many others. Thus we also need to make sure science supports knowledge democracy and epistemological pluralism

[Ramos, 2020].

4 - WISE RAGE

Most societies suffer from structural inequalities and structural violence of some kind. Neoliberalism has had the effect of hollowing out the middle class and creating hyper inequality in many parts of the world, amplifying class / caste disparity everywhere.

COVID-19 has shined a spotlight and exposed these inequalities. I am fortunate to live in a country like Australia with universal health care, but these were political choices and efforts by Australian citizens in the 1970s and 80s, not the product of random chance. We hear horrifying stories from other countries where hospitals are overwhelmed and those infected cannot get proper treatment. Once out of hospital, many have been hit by absurd medical bills.[6] The lack of equitable health care, combined with the treatment of minorities and people of color and economic for millennials has added to the pressure cooker of the lockdown.

From the Chrysalis "wise rage" against injustice is born. Wise rage is rage through peaceful and wise means. Rage erupted with full force after the killing of George Floyd. Black Lives Matter harnessed this rage in a constructive way in response. [7] The global response and solidarity to BLM is significant, as a global rainbow coalition (multi-ethnic / intersectoral) is proclaiming that this type of structural violence is not acceptable. Wise rage is, importantly, wisdom about and rage against the structural dimensions of injustice. This is why, when answering the questions of who killed George Floyd, Inayatullah argues that "structures" are the critical determinants.[8] From the Chrysalis many are more than ever challenging the many inequalities and inequities people face, economic, racial, gender based, whether it is "us" or "them" who is suffering, with a deepened sense that "we" are indeed "them".

5 - GREEN INDUSTRIAL TRANSITION

Trillions have been spent propping up economies in the early stages of the pandemic. As the pandemic has driven an economic crisis, there has been knee-jerk spending by nations everywhere trying to rescue economies teetering on the edge of collapse. The pandemic is driving a joblessness crisis the likes of which we have not seen since the Great Depression.[9]

At the same time we are faced with the most epic challenges we have ever faced—in drawing down carbon emissions and addressing the broader ecological crises. We live in a world with many mouths to feed, but we are butting up against ecological limits. From the Chrysalis emerges more clarity that we need a Green Industrial Transition which both creates jobs and drives down carbon emissions. The idea for a Green New Deal has been around for a while, and it has taken a variety of forms in various countries.[10] These are solutions that have been developed in many different places that can achieve both economic stimulus, job creation and industrial transformation to draw down carbon. In Australia the Beyond Zero Emissions NGO has launched a well researched Million Jobs plan to draw down carbon.[11] The coming years will need both job creation strategies and dramatic investment in energy transition, and the case for this is now strong. Neither can happen with just industry led or even community led efforts. It will require political-economic-community coordination of great scale and strategic clarity.

6 - ECONOMIC RESILIENCE

Under neoliberalism the past 30 years has created a new "precariat" class, a workforce that lives in continual economic uncertainty with gig jobs and short term contracts. Under "normal" conditions the effects of this were hidden to many. The pandemic has taught us that this, and our hyper leveraged credit based economy, is much more fragile than we thought. Airlines out of business, restaurants and other businesses in ruins, and millions upon millions unemployed. In reality we can't totally blame neoliberalism for an economic crisis when previous pandemics have also created economic crises. However the particular way in which neoliberalism combines with the pandemic shows the limits to an economy where people no longer have savings, hold sky high mortgages and loans, and where the state and welfare have retreated and dwindled.

We have also seen that some of the state responses to the economic crisis looks like an emergency version of universal basic income (UBI).[12] This was a knee jerk response to avoid economic collapse. But more broadly and looking into the future, how many other crises will we face? From the Chrysalis is an emerging understanding that we need a resilience approach to the economy, able to support people in a variety of ways. UBI is one possible solution - whatever happens people will have economic support. As well, a real sharing economy can unlock idle social energy and resources. This can include new local and trans-local currencies designed to tap and circulate social energies and talents. Localizing economic opportunities can help, as can leveraging our global design and knowledge commons. All these can support livelihoods amid the turbulence and shocks that we are increasingly likely to experience this century.

7 – COSMO-LOCALISM

We had been told globalization was inevitable. Questioning it was attacking a sacred cow. Suddenly, in the pandemic national borders are closed, international air travel is practically gone. We no longer commute to work, we work from home. Global supply chains are disrupted. At the same time the world is very close. Everybody is on zoom or similar platforms. Knowledge is ubiquitous and shared. Between homeschooling the kids and lunch, sneak in a call with a colleague in Minsk, London or Mumbai. The pandemic has altered spatiality in various ways. It has reduced physical movement to the local. It has reduced movement across national borders. It has accelerated global connected-ness via web conferencing. And the world experiences itself as a unit, as the effects of the pandemic are planetary and ubiquitous.

In short, the pandemic has made us "cosmolocal", both planetary in digital scope but localized in physical scope. This cosmo-local turn has come quicker than anticipated - but driven from an unexpected source, a virus. P2P-driven and commons-oriented citizen groups have stepped in, showing the vitality of the open source and commons movements, as well as their expertise, capacity for mobilization, and global-local scope. This includes open source medical devices, open data and social networks for COVID-19 containment, open knowledge testing, vaccine production, open mutual aid and localised coordination systems, rigorously documented by Michel Bauwens at the P2P Foundation.[13] From the Chrysalis emerges cosmolocalism as a mainstream social form, and we can expect this shift to strengthen in an era where global trade and travel can no longer be taken for granted, but digits flow ever more fluidly.

8 - CRISIS OF TRUST

Surveillance capitalism and state surveillance has destroyed peoples trust in relational platforms, when we need it the most (Slaughter, 2020). Just when we needed trust in social networks and the sharing of personal information (for example to track COVID-19), platforms like Facebook are losing credibility. In Australia where I live the government developed an app that helps with tracing and containing the virus. However many people were so skeptical that their data was being used by large corporations being employed as third party suppliers, or that it was a Machiavellian play on the part of the state, that the uptake of the app was much lower than required to be a useful tracing platform. China's use of data to control citizens (social credit system, firewall, etc) is well established and this example has corollaries in many parts of the world, e.g. NSA surveillance in the USA and the Five Eyes (Snowden, 2019).

From the Chrysalis is an understanding that in order to harness the strengths of social networks and the use of apps that can do micro tracing, we need to fundamentally reimagine our relationship to the internet and data. Relational data needs to either be added into public trusts (state regulated), data cooperatives, or owned and controlled outright by those that create the data (Nycyk, 2020). Rebuilding this trust can then allow more people to use sophisticated app tools that can help the right people solve social problems, far beyond COVID-19 and through the 21th Century.

9 - RELATIONAL HEALTH AND WELLBEING

The pandemic has created asymmetrical home structures. People who were single are now more single, many suffering isolation. Those people with young families and in lockdown or homeschooling face intense pressure to hold jobs and home-make (I know first hand what this is like with two young kids). Incidences of domestic violence[14] and mental health problems are up.[15] Personally, this has underlined for me the importance of extended family and friends, who are as important as the people we are living with every day. The biggest impact on my two children has been the inability to see friends and family - upsetting for both of them. As a parent I have tried to be their "friend" as much as possible (not just play the role of the parent), but it is a challenge.

From the Chrysalis is new clarity on family structure. New questions have emerged. Can we acknowledge the limits of the nuclearisation of the family? Can we design or coordinate larger groupings (pods) to be part of during future crises? What does relational health look like in a time of crisis? (Milojević, 2020) What are the new relational forms and structures that could engender better health and wellbeing in such situations? From the Chrysalis new relational structures may emerge that are more viable within the context of challenges we face.

10 - THE INNER GAME OF EPIC TIMES

The pandemic has driven a movement inwards: nations into themselves, communities into themselves, families into themselves, the planet into itself. Yet the most felt movement inward is our subjective experience. Many of us have also been thrown into a personal movement and moment of crisis. Can this be a Chrysalis moment, and what does this mean for each of us?

For me, I lost half a year of anticipated work in a matter of a month. I came back from a workshop in Mexico City and was in quarantine with my family for 2 weeks, and then in a strict social lockdown imposed on all of the state I live in (Victoria) for 3 months. It was a weird moment. It took some time to just process and accept the changes. It then became more clear that this moment had a lot of challenges but also some opportunities. Magic time with my kids, Spanish lessons for my son, a stronger exercise routine and getting fit.

There were also some ideas and projects where I had the inner story that I was "too busy" to do them. Courses I wanted to run, blogs and books to write, all require time and effort. This requires letting go of some things, to begin to do the new. Would I take the opportunity to do those special things I've told myself I would do?

The inner Chrysalis takes patience, letting go of old patterns, accepting the present, and push, out of the Chrysalis. We live in Epic Times. What new patterns is the era asking from us?

CONCLUSION

Finally, from the Chrysalis is a greater appreciation that social structures and systems matter. Public health, our economies and the ecological health of the planet are all commons - we mutually depend on them for our health and wellbeing. We're in this together. One critical structure and commons we'll need moving forward is a "global foresight commons" (Dumaine, 2010). COVID-19 will not be the last challenge humanity will face. In fact, we may see this pandemic as an early road test for the 21st century. Can we really afford to be unprepared for the next shock? Can we really accept zombie-walking into climate catastrophe? Out of the Chrysalis, can the post COVID-19 world embody anticipatory governance and participatory futures (Ramos, 2015, 2020) - shared global systems and structures to anticipate change, prepare for change, mobilize and adapt in the face of change. It is with our futures at stake that we need to lean in, embrace our ability to think futures and adapt in ways our children's children will be proud of. Wings out - lets fly!

*Many many thanks to reviewers and critical friends for constructive comments which improved the paper: Reanna Brown, Sohail Inayaullah, Peter Black, Mick Byrne, Mel Rumble, Gareth Priday, Andrew Ward, and many others.

REFERENCES

Benecke, O., & DeYoung, S. E. (2019). Anti-Vaccine Decision-Making and Measles
Resurgence in the United States. Global pediatric health, 6. https://doi.
org/10.1177/2333794X19862949

Dumaine, C. (2010). On a Global Foresight Commons. Seed Magazine. http://
seedmagazine.com/content/article/on_a_global_foresight_com-mons/

Galtung, J. (2009). The Fall of the US Empire and Then What?: Successors,
Regionalization Or Globalization? US Fascism Or US Blossoming? Transcend University
Press.

Hamilton, C. (2007). Scorcher: The Dirty Politics of Climate Change. Black Inc. .

Inayatullah, S. (1998). Causal layered analysis: Poststructuralism as method. Futures,
30(8), 815-829.

Laville, S. (2019, March 22). Top oil firms spending millions lobbying to block climate
change policies, says report. The Guardian. https://www.theguardian.com/business/2019/
mar/22/top-oil-firms-spending-millions-lobbying-to-block-climate-change-policies-
says-report

Milojević, I. (2020, May 11). Minimising Conflicts Amidst The COVID-19 Pandemic, Journal
of Futures Studies. https://jfsdigital.org/2020/05/11/minimising-conflicts-amidst-the-
covid-19-pandemic/

Nycyk, M. (2020). From Data Serfdom to Data Ownership: An Alternative Futures View of
Personal Data as Property Rights, Journal of Futures Studies, 24(4), 25–34. DOI: 10.6531/
JFS.202006_24(4).0003

Ramos, J. (2014) Anticipatory Governance: Traditions and Trajectories for Strategic
Design, Journal of Futures Studies, 19(1), 35-52.

Ramos, J. (2015). Liquid democracy and the futures of governance. In Winter, J and Ono,
R, (Eds) The Future Internet: Alternative Visions. Springer (pp. 173-191).

Ramos, J., Sweeney, J. A., Peach, K., & Smith, L. (2019). Our futures: by the people, for the
people. Nesta. https://media.nesta.org.uk/documents/Our_futures_by_the_people_for_
the_people_WEB_v5.pdf

Ramos, J. (2020). Four Futures of Reality. Journal of Futures Studies, 24(4), 5-23. DOI:
10.6531/JFS.202006_24(4).0002

Slaughter, R. (2020). Confronting a High-Tech Nightmare: A Review of Zuboff's the
Age of Surveillance Capitalism, Journal of Futures Studies, 24(4), 99–102. DOI: 10.6531
JFS.202006_24(4).0010

Snowden, E. (2019). Permanent record. Macmillan.

NOTES

1- The jury is still out but women leaders seem to be doing a better job of dealing with the crisis. See https://www.nytimes.com/2020/05/15/world/coronavirus-women-leaders.html

2- As Peter Black pointed out to me, in the case of Vietnam, they acted quickly and early as they understood they did not have the resources to manage society wide infections. See: https://theconversation.com/vietnams-prudent-low-cost-approach-to-combating-covid-19-136332

3- See: https://www.theguardian.com/business/2019/mar/22/top-oil-firms-spending-millions-lobbying-to-block-climate-change-policies-says-report

4- See: https://awayforward.undp.org/

5- See: https://www.sciencealert.com/the-five-corrupt-pillars-of-climate-change-denial

6- See: https://www.theguardian.com/commentisfree/2020/jun/16/coronavirus-hospital-bill-healthcare-america

7- Mahatma Gandhi believed in using anger toward wise ends. See: https://www.youtube.com/watch?v=fDPc4CisPJQ

8- See: https://www.facebook.com/ProutRev/posts/224815765840648?comment_id=225105209145037

9- https://www.worldbank.org/en/news/feature/2020/06/08/the-global-economic-outlook-during-the-covid-19-pandemic-a-changed-world

10- https://en.wikipedia.org/wiki/Green_New_Deal

11- https://bze.org.au/the-million-jobs-plan/

12- https://www.undp.org/content/undp/en/home/blog/2020/the-need-for-universal-basic-income.html

13- See: https://wiki.p2pfoundation.net/Category:Corona_Solidarity_Initiatives#Tools ; https://wiki.p2pfoundation.net/Category:Corona_Solidarity_Initiatives#Data ; https://wiki.p2pfoundation.net/Category:Corona_Solidarity_Initiatives#Testing_Kits ; https://wiki.p2pfoundation.net/Category:Corona_Solidarity_Initiatives#Mutual_Aid

14- https://www.theage.com.au/national/victoria/new-reports-of-family-violence-spike-in-covid-19-lockdown-study-finds-20200607-p55096.html

15- https://www.theage.com.au/national/victoria/new-reports-of-family-violence-spike-in-covid-19-lockdown-study-finds-20200607-p55096.html

HOW TO KEEP A FUTURE PERSPECTIVE IN A CRISIS

Karen Morley

In our mid-covid world we're grappling with what leadership is and could be in the future. There's plenty of despair and frustration. At the same time, many are looking to use the opportunity to create a better, fairer and more inclusive future: the World Economic Forum's 'The Great Reset' project is just one example.

THE PAIN OF LEADING IN A CRISIS

Yet, how do we create a world of growth and abundance, when it feels like we're in a world of pain?

Most leaders I speak with want more certainty, much of their planning attention is focused on tomorrow. They want and need to feel less pressure. They're working too hard; work seems harder and more complex now. And the downside of being safe in lockdown is the sense of restriction it imposes. A better future is on everyone's minds, yet seems a luxury for later.

Rowan was promoted two levels up to bring about cultural change in a non-performing division of her organisation. Lockdown commenced the next day. Half of her people were immediately reassigned to covid-related work. Rowan created a sense of order for the remaining teams, while still expected to deliver the full result. And just when it looked like there'd be a chance to settle into a business-as-usual approach, a larger organisational restructure looms. The threat of massive change is unsettling to say the least.

Cue high demand, uncertainty and stress. It all feels exhausting and relentless.

Glimpses of light at the end of the tunnel are dimming rather than brightening for Rowan. As we work our way through waves of of covid lockdowns, hope that things will revert quickly to 'the new normal' is dissipating. This is a long haul.

Cognitive strain results from too much effort and the existence of unmet demands, such as Rowan and many others are experiencing. Strain increases vigilance and suspicion. It decreases comfort, intuition and creativity. As we know from the work of Daniel Kahnemann (World Economic Forum, 2020) , high levels of demand and effort, exerting self-control to stay on task, and intense concentration all deplete energy.

HOW TO AVOID THE PAIN

How to create desired futures amidst this uncertainty and complexity? It comes down to three fundamentals for leaders:

- Paying attention to what's most important,
- Feeling aligned with a sense of purpose, and
- Maintaining energy and a sense of vitality.

The superpower that underlies these capabilities is psychological flexibility. Psychological flexibility increases the quality of decisions, and helps manage composure and wellbeing.

Psychological flexibility (see Figure 1) is the "ability to be present in the moment with full awareness and openness to our experience, and to take action guided by our values" (Harris, 2009).

Figure 1: Elements of psychological flexibility

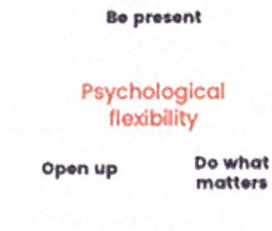

Be present

Psychological
flexibility

Open up   Do what
matters

Being present means being fully conscious and aware, which means managing attention. Attention is that most precious of resources for leaders; according to Ron Heifetz (Heifetz and Laurie, 2001), disciplined attention is the currency of leadership.

When your attention is focused it's possible to see yourself in your context, to be in contact with what is going on around you. Under usual circumstances Rowan was especially competent at this. The new challenges, relentless pace and long work hours in her new role meant that capacity was often spent. Thoughts became a staccato blur of what needed to be done, what hadn't been finalised, prioritising and reprioritising on the fly. Rather than feeling focused, Rowan was increasingly confused, even at times somewhat dazed.

When what we do aligns with purpose, we're doing what matters, and from that flows a sense of vitality. Being guided by values develops meaning and purpose. Otherwise we feel lost, adrift in the overwhelming ocean of options.

Opening up means accepting reality for what it is, without denying it or feeling stuck in it. We're not fused with the current reality, or the one 'right way'. We are open to change, adaptation and alternative ways of thinking.

HOW TO INCREASE PSYCHOLOGICAL FLEXIBILITY

Psychological flexibility for leadership can be increased by consciously shifting perspective.

As an avid travel photographer – when such a thing was possible - I always explored with my camera at the ready. The way that I use my camera helps me more rapidly make sense of the drama and chaos I experience when visiting new countries. Two key options give me the chance to both give up my perspective and take new perspectives. I manage my perspective, and the amount of complexity I deal with, by framing and zooming. I can frame my shots to heighten or reduce the familiarity of information around me. I can zoom my lens to examine things in more or less detail, to narrow or widen the scope.

This metaphor has proved a useful one to help navigate complex, unfamiliar territory. By increasing or decreasing, narrowing or widening my shot, I can manage the perspective I am taking.

Zooming and framing gives four ways to get perspective, to manage psychological flexibility: Endorsing, Examining, Enlarging, and Exploring (see Figure 2 below).

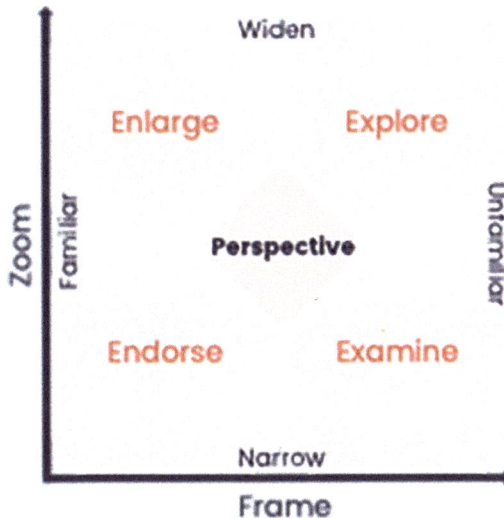

A narrower frame, focusing in on the familiar, helps when complexity is high. Endorsing what I know helps to avoid overwhelm, and to recharge. It's a retreat to the safety of the known.

Mindfulness is a great foundation practice. Focus in on this breath, this sensation. As a practice it provides a familiar way to manage attention and create calm.

Other tactics we used for increasing Rowan's sense of ease:

- A clear, repetitive cadence for her day, to reinforce familiarity,
- A visual display, in her case a mindmap, of what's known, agreed, and what's left to do.

In Aditya's case, what he needs to change is clear. How he needs to change is also clear. Why others need him to change is loud and clear. What Aditya wrestled with was his own motivation to change. He's not fully committed to the value of the change, given the energy it requires.

On the upside, he was open to seeing things differently.

We started by framing using his purpose and values; we kept the lens familiar. We focused on doing what matters, to him. Without this, nothing else will make the right kind of sense. We examined how he could live his purpose and values in the new, unfamiliar territory. He could feel his resistance softening. This gave him a sense of renewed focus and energy.

Other tactics that helped Aditya examine new perspectives:
He primed his day to attune his engagement: he used catchphrases and reminders to reinforce his purpose, to switch off, to be compassionate to himself and others
He tracked and primed his mood: in a good mood, he would access his intuition and it would feel easier.

THE POWER OF SHIFTING PERSPECTIVE

Robyn is another good example of the power of shifting perspective. Her responsibility for the organisation's crisis response to COVID-19 found her stuck fixing daily crises. While in a sense it was why the role existed, she was also aware that their approach needed to be much more systematic.

She thought a couple of members of the crisis response team lacked systemic thinking capability and that the crisis-focus fed their sense of self-importance. She felt responsible for making sure things were done 'the right way'. She felt let down by her colleagues.

The approach we took was to move to enlarge the way she saw the situation. She sought a perspective that would be more workable; one that gave rather than sapped her energy, that created rather than reduced options for everyone.

Viewing the same situation from multiple positions - I, you, and we - helped to increase her flexibility.

She was able to shift out of first position, 'I', 'me', 'my' perspective, and move into third, 'we', to see more of the interplay between herself and her colleagues. Plotting the dynamic of interactions allowed patterns to become clear.

Robyn was able to shift into second position to imagine the perspectives of her 'problem' colleagues. She humanised them by thinking about their needs and interests, and what she knew about their personal circumstances. Her empathy for their experiences immediately increased her compassion. They stopped being 'the problem'.

By keeping the frame narrow while widening the lens, she widened her view and in doing so, freed herself from an unhelpful perspective.

Exploring requires the greatest shift in perspective. There's no better approach than Sohail Inayatullah's Causal Layered Analysis (Inayatullah, 2009). It provides a comprehensive and integrative way to explore multiple perspectives and levels of analysis.

QUESTIONS TO INCREASE FLEXIBILITY

A final tactic that helps to keep an open mind, avoid the trap of certainty, and explore new territory is to ask good questions. Here's a few based on my experience, and Jennifer Garvey-Berger's work (Garvey Berger, 2019):

- What don't I know about this situation/person? What might I learn from this situation/person?
- What do I believe? How might my thinking be wrong/limited?
- What's another way to think about this? And yet another? And still another?
- How does our disagreement help us to increase the possibilities?
- What can I enable?

These questions help shift perspective, which increases psychologically flexibility; it is an absolute must for a world made more complex and where there are no easy answers. The more flexible you are in your thinking:

- The less stuck you feel.
- The less 'fused' you are with any one way of doing things, which opens up multiple options for the future, and
- The easier it feels.

In the midst of our covid crisis, you can balance your future focus with day-to-day realities by increasing your psychological flexibility. You'll be able to pay attention to what matters most, feel aligned with your purpose, and retain your vitality.

AUTHOR

Dr Karen Morley is an Executive Coach, an authority on leadership coaching, and a thought leader on gender and inclusion. She has held leadership roles in the public sector and higher education. She helps leaders understand the value of inclusive leadership to organisational as well as social outcomes. She is the author of Beat Gender Bias: How to play a better part in a more inclusive world; Lead like a Coach: How to Make the Most of Any Team; and Gender-Balanced Leadership: An Executive Guide. Find out more at www.karenmorley.com.au

NOTES

Garvey Berger, J. *(2019). Unlocking Leadership Mindtraps: How to Thrive in Complexity.* Stanford Briefs.

Harris, R. (2009). *ACT Made Simple.*New Harbinger Publications.

Heifetz, R.A. & Laurie, D.L. (2001, December). 'The Work of Leadership', *Harvard Business Review*, 131-141.

Inayatullah, S. (2009) *Causal Layered Analysis: An Integrative and Transformative Theory and Method.* In J. Glenn & Gordon, T. (Eds.) Future Research Methodology, Version 3.0. The Millennium Project.

World Economic Forum, (2020). *The Great Reset*. https://www.weforum.org/great-reset/

NARRATIVE FORESIGHT AND COVID-19:

Successes And Failures
In Managing The Pandemic

Ivana Milojević & Sohail Inayatulla

Journal of Futures Studies, March. 2021, 25(3): 79–84

I n this article, taking a text-based discourse approach (Shapiro, 1992), we outline narratives used to manage the COVID-19 pandemic and argue that some have been more and some less helpful for the current and future pandemic preparedness or shift to not only 'new' but a 'better normal'.

This work develops on earlier work by Milojević (2021, in press) where she focused on narrative foresight frames - the stories individuals, organizations, states and civilizations tell themselves about the future. It linked these narratives to futures fallacies, or detrimental thinking patterns about the future. The text selected were based on being public sector futures-oriented responses to COVID-19, that is, "key narratives in circulation during the implementation of governments' strategic objectives and the realization of visions of a 'pandemic-free' society (Milojević, 2021, in press).

This essay further develops the argument and organizes these narratives in terms of the discourses of blame, surprise/denial, exceptionalism, and alternatives of global solidarity, planning and social inclusion.

However, prior to these conclusions, we first explore the context of public policy responses: the rational-analytic versus the polis.

THE NARRATIVE CONTEXT OF PUBLIC POLICY RESPONSES

In her influential *Policy Paradox: The Art of Political Decision Making*, Deborah Stone outlines two basic models for political decision making (Stone, 2012). The first is the rational-analytic model. This model is based on the following assumptions:

> Reason forms basis for personal and government decisions. Facts, data, and information are neutral, and can settle conflicts. Individuals are rationally self-interested utility maximizers. They try to minimize costs and maximize benefits. Decision makers evaluate the costs and benefits of each course of action as accurately and completely as possible. The essence of rational decision-making is to tally up the consequences of different alternatives and choose the one that yields the best results. (Stone, 2012: 260)

The polis model, on the other hand, more closely represents the way we make and understand public policy (Stone, 2012). This model is based on the following assumptions:

> Policy is about storytelling, ideas, and argument. Community is the major unit of composition with ideas, wills, goals etc. outside of the individual. There is a public interest beyond individual interests. Most policy problems are commons problems. Influence sometimes verging on coercion, cooperation, and loyalty are the major forms of interaction. Groups and organizations are the building blocks of the community. Information is never perfect. Some resources are scarce and rivalrous, but many are anti-rivalrous and abundant. (Stone, 2012: 32)

The first approach focuses on "cost benefit analysis", while the second focuses on "hidden storylines", commonly in the form of stated goals as "inspirational visions of a future, hoping to enlist the aid of others in bringing it about" (Stone, 2012: 252). In this latter approach, it is understood that the way a problem or an issue is framed critically influences the way alternative futures and solutions are constructed.

For example, during the global financial crisis over a decade ago, the *Financial Times* (Yergin: 2009) reported that at its heart this was a narrative crisis. How one creates national policy and strategy depends on the story one uses. Depending on the narrative used – i.e., a mortgage crisis, a banking crisis, a geo-political crisis of the shift to the Pacific (higher savings rates), a financial crisis, or even a crisis of capitalism – different strategies are created (Inayatullah, 2010). Some are shallow and short term oriented; others are deeper leading to foundational changes. Ultimately, in this example, solutions to deal with the deeper crisis (of capitalism) were eschewed, and Wall Street was saved at the expense of Main Street. Through massive spending, China also helped to save the world economy, and all returned to normalcy. The window of a possibility of structural change did not materialize.

We are in a similar turbulent situation today. As during the French Revolution, time is plastic; we have entered uncharted waters. What is the best national policy for dealing with COVID-19? Will the virus mutate and become even more dangerous? Will the vaccination strategy succeed? How severe or how long should lockdowns/quarantines be? It may be that once the crisis nears its end, many will be tempted to go back to the world we knew i.e., one where nature is still seen an externality, and profit is the core focus. However, as with the earlier financial crisis, this is also the opportunity to create a different world, to create structural changes in the global health system, in food safety, to begin with. As biosecurity expert Peter Black argues, "Historically, pandemics have forced humans to break with the past and imagine their world anew. This one is no different. It can become a portal, a gateway between one world and the next" (Personal email, 6 April 2020).

What we do from here on - in response to COVID-19 pandemic and other challenges we currently globally face - will be decided by the narrative we use. It will also be decided by answering the following question: How much do we wish to change? As seen from many debates in relation to COVID-19, some people want to "go back to normal", yet others are still in various forms of denial in relation to the new reality. Parallel to this, various groups are promoting solutions focused on "changing the world radically" based on the worldviews and metaphors they employ. Here, we have seen the polarisation between those wishing for more government control, even repression, and those wishing to use this crisis to create a more inclusive, democratic, ecological, and benevolent world. Finally, each public policy sector has introduced various sets of reforms in attempts to address the crisis. These too are dependent on the framing of the issue, as well as the social, historical, and cultural context of each respective society.

RATIONAL VS POLIS MODEL FOR POLICY MAKING

If the rational model for policy making had been the one best explaining COVID-19 pandemic preparedness and best responses, we would have had a different set of countries leading the way here. For example, in the 2019 *Global Health Security Index (GHSI)*, an assessment of 195 countries' capacity to face infectious disease outbreaks – compiled largely by the US-based experts – it is the US which is ranked first in terms of overall preparedness score, followed by the UK, Netherlands, Australia and Canada (Cameron et al., 2019). Considering the devastating COVID-19 death rate and other policy failures in the US, the authors of the GHSI have since provided a further elaboration as to the "significant preparedness gaps" in the US (GHSI, 2020):

> The United States' response to the COVID-19 outbreak to date shows that capacity alone is insufficient if that capacity isn't fully leveraged. Strong health systems must be in place to serve all populations, and effective political leadership that instils confidence in the government's response is crucial.

In addition to the pandemic preparedness, the stories and metaphors which circulated within societies provided a specific context for public policy responses. In broad strokes, we could argue, that due to the individualism and market orientation of societies or better say political leaderships in countries such as UK and US, the narrative framing the response was the one of individual responsibility and techno-medical solutions (vaccination, cure). This framing is based on a particular conservative political worldview, which prioritises individual over social responsibility (Lakoff, 2011). It further prioritises the narrative of 'letting the market decide' over science, and short-termism/immediate gratification storylines over prevention/long-term outcomes.

While perhaps helpful for other social problems, the narrative frame – trust the market - has fallen short for the pandemic. Arguably, collectivist societies, as well as collectivist narratives/measures taken in western societies, coupled with reliance on science, have, so far, resulted in much better outcomes. Before we proceed with this argument any further, it is important to distinguish collectivism vis-à-vis totalitarianism, given how often these two social and political models are conflated. In a nutshell, what we assume under collectivism: primary is social responsibility – i.e., this is the consideration of how one's individual actions are impacting others and measures taken for the benefit of most, including the most vulnerable members of society. This contrasts with 'totalitarian model' of policy making, wherein:

> A central government produces slanted information predominantly aimed as a means of social control and tightly controls all news/information. Citizens, including 'elites', accept government propaganda, act like puppets, and do not decide for themselves. (Stone, 2012: 323)

While totalitarianism and democracy are mutually exclusive, it is entirely possible to have collectivist narratives and measures in the context of democratic societies. One example is New Zealand, where the Prime Minister was decisive, utilized evidence-based policies and WHO strategies, all the while ensuring that she had an overall shared narrative, what she called, "A team of five million" (Smith, 2020). Its neighbour, Australia, followed New Zealand's lead, in protecting the collective (i.e., some twenty-five million people) with the early and, some would argue, rather harsh closing of borders. The metaphor used early on was that of "we are all in this together" (Dennis, 2020). While the policy of closed borders is highly controversial, the collectivist focus has resulted in several phases wherein there has been an almost complete elimination of the virus. As of 14 December 2020, Australia has gone ten days without a locally acquired case of COVID-19. In narrative terms, the decision was made to prioritise "lives over lifestyles". Long-term thinking and modelling played an important role. For example, in March 2020, the Australian federal government was preparing for 50,000 deaths in a best-case scenario and 150,000 deaths in the worst-case scenario (Davey, 2020). Largely due to various measures taken, as of 14 December 2020, Australia had recorded 908 total deaths from COVID-19, and 28,031 of total cases (Government of Australia, 2020). Eight hundred and twenty of those cases were in one Australian state, Victoria, largely because of the mismanagement of quarantine measures. Victoria thus first became a "cautionary tale of a second wave which killed hundreds and shattered the economy" due to several oversights in managing the pandemic. It later also became a "success story of a state which brought daily infections down from the high hundreds to zero" (Murray-Atfield, 2020). The success came despite competing narratives aiming to avert the collectivist approaches which included severe lockdowns. Protests calling on the Victorian premier Daniel Andrews to "let us out" and "let us work" and framing him as a totalitarian leader (i.e., 'Chairman Dan', and 'Dictator Dan') failed. Instead, a formula of "strong political leadership, community engagement and public health measures" succeeded in eliminating the virus. The narrative used here, instead of "individual responsibility", "control", "management", "mitigation", "light touch" (Moody, 2020) "flattening the curve" and so on, as used in many comparable western countries, was that of "aggressive suppression" instead. "If you do not crush this virus, it could crush you" was the narrative expressed by the Victorian Chief Health Officer (Murray-Atfield, 2020). This storyline paved the way for the community's acceptance of difficult measures.

In addition to New Zealand and Australia, a similar strategy of suppression/ elimination has been pursued by a limited number of countries/jurisdictions, including China, Hong Kong, Taiwan, South Korea and Fiji (Murray-Atfield, 2020). While there are many differences between policy measures implemented in these countries (beyond the scope of this article), all have employed communal solutions to the issue of community transmission based on the collectivist worldview. These nations are amongst those which have been ranked as the most successful globally in dealing with COVID-19, as of December 2020 (Chang, 2020). In addition to investment in public (i.e., collective) health infrastructure, social cohesion (inclusive of little inequality and a lot of discipline) has been a major factor behind the cohesive response of the country. This in turn has led to greater success in managing the pandemic (Chang, 2020).

PREPARING FOR THE FUTURE

But what are the implications of the previous argument – the relevance of narrative and metaphor within the polis model of political decision-making – for the future, for alternative futures?.

Clearly while there are many lessons from COVID-19, the most important one appears to be being adequately prepared for the future. At a basic level, this means not just having the ability to read emerging issues and weak signals but also being able to rapidly respond to these signals. More, advanced futures-preparedness means that foresight is institutionalized into one or multiple branches of government. Ultimately, of course, futures-preparedness means a citizenry that is futures literate (Miller, 2018). Returning to narrative, what metaphors and stories can help us move from being unprepared to being more prepared for the future, alternative futures?.

In previous work, we argued that the multiple narratives used to manage COVID-19 could be organised across two variables, those that hinder and those that assist (Milojević, 2021, in press). We now categorize these approaches into meta-narratives – once again, those that hinder and those that assist. Three that hinder are: blame, surprise/denial and exceptionalism. On the other hand, those that assist are global solidarity, planning and social inclusion.

FROM BLAME TO GLOBAL SOLIDARITY

The first unhelpful position is based on electoral politics with the goal of gaining political capital by blaming others. The narrative used, by, for example, the former President of the US, Donald Trump has been, "the China virus" or "kung flu." Blame can lead to a situation of a "battlefield" where the troops are rallied to fight the virus. The nation is seen as an organism, fighting the foreign virus. In addition, after blame, the worldviews of "herd immunity" and "natural selection" were used. This approach reduced preparedness and has resulted in nearly 350,000 deaths from COVID-19 in the USA by the end of 2020 (Bryant Miranda, 2021).

In contract to these narratives, there have been alternatives such as: "same story, different boats", "global solidarity", "viruses know no country", and "all lives matter." It is this second set of narratives, we argue, that is needed to be more adequately prepared for the future.

FROM SURPRISE AND DENIAL TO PLANNING

The second not so helpful frame or meta-narrative has been one of surprise. In this frame, the narrative has been, "who would have thought," "sit back and wait for the avalanche", and "never before" or a fatalistic "act of God". Linked to this approach is denial as in the narrative of it is "just the flu". These narratives ensure a lack of preparedness and lack of decisive action.

In contrast are the narratives of "time is running out, use it wisely," "pandemics are as certain as death and taxes", and "man vs microbe" – a part of our evolutionary history and thus not a surprise. As argued in previous work (Milojević 2021, in press), challenging surprise/denial are also narratives such as "a new disease, a new approach" and "responding to signals amidst the noise".

FROM EXCEPTIONALISM TO SOCIAL INCLUSION

The third frame or meta-narrative that hindered adequate preparedness and response has been exceptionalism, i.e., everyone else but me or my tribe or group. The most vulnerable (who are not 'us') are to be sacrificed via "only those with pre-existing conditions" (sick and elderly) narrative. The language used has been "not me, not us," or "out of sight, out of mind." Singapore, for example, had been a success story but it was remiss on COVID-19 strategies for poorer and neglected migrant workers. Their harsh working conditions – cramped, lack of access to medical care, lack of information on COVID-19 measures – led to an outbreak which then spread. This was also true for Sweden. (Gustavsson, 2020). The nation eschewed strict quarantine for trusting its citizens, but its policies did not create adequate safeguards for those in elderly homes and migrant communities, and thus the nation is ranked poorly in comparison to its neighbours.

An alternative and more futures-prepared narrative is that of "all of us are vulnerable" and "all in this together."

CONCLUSION

Narrative (Milojević and Inayatullah, 2015) thus as we have argued throughout this paper is decisive in which futures emerge and which do not.

The narratives and metaphors used to inform policy-based decisions, as per the polis model, seem to have trumped pandemic preparedness in terms of resources and systems previously put in place. As argued by Deborah Stone, political reasoning always involves "metaphor-making and category-making, but not just for beauty's sake or for insight's sake" [Stone, 2012: 12]. Rather, it is a "strategic portrayal for persuasion's sake and, ultimately, for policy's sake." [Stone, 2012: 12] This is about shifting the discourse to future pandemic preparedness using approaches that work. These we have argued tend to be collectivism using evidence-based science within a narrative of inclusion, taking the New Zealand narrative of a "team of five million" to a planet of eight billion people. We close this essay with a warning i.e., COVID-19 may be a portal to a new world, but it is certainly a warning to prepare for a dangerous world ahead and do our best to ensure that the Age of Pandemics is short lived (Inayatullah and Roper, 2020).

ACKNOWLEDGEMENTS

A significant part of research by Dr. Ivana Milojević reported in this article was supported by the First Futures Research Grant, awarded by the Prince Mohammad Bin Fahd Center for Futuristic Studies (PMFCFS) and the World Futures Studies Federation (WFSF). Its content is solely the responsibility of the authors. The research paper is based on a keynote speech by Ivana Milojević at the Philippine Society for Public Administration International Conference, Public Administration Towards a Better Normal: Paradigms, Policies, and Perspectives, October 23, 2020

REFERENCES

Bryant, M. (2021, January 3). US braces for post-holiday Covid surge as death toll nears 350,000. *The Guardian*. https://www.theguardian.com/us-news/2021/jan/02/us-coronavirus-covid-cases-death-toll-holidays.

Cameron, H., Georghiou, L., Keenan, M., Miles, I., and Saritas, O. 2006. *Evaluation of the United Kingdom Foresight Programme Final Report.* PREST, Manchester Business School, University of Manchester.

Chang, R. Hong, J., and Varley, K. (2020, November 30). The Best and Worst places to be in COVID: U.S. Sinks in Ranking. Bloomberg.https://www.bloomberg.com/graphics/covid-resilience- ranking/.

Department of Health, Australian Government (2020, December 14). *Coronavirus current situation and numbers.* https:// www.health.gov.au/news/health-alerts/novel-coronavirus-2019-ncov-health-alert/ coronavirus-COVID-19-current-situation-and-case-numbers.

Davey, M. (2020, June, 21). A peek into the future: how worst-case scenario coronavirus modelling saved Australia from catastrophe. *The Guardian* https://www.theguardian.com/australia- news/2020/jun/21/wildly-off-base-how-did-australia-get-its-coronavirus-modelling-so- wrong.

Denniss, R. (2020, October 1). Thank you, Victoria – Australia as a whole is healthier and wealthier because of you. *The Guardian* https://www.theguardian.com/commentisfree/2020/oct/01/ thank-you-victoria-australia-as-a-whole-is-healthier-and-wealthier-because-of-you.

GHSI. (2020, April, 27). The U.S. and COVID-19: Leading the World by GHS Index Score, not by Response. *Global Health Security Index News.* https:// www.ghsindex.org/news/the-us-and-COVID-19-leading-the-world-by-ghs-index-score- not-by-response/.

Gustavsson, J. (2020, December 15). COVID-19 and the failure of Swedish Exceptionalism. *The Dispatch*. https:// thedispatch.com/p/COVID-19-and-the-failure-of-swedish.

Inayatullah, S. (2010). Emerging world scenario triggered by the global financial crisis. World Affairs: The Journal of International Issues. 14(3), 48–69.

Inayatullah, S., and Roper, E. (2020, July 28). Let's Get Flexible: Brisbane Grammar School Navigates the COVID-19 Crisis. *Journal of Futures Studies.* https://jfsdigital. org/2020/07/21/brisbane-grammar-school/.

Lakoff, G. (2011, February 19). *What Conservatives Really Want.* https://georgelakoff. com/2011/02/19/what-conservatives-really- want/.

Miller, R. (Ed.) (2018). *Transforming the Future: Anticipation in the 21st Century.* Routledge and UNESCO.

Milojević, I. (2021). COVID-19 and Pandemic Preparedness: Foresight Narratives and Public Sector Responses. *Journal of Futures Studies.* 26(1), 1-18.

Milojević, I., and Inayatullah. S.(2015) Narrative Foresight. *Futures*. (73), 151- 162.

Moody, O. (2020, June 4). Light touch cost us many lives, Swedish scientist says. *The Times* https://www.thetimes.co.uk/article/light-touch-cost-us-many-lives-swedish-scientist-says- 6qv7q7d5g.

Murray-Atfield, Y. (2020, November 17). What can South Australia learn from Victoria's coronavirus outbreaks and response? *Australian Broadcasting Corporation*. https://www.abc.net.au/news/2020-11-17/what-can-sa-learn- from-victorias-coronavirus-response/12887972.

Murray-Atfield, Y. (2020, November 5). Coronavirus second waves are crashing into Europe. What will their lockdowns achieve? *Australian Broadcasting Corporation*. https://www.abc.net.au/news/2020-11-05/coronavirus-COVID- 19-europe-second-wave-melbourne-vic-compared/12839600.

Shapiro, M. (1992). *Reading the Postmodern Polity: Political Theory as Textual Practice*. University of Minnesota.

Smith, N. (2020 August 3). A Team of Five Million. How New Zealand Beat Coronavirus. https:// www.directrelief.org/2020/08/a-team-of-5-million-how-new-zealand-beat-coronavirus/.

Stone, D.(2012). *Policy Paradox: The Art of Political Decision Making*. Norton.

Yergin, D.(2009, October 21). A Crisis in Search of a Narrative. *FT* https://www.ft.com/content/8a82d274-bda9-11de-9f6a-00144feab49a.

REGIONAL
& NATIONAL
RESPONDS
STUDIES

COVID-19 AND THE FUTURES OF PAKISTAN:

Inclusive Foresight and Innovation

Sohail Inayatullah, Puruesh Chaudhary,
Syed Sami Raza and Umar Sheraz

SOHAIL INAYATULLAH – USED FUTURES AND ALTERNATIVE SCENARIOS

It was late January when four Pakistanis studying in China tested positive to the novel coronavirus (SARS-CoV-2), which causes the disease known as COVID-19. Internally, the country reported its first two COVID-19 cases on February 26, 2020, both of which had returned from Iran. Pakistan, as of April 29, had reported 14,885 confirmed cases with 3,425 recoveries and 327 deaths.

While the pandemic continues to spread, Pakistan faces other critical issues as well. For example, from 8 July to 12 November, there were 47,000 confirmed cases of dengue with 75 deaths. Moreover, twenty-four percent still live below the poverty line.

While in Islamabad in early March, I asked the guard at the SafaGold Mall why he did not have hand sanitizer or temperature scanners, as I had seen in Singapore. He stared at me with a puzzled look. I explained to him that COVID-19 was on its way to Pakistan. Another guard came by, and soon we had a conversation that went nowhere: they were ready for the Taliban and other extremists, not a virus. Geopolitics and the long war on terror had framed the national narrative. A virus is not an enemy, cannot be imprisoned, nor does it provide the opportunity to create patriotic songs that focus on national sentiments.

But the inter-generational memory of pandemics is there. A few years back, while asking about my mother's family history, she told me that she had never met her grandmother. I was surprised and asked why; she told me she died in her late teens from the plague. The last plague epidemic in British India broke out in 1896, imported from Hong Kong.[4] Eventually, over a 31-year period, 13 million died.[5] As the British attempted to control the plague, riots broke out across the country. [6] What will happen this time if COVID-19 spreads? Moreover, is Pakistan at all prepared for such a spread?

Futurist Puruesh Chaudhary writes that not just COVID-19 but also climate change, internal and external debt, and other crises are coming. "In my work with Agahi and the Pakistan State of the Future Index, we suggested that a pandemic could re-occur in Pakistan. When we published a policy exercise, 'The Future of Possibilities' in 2019[7], participants identified the emergence of a pandemic that could severely impact the country's future." However, futures work is still not seriously used in the corridors of institutional power. They are focused, as are most governments, on actions that ensure votes in the next elections.

Currently, Pakistan, like the rest of the world, is engaged in the "hammer and dance"[8] strategy – that is, hit the pandemic hard with lockdowns and then as economic livelihood, mental health and travel become more important, go back and forth between restrictions and movement. However, the strictness of these lockdowns is being challenged, especially by the religious right.

Modeling remains unclear how many Pakistanis could potentially be affected by this virus. Chaudhary writes: "A huge population (nearly two hundred million), inadequate health care systems, capability gaps, lack of accountability, and our failure to imagine multiple possibilities is our biggest misfortune. There is a pattern to how Pakistan responds to crises, and this outbreak is no different. Many of the nation's leaders are still rehashing used futures." There is also complacency and a feeling of lack of agency. As a security guard commented: "What can we do about the Coronavirus? One can die of a heart attack. Death is inevitable, and it could come at any time.[9]

So, given the current crisis, what is next? While we certainly cannot say what will happen, we can outline probable futures.

THE SAVIOUR

In the first future, it is external – another nation attacking or saving- that is paramount. Once it was, the USA was saving Pakistan. Now it is China with its face masks and public health strategies.[10] A year from now, it will be China that helps Pakistan recover from financial collapse. The International Monetary Fund will come to the rescue later. Five years from now, it may be a different country. But Pakistan will remain the child, always waiting for the elder to save him/her.

THE REVENGE

While forty years ago, the maulvis (clerics) occupied a minor space in Pakistani politics, today they are central to how reality is perceived. Their insistence on doing nothing, not allowing masjids to be closed, on using ignorance as a defense becomes the final straw. As one recently said: "Today, you all will shake each other's hands before leaving the mosque. Perform namaz (prayers) standing shoulder-to-shoulder and ankle-to-ankle in the rows! If anyone amongst you contracts Coronavirus, shoot me in the middle of the street, and you will not be punished for that!"[11] Said another: "It is all in the hands of Allah … we should fear God, not a pandemic."[12] Worse, the Pakistani state is unable to resist the power of the clerics. Indeed, "Even as the pandemic spread to the country, Pakistani authorities allowed tens of thousands of Islamic clerics from around the world to congregate for three days outside the eastern city of Lahore. Some 200 of the clerics are now quarantined at the site of the gathering, a sprawling compound belonging to an Islamic missionary group, Tableeghi Jamaat."[13]

Eventually, the religious right is forever banished to a peripheral role in politics. Progressive values once again take hold; it will no longer be fact versus faith, but a nation focused on science, technology, and inclusive economic development.

EVERYONE IN A DIFFERENT DIRECTION

Pakistan's vision of the future is clouded, there is no unified identity. Me, myself and my tribe are most likely to dominate the agenda. Fragmentation will be the reality. Over the next six months, we can anticipate riots throughout the nation as poverty worsens and conflicts between the religious right and others increase. This will most likely lead to direct military rule, a return of to the civilian-military pendulum of governance.[14] The military will impose law and order. This will continue over the next few years. Looking back, Pakistan's response was "too little, too late." Power politics, poverty, and traditional ways of seeing the future were all complicit.

PURUESH CHAUDHARY – TECHNO PAKISTAN AND THE AWAKENING

In this future, the young make a massive push towards the digitalization of the economy. The 4th Industrial Revolution creates real change. Entrepreneurs and small business owners increasingly rely on using technology to enhance productivity and consumer experience, setting a better balance between work and life. This group of energetic young Pakistanis enables meaningful economic opportunities. 5G technologies create more jobs. They are not only leading a movement on flattening the curve but also paving the way for a future-centric ecosystem. Baby boomers and Gen X see the shift and join the bandwagon. Notions around platform cooperativism gain momentum. Ministries and regulators start using a systems-based approach to integrate databases for anticipatory governance. Imagination and creativity become the core function for all future R&D investments.

As technologies continue to transform, geopolitics becomes less of a defining factor, and public health and equity become foundational. Political parties work together as the national emergency is so grave, during, and after COVID-19. No-one can go it alone. Landlordism and the military become far less important. Instead of nationalism, South Asia and regionalism become defining. Instead of searching for enemies, Pakistan searches for partners, within and without. Women gain inequity, as do the poor.

SYED SAMI RAZA – DOOM AND GLOOM

The people are depressed. PTSD cases increase. At present, the people don't believe that the government can control the pandemic or that it is at all serious about doing so. This situation of doom and gloom exacerbates. Some of the reasons include the political and economic situation in the country. On the political level, the people feel helpless because they have tried several political parties and not a single one delivered. In this future, trust in party politics is lost.

On the economic side, severe depression has already started. We know from the global economic depression of the late 1990s as well as from the depressions of the post-war and interwar periods that it takes quite some time for the economy to pick back up again. This time the depression will be greater as it is global in scope. All production channels worldwide have come to a stop. It could take years before the depression is over, but by then, it will have left the local economy of the country devastated. The industrial and services sector will shut down. It will take years for systems to get going again. By then, hundreds of thousands of people in the private sector will have lost jobs. Unemployment, poverty, and crime rates will increase. Global production will also shut down, and therefore there won't be enough resources to fulfill local needs. Violence against women will also dramatically increase.

The economic depression will not just to deepen because of the pandemic, but also because of the increasing control of information. The establishment of the Command and Control Authority and government's control over information is already raising suspicions among the people of the increasing power of the state. Information control will be used in calculating ways. It will be used as a way to bring in donations, aid, debt rescheduling, waivers, and so forth.

In this future, the legitimacy of political leaders, the Army, and the economy disappears. However, the nation does not break apart as all are too tired to resort to any dramatic action. Doom decreases the capacity to act.

UMAR SHERAZ – COMPETING NARRATIVES AND SOLUTIONS

Narratives have huge persuasive power and strongly influence how people and nations think and act. Flawed historical narratives seduce nations into thinking, creating value, and justifying a particular course of action. The course of Pakistani history, present (and eventually the plausible future) has consistently fixated around two narratives. The first narrative is that of war. We are a nation that has always been at some sort of war. Our neighbor across the border has been our favorite punching bag, but we have forever been at war with more than them: the war against the infidels (Jihad), the war against terrorism, war against inflation, against corruption (Ehtesaab) and war for change (Tabdeel). It comes as no surprise, then, that current efforts against the coronavirus have been anointed the "War against COVID 19". In a recent interview, Dr. Peter Black discussed how the usage of the war metaphor discounts or limits the number of options that become available to address the challenge.[15] Sadly, the biggest casualty of war is the human capital, which then becomes the fuel of the engines of war.

The second narrative is the term "opportunity," and I cannot think of any time in recent memory when any Pakistani leader has not talked about the "opportune moment" to act as the nation is "at a crossroads." This, in itself, is problematic as people who see opportunities eventually become "opportunistic." Once that happens, there is scant regard for alternative ways of thinking, and they eventually become the monster that they set out to fight. At a time when the leading thinkers discuss a global reset button, the narratives instilled in our national psyche remain the biggest hurdle in the whole nation coming together and moving towards a unified vision, a preferred future.

COUNTER-NARRATIVES FOR A PREFERRED FUTURE

The foreseeable future will be driven by these two narratives of opportunity at once a narrative has taken hold; they can be very difficult to shake off, at least until an even more compelling counter-narrative is introduced. Instead of war metaphors, there are other narratives that are much more useful for us in thinking about our preferred future. We could talk about the "Coronavirus movement," similar to the Pakistan movement, which united all and sundry towards a common goal and cause. The other change in the narrative could be putting "Pakistanis before Pakistan," instead of the other way round. "Opportunity" needs to be replaced by the possibility to accommodate other world views, experimentation, and backup plans in case of failure. The goal would be to make a post-corona Pakistan more humanitarian, rather than a victim of opportunistic wish lists. There is already a narrative that says that Pakistan is considered one of the most generous societies in the world – what is called the Law of Generosity. "We Pakistanis believe that one good deed begets another, and perhaps our generosity will spread faster than the virus. Armed with the unwavering belief that humanity at large will benefit, we are trying our best to provide a cushion to those who need assistance – and hope to those who need hope."[16]

ACTION PLANS FOR A PREFERRED FUTURE

At the systemic level, there are a few things that need to be sorted out in the march towards a preferred future.

The coronavirus is exacting a heavy toll on health systems and personnel. In Pakistan, there is a different kind of predicament: there are about 85,000 "missing" "doctors-in-law" in Pakistan.[17] These 85,000 female doctors have completed their medical education at the expense of the state or privately, but they are not part of the medical workforce in Pakistan. They are victims of the "trophy wife" phenomenon. If only 50 percent of these doctors are mobilized, 70 percent of health issues of people in low-income communities can be resolved. Unfortunately, this is an issue that has not been voiced in the current drama, which is a criminal mistake made by the media and intellectuals. Our medical pipeline is bleeding profusely, and applying a tourniquet quickly is the first step in rehabilitating our medical system, which will be under tremendous stress and short of professionals in the Corona Movement.

The current Prime Minister came to office with the slogan of universal quality education in the country, for all. The plan ran into issues with all stakeholders and just seemed to have fizzled out like any other electoral promise. The current predicament has brought all sorts of education systems in Pakistan (Montessori, Madrassa, government, elitist, right-wing) to a standstill and forced them to move online. As all education systems are now looking toward the government for direction and assistance, this the right time to make sure all educational systems are on the same page. This will bring the poorest of the poor in Madrassas and government schools on par with elitist schools in a uniform curriculum and uniform code of quality and pave the way for a unified vision of the future.

As a general rule, governments around the world have failed the poor and the underprivileged. This is starker in developing countries like Pakistan, where the bottom of the food chain has been left to fend for themselves. Seventy percent of Pakistan's economy is informal and undocumented. In these times of hardship, it is the networks of trust and informal networks of mutual assistance that have held the fabric of society together. A witch hunt against these networks was initiated in the aftermath of 9/11, with no clear evidence of financial wrongdoing. Twenty years later, it is time to honor and legitimize these networks.

Move the ideas of pro-poor foresight and frugal innovation from the level of slogans and academic discourse to real-life practice [Kapoor, 2001].[18] COVID-19 has laid bare the fact that foresight and innovation tend to happen for those who can afford it. Both institutions have been found wanting in this time of global strife. In a post-corona world, this needs to change. More inclusive models of foresight and innovation need to be experimented with and embraced.

ABOUT THE AUTHORS

Dr. Sohail Inayatullah is the UNESCO Chair in Futures Studies, at Sejahtera Centre for Sustainability and Humanity, Malaysia, Professor at Tamkang University, Taiwan and Associate Professor, Melbourne Business School, the University of Melbourne. He can be reached at sinayatullah@gmail.com.

Puruesh Chaudhary is a futures researcher and strategic narrative professional. She is the Founding President of AGAHI.

Dr. Syed Sami Raza is an assistant professor in political science at the University of Peshawar. He is the editor of the Journal of Review of Human Rights.

Umar Sheraz is the blog editor of the Journal of Futures Studies and can be reached at umar_sheraz@yahoo.com. He works at the Centre for Policy Studies at COMSATS University Islamabad, Pakistan.

REFERENCES

Government of Pakistan (2021). Realtime Pakistan and Worldwide COVID-19 situation! http://covid.gov.pk/.

WHO (2019, December 12). Dengue Fever: Pakistan. https:// www.who.int/csr/don/19-november-2019-dengue-pakistan/en/.

Asian Development Bank. (2021). *Pakistan: Poverty*. https://www. adb.org/countries/pakistan/poverty

Medical History of British India – National Library of Scotland. (2007). Disease: Plague. https://digital.nls.uk/indiapapers/plague.html.

Seal, S. (1960). Epidemiological Studies of Plague in India. *Bull World Health Organ*. (23(2-3): 283-292.

Klein, I. (1988). Plague, Policy and Popular Unrest in British India," *Modern Asian Studies*. 22 (4): 723-755.

Chaudhary, P. (2019). Pakistan 2029 – Policy Exercise. Pakistan State of Future Index. www.academia.edu/41497049/Pakistan_2029_-_Policy_Exercise.

Pueyo, T. (2020, March 23). Coronavirus: The Hammer and the Dance. https://medium. com/@tomaspueyo/coronavirus-the- hammer-and-the-dance-be9337092b56

Shams, S. (2020, March 18). Coronavirus: Is Pakistan taking COVID-19 too lightly? https:// www.dw.com/en/coronavirus-is- pakistan-taking-COVID-19-too-lightly/a-52824403.

Gannon, K. (2020, March 29). China sends medical aid to Pakistan to combat virus outbreak. https://abcnews.go.com/International/wireStory/china-sends-medical-aid-pakistan-combat-virus-outbreak-69851504.

THE ISLAMIC WORLD AND COVID-19 FUTURES

Sohail Inayatullah

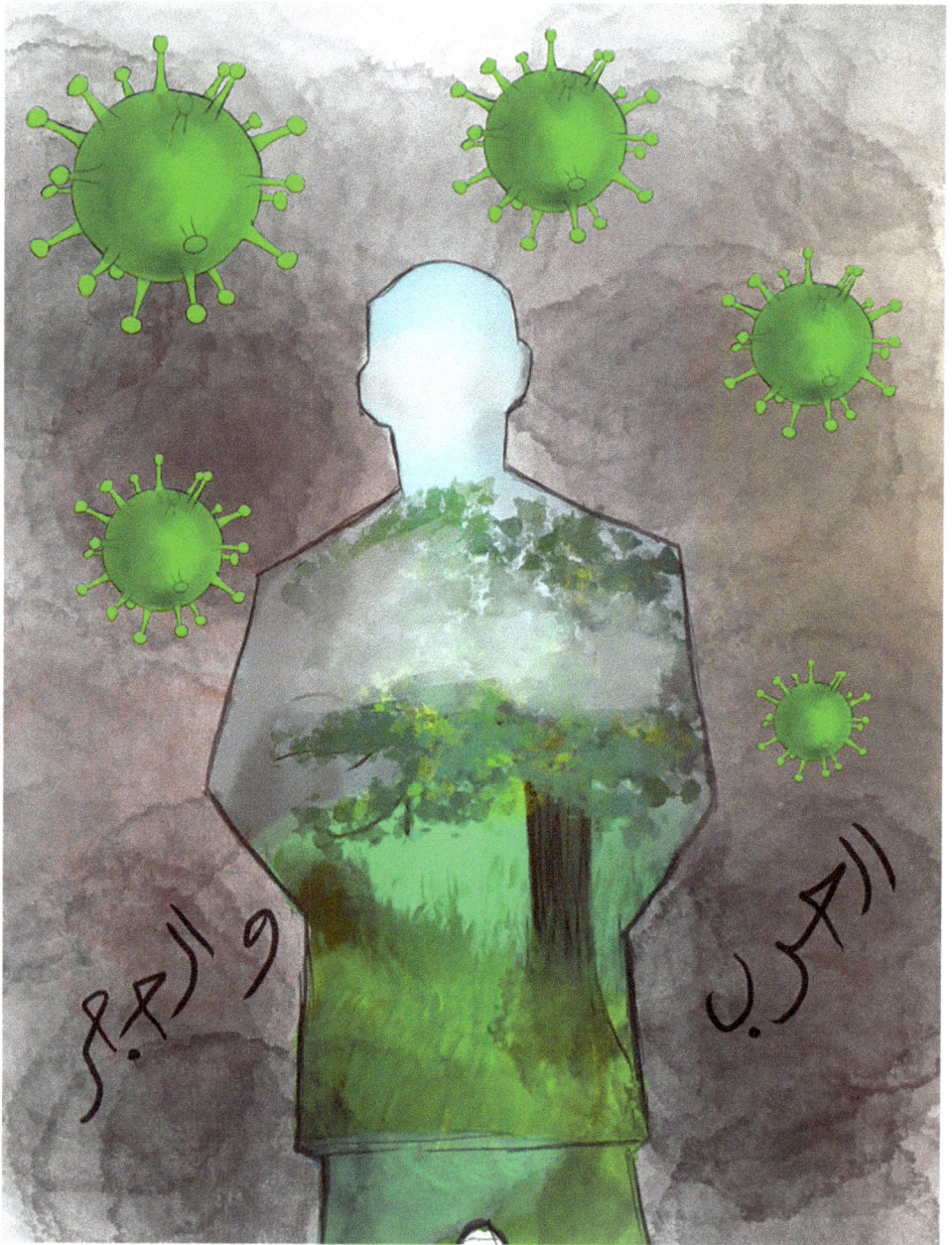

Illustration: Manar Husainemail

No part of the world has been left untouched by the path of COVID-19. Nations and regions have responded differently. East Asia was quick to implement lockdowns, social distancing, hand washing and other recommendations of the World Health Organization (WHO). Tracing, the use of AI and apps have all been helpful. Australia and New Zealand have successfully suppressed the virus. They are keeping borders closed at this stage, though they are likely to adopt a traffic light model of opening (green, orange, and red zones of travel).

However, in many parts of the Asian and African continents, WHO preventive measures might be difficult to carry out. Consider the case of Egypt. Egypt's statistical agency, the Central Agency for Public Mobilization and Statistics (CAPMAS), reported that 32.5 percent of the total population falls below the poverty line (estimated at approximately $46.6, monthly) in 2017-18. *The Middle East Eye* of April 16, 2020 quoted Samira Outt, a street vendor, as saying "If I catch the virus, I will die. And if I don't work me and my children will die also, but out of hunger. So it is the same."

In an earlier work that explored the futures of a COVID-19 world, four scenarios were identified (Inayatullah and Black, 2020). These were: In the first scenario, "Zombie Apocalypse," fear and panic rule as markets crash and nations fracture. The second, "The Needed Pause," anticipates that a year or so of lockdowns leads to speeding up in late 2021, once a vaccine and a cure make the world safe again. Humanity is then back to business-as-usual. In the third scenario called "Global Health Awakening," the crisis leads to the 5p health model: precision, prevention, personalization, partnership and participation. The gains from working and staying at home –cleaner skies and cities, flexible work, slowing down, and the healing benefits of pausing– are not forgotten. Global cooperation, science and artificial intelligence lead to dramatic innovation. The world is transformed. In the fourth scenario, "A Great Despair" ensues. Walls appear, globalization disappears, and the virus mutates. Even though a vaccine is found, the vulnerable do not recover. A decade is lost in meeting the UN Sustainable development goals.

BUT WHAT OF THE ISLAMIC WORLD?

As the Muslim community encompasses a vast region stretching from Jakarta (Indonesia) to Tanja (Morocco), and includes diverse languages, cultures, religions and political systems, anticipating its futures demands a context-sensitive approach. From an Islamic point of view, WHO preventive measures and guidance do not contradict Islamic teaching regarding pandemics. Prophet Muhammad (PBUH) advised: "If you hear of an outbreak of plague in a land, do not enter it; if the plague outbreaks out in a place while you are in it, do not leave that place." [1]

The following are four possible futures: (1) The changing of the guard; (2) the revolution of the youth; (3) Hold the line; and (4) The new planetary Ummah.

THE CHANGING OF THE GUARD

The pandemic creates a seismic change in the geopolitics of the region: Iran sinks – its leadership claims disappear. Saudi Arabia loses its status as the protector of the Holy Sites and the pilgrims due to border closure. Its Legitimacy is further weakened by the steep drop in oil prices. There is a power vacuum. It is far from clear who leads the Islamic world. As the western world reels from the seven-year depression and oil-exporting nations succumb to waves of poverty, nations, which are not saddled with the resource curse, rise. Will it be Turkey? Indonesia? Or Malaysia? The core metaphor for this future is: "Behind every dying Caesar, there is a new one." To articulate this scenario, we present a day in the life of Udday, an Iraqi soldier.

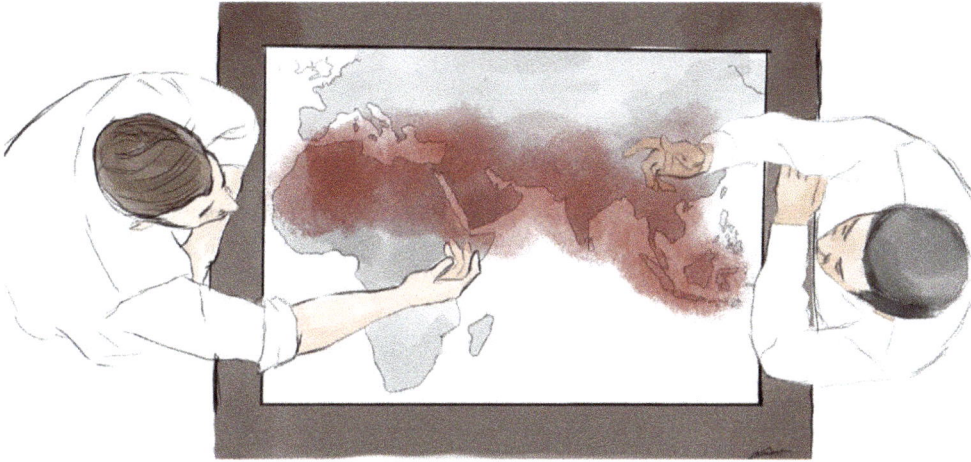

Illustration: Manar Husain

Udday, an Iraqi soldier, is stationed at a border outpost in Diyala Province along the Iranian border. He returns home after months of work in harsh circumstances. He sits down with Zainab, his daughter in the seventh grade, to help with her homework. She is in the process of putting together a digital poster with a title "Turkey: Our reliable ally."

Zainab explains: "I need three points that demonstrate Turkey's support of Iraq and the Ummah. See, I have already collected some information about how Turkey liberated Iraq from Iran's control. I have also prepared excerpts from Turkey's plan to rebuild our economy."

Proudly showing her work to her father, Zainab adds: "If you can help me with the last point, then my task will be completed. The teacher says we have to use an example that illustrates Turkey's role in leading the Ummah."
Udday eyes his wife, Zahra, and sighs "Subhana Allah! The very spot where I am stationed used to be a transit point for Iran's military leaders. Militias, military supplies and trade goods moved freely through our border. We were the corridor all the way to Syria and Lebanon. Now military supplies and most goods come from Turkey."

Zahra responds: "pandemics have the potential to change history. One would wish to see the end of this state of clientelism, but we are still far from it."

In the evening, the family picks the newly released film of Sultan Muhammed Al-Fatih, already dubbed in several languages including Arabic. Their Ottoman table is filled with Turkish tea and Baklava.

THE REVOLUTION OF THE YOUTH

The pandemic – in addition to crises caused by climate change in the decade ahead – results in great decimation, especially in territories already suffering the politics of unelected leaders. No vaccine or cure is found and the virus mutates. Poverty and ill-equipped health services with a lack of preventive action eventually lead to millions of deaths in the Islamic world. Acceptance instead of a transformative strategy becomes the norm. As one Pakistani guard commented: "What can we do about the Coronavirus? One can die of a heart attack. Death is inevitable and it could come at any time.[2] COVID-19 is but the will of Allah."

The youth points out: "While the emergence of the virus was not in human control, the management of the pandemic certainly is. ...Prophet Muhammad advised a man who did not tie his camel because he trusted in God: "tie the camel first and then trust in God".[3]

Even as many veer toward surrender, we can anticipate the youth revolt. As the old die, the power of youth becomes defining. They lead. Tying their camel through both the use of new technologies and development of solidarity with other oppressed groups, they lead the way. The Arab Spring returns with a vengeance. Their uprising is also a health care revolt, as the epidemic exposed the fragility of the health sector and the callousness of many governments towards the basic needs of their populations. As well, the lack of trust in governmental and international organization led to the spread of conspiracy theories – that COVID-19 was a hoax – which again led to system failure (Shakra, 2020).

Zooming in on Egypt, the poetry that was recited in victorious tones in Tahrir Square in 2011, as if the Kali Yuga was over, is back in circulation in hushed tones. People now listen to it or recite it knowing that their grievances have deepened and widened. Hisham Al-Jakh's Joha is one such poem that decries life in Husni

Mubarak's era. Composed in April 2010, Joha goes over many indignities forced upon the people, the watan (nation-state) and the Ummah:

> It is a ridiculous feeling
> When you feel that your watan is something weak
> Your voice is weak
> Your opinion is weak
> When you sell your heart and body
> When you sell your pen and name
> And they do not cover the cost of bread
>
> ...
>
> And it is a ridiculous feeling
> To be a symbol of beggary
>
> ...
>
> I am the owner of the house
> Alive... but useless
>
> ...
>
> Our dignity is insulted
> And the bite comes with humiliation
> What does this mean... when rice husk, a treasure being burned
> And when the Ummah's oil, a treasure being looted
> ... when your executioner crushes his own children
> What does it mean to be jailed for four years as a preventive measure?
> What does it mean to raise our hands welcoming invaders?
>
> ...
>
> Tell me, why don't you feel our being and its preciousness?
> I was going to gift you its sweetness [Al-Jakh, 2017: 63-67].

Instead of the sweetness of life in freedom, dignity and social justice promised by the so-called Arab Spring, bitterness is what people have reaped. Those who compose poetry of the streets keep reminding people of other futures they claim to read from peoples' faces. Tamim Al-Barghouti's "A-Dawla" (The Nation-State, 2016) weaves a parable of power, politics, fear, solidarity and resistance: a hyena attacks at will a flock of gazelles that runs away each time it senses danger, until a fawn unthinkingly decides to fight back. The poet invites his listeners to imagine what would happen if instead of running away out of fear, the flock runs into their attacker. His line "If only the flock changed its direction/All would survive" can constitute the litany of this future. In this future, the young people, infuriated by the obscenities of power, take to the streets, the virtual and the real ones, to demand once again freedom, dignity and justice. People yearn for their voices to be heard and their right to self-determination. They are aware of the brutality of the government's response; yet, they know that communities suffering injustices are all over the globe and work to create a vast network of solidarity that strengthens their fight against oppression.

The core narrative in this future is: In tune with the streets, we will sing and heal. To articulate this scenario, we have a glimpse into the life of Fahima, a nurse and a poet.

Fahima, a twenty-four-year-old nurse, who is employed in a hospital in Boulaq Ad-Dakrour in Giza, returns home after a hard day at work. The working conditions have been beyond bearable for a long time. She checks her YouTube account and sees that her poem in which she compares Egypt to a large collapsing hospital has gone viral. Mahmoud aka MaD, a 19-year- old rapper gets in touch with her asking for her permission to turn the poem into a song. He tells her of his intention to invite other artists, from Mali, the US and other places, to collaborate with him on a project of the large hospital the world has become thanks to the power-addicts. Fahima does not like rap music. She would have rather avoided anything connected with music, especially Western one; yet, she accepts Mahmoud's offer and welcomes the opportunity of working with him. Fahima understands that she needs to reach out to and even learn from other fellow-workers for the same cause. Fahima reads dozens messages notifying her of work to be done in preparation of upcoming protests. She feels exhausted; yet knows that the battle is about to begin. She wonders about her ability to keep it up, but then reiterates the proverb "Forced by circumstances, rather than led by courage." In their sit-in planned for next week, she will wear a mask on which she has stitched "I demand sanity."

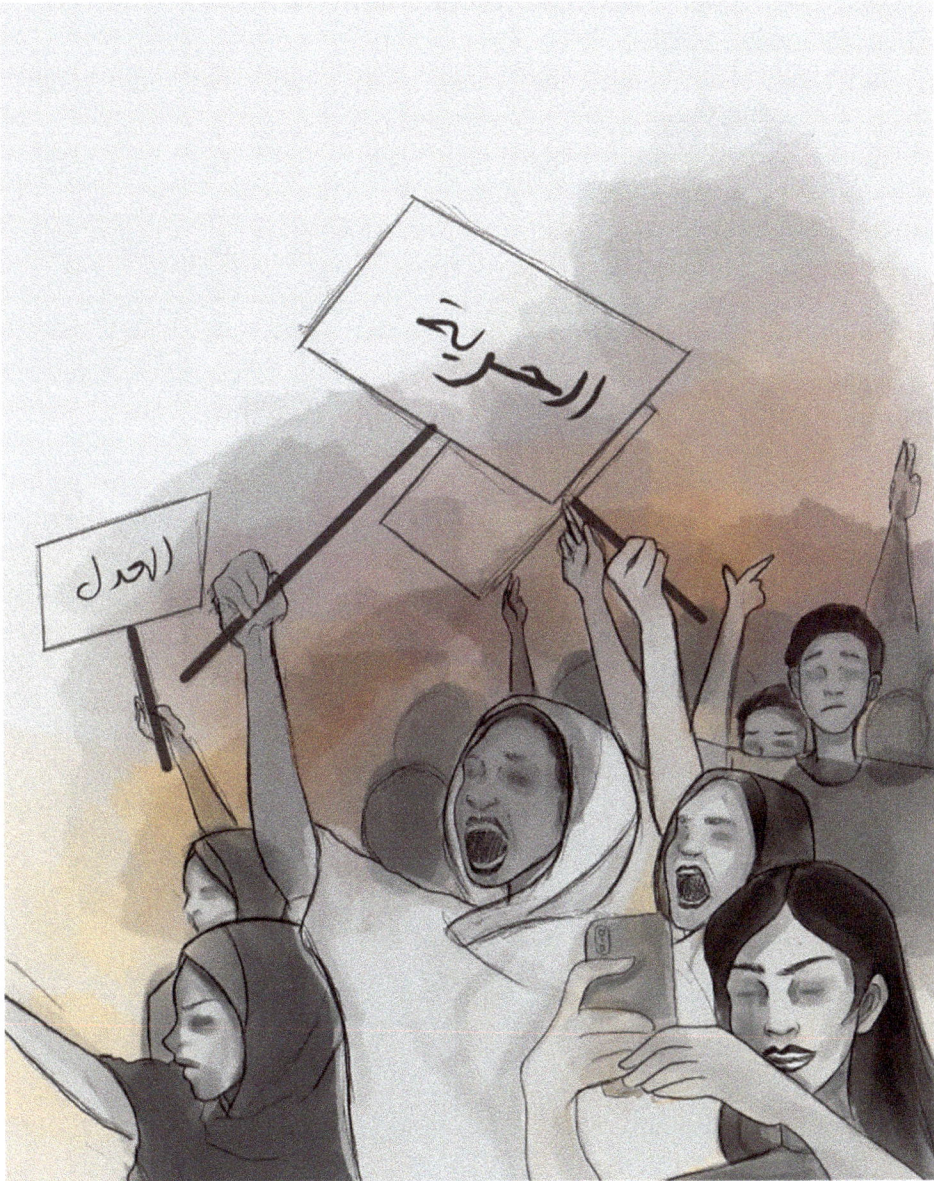

Illustration: Manar Husain – manarhusain17@gmail.com

The demographic challenges as well as the relationship between the youth and civil conflict render this scenario possible, as the following tables illustrate (Financial Times, 2020).

The youth bulge in the Middle East

Total population of selected countries* by age and sex, 1960-2020 (m)

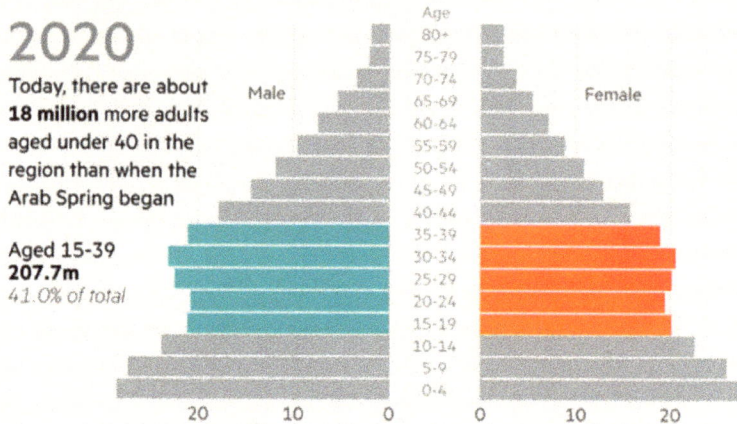

2020

Today, there are about **18 million** more adults aged under 40 in the region than when the Arab Spring began

Aged 15-39
207.7m
41.0% of total

The following table explores the relationship between age structure and intra-state conflict (Cincotta, 2018).

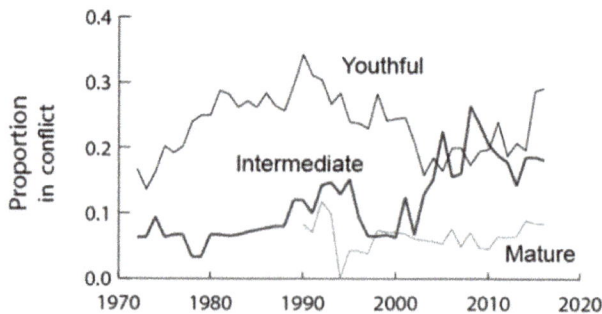

Figure 1. *The proportions of three age-structural groups (youthful, intermediate, mature) in intra-state conflict, 1972 to 2016.*

HOLD THE LINE

Powerful nations in the Islamic world safeguard as much as they can of their power and influence, given the instability in the world economic system. They do their best to continue the status quo. Fearing the revolution of the youth, they offer economic aid to poverty-stricken Muslim nations led by governments perceived as allies. In an attempt to preserve the status quo, the pandemic is used to suppress any form of dissent. Preventive measures are implemented in the name of public health; yet they serve the purpose of deepening control over the population. The metaphor is: still chained to the past.

We describe a day in the life of Jawad, a journalist and a dissenter.

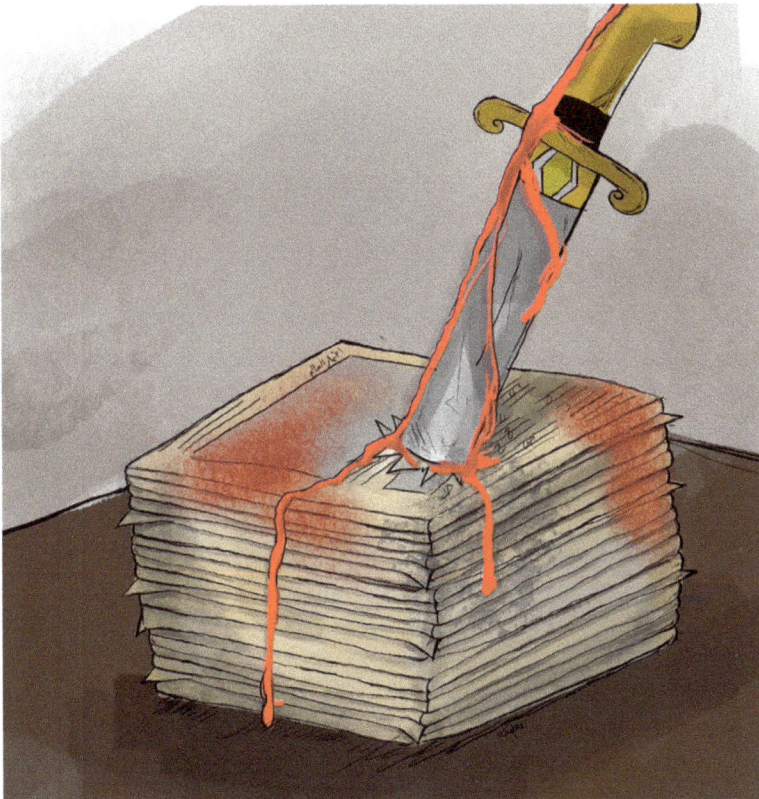

Illustration: Manar Husain – manarhusain17@gmail.com

Jawed, a freelance journalist in The Ummah newspaper, glimpses at the message he receives from the ministry of health. Again it notes prayers at mosques are not allowed until further notice. Jawed understands that so much of daily life has changed with the COVID-19 pandemic. Yet, realizing that the world has to learn to live with it, governments all over the world have introduced ethical and legal norms to regulate life during the pandemic. Some of these norms have lingered despite the end of the crisis. Moreover, many decisions seem to be out of sync with his government's declared intention of protecting citizens. Jawed wonders "Why do mosques continuously swing between opening and closure?"

Jawed composes the number of his best friend and tells him that he has been laid off again. His boss claims that the reason is loss in advertisement revenues and the necessity to reduce the number of staff. Yet, he suspects that his recent articles that question decisions taken by his government cost him his job. Jawed tells his friend to keep him in mind if he hears of any hiring. Before hanging up, he tells his friend: "remember I am a freelance worker in unfree territory, so I can carry bricks too."

THE NEW PLANETARY UMMAH: SCIENCE AND SPIRIT

Research in the late 1990s reveals a shift in the Islamic world: the Ummah with capital U has shown signs of moving toward syncretic Islam. This shift was noticed by Bin Laden and others, who worked hard to end it through bringing believers back to the Wahabi fold. They failed. Fed up with geopolitics, ruthless leaders, and false clerics, Muslims dive deep into spirit. Rumi and his teachings become more important than ever. The Islamic renaissance of science and spirit leads the way in a post-pandemic and post-depression world.

This is the most idealistic scenario. The metaphor is: Call me by my true names

Below is a description of a day in the life of biochemist Malika.

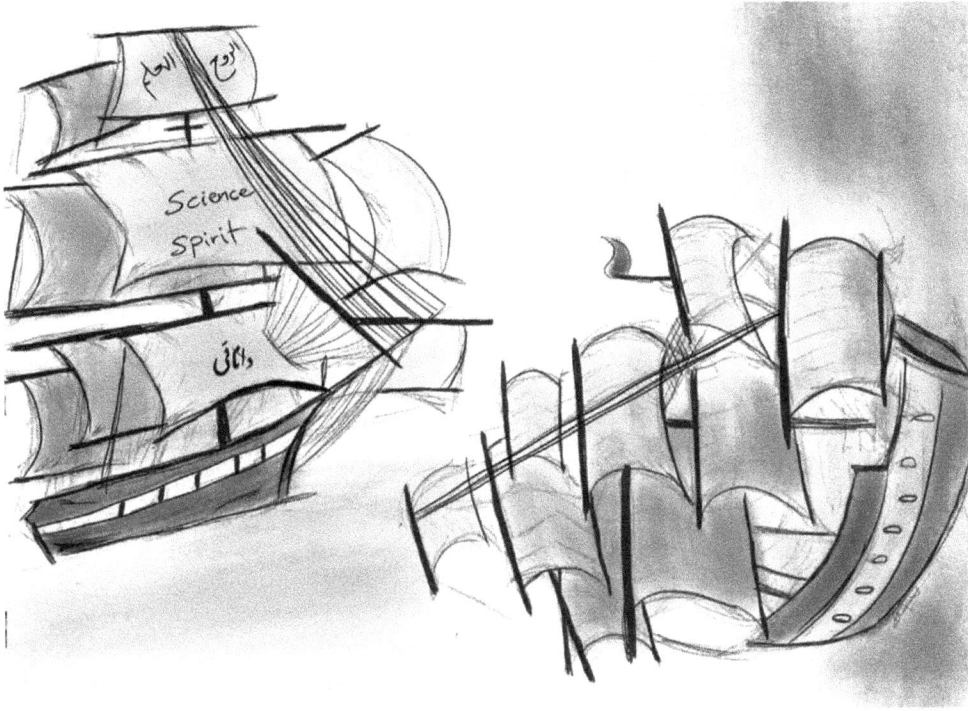

Illustration: Manar Husain – manarhusain17@gmail.com

Malika Nas, a thirty-two -year old researcher in biochemistry and professor of creative methodologies in Ibn-Arabi pluriversity in Fes, is getting ready to pay a visit to her mother, Asma. Malika looks forward to the conversation with her mother, the gathering at the rooftop, the ritual tea after 'Asr prayers and the Qarawiyyin view. At home, Asma is excited about her daughter's visit. While washing spearmint and sage leaves, she thinks back to the time when she felt misunderstood. Her parents used to feel suspicious of digital technology, while she grew up considering it an integral part of life. Asma remembers her vow to do her best to bridge the gap between her and her children when generational differences make communication difficult. Yet, what Malika and her generation have come up with is something that goes against human nature and probably even against Islamic creed. Malika, for instance, speaks of all species making up the larger biosphere as umam (communities; plural of ummah) whose general well-being should be promoted. When Asma pointed out that the term community for non-human species was misplaced, her daughter quoted Chapter 6, Verse 38 from the Qur'an.

Asma realizes that she ignores many important aspects of her religion, yet, she still worries about her daughter's worldview that smells of an identity crisis. Asma decides to tackle again this topic over tea, smiling over the irony of having been accused of the same transgression by her parents. Ah, water has been simmering for a while.

After catching up on the latest news with her daughter, Asma spoke her mind: "You know, Malika, before you were born, the Internet revolution enabled the human race to be connected. We were exchanging information and learning from each other but we were also fighting and sometimes even hating each other! The fighting was inevitable because we insisted on being who we are. We had to resist being kneaded into something wholly alien to where we come from. Such is, anyway, human nature: people crave power and impose their norms on those deemed powerless. I feel that your generation's talks about the planetary Ummah is a major abdication of who you are."

Malika nods and says "Your generation started the important work of putting in place the infrastructure for planetary connection. Yet, your understanding of identity and power as well as privileging the human species led to impoverished politics and impoverished economics and ethics! All what my generation is doing is to extend our identity, reimagine power and engage deep communication with the common biosphere. The results have changed our consciousness. Probably the pandemic outbreak during your time opened our eyes and hearts to the moral debt we owe to each other and to all the creatures with whom we share our planet. Already at the turn of the millennium, neuroscience questioned the understanding of human nature as driven by self-interest and selfishness. Today, we know that terms, such as "interbeing," coined by the Vietnamese poet Thich Nhat Hanh, I think in the 1960s, is not just a flight of fancy but a scientific fact. It is funny, during his time people found Thich Nhat Hanh's ideas esoteric, today when I read "Call me by my true names," where the poet is the bud on a spring branch, the tiny bird, the vulnerable and the powerful, that's me.

Asma sighed: "Were we that wrong?"

Malika: "And if so, then the wound is the place where the light enters you, as Maulana Rumi says. So you gave us the infrastructure, knowledge and the wound that allowed light in. We can't thank you enough."

NEXT STEPS

To create this transformative future, the following steps are necessary:
A shift in perception: The past does not define us, as both the past and the future are equally important. As William Wordsworth poetically put it: "Past and Future are the wings/On whose support, harmoniously conjoined/Moves the great spirit of human knowledge."

- Educational institutions teaching futures literacy
- Confidence in the Islamic world translates into liberation from resorting to the past for defensive purposes and the conviction to use the future to create. Instead of sighing over perceived golden periods or crumbling under the weight of the colonial and neo-colonial wounds, the past can serve as a springboard to imagine future possibilities.
- Massive investment in science and technology
- Leaders who put the Ummah first, and the nation second. Incentives to do this are created. These could be in the form of awards bestowed on leaders who serve their Ummah.

Which scenario will gain traction? This is too difficult to say at this point. Certainly, if life goes back to Business-as-usual, "hold the line is most likely." If we undergo a long recession or depression, then the "Revenge of the youth" is most likely.

However, as the writer Arundhati Roy argues, COVID-19 does not have to be a war, it can be a portal into a better world. Can the Ummah enter through this portal and transform itself and the world into a place where pandemics provide a historical opportunity for soul rejuvenation and planetary justice? If the Ummah does, then a new dawn of science and spirit rising is possible.

Illustration: Manar Husain – manarhusain17@gmail.com

AUTHORS

Khadija El Alaoui, College of Science and Human Studies, Prince Mohammad Bin Fahd University, khalaoui@gmail.com

Sohail Inayatullah, Professor, Tamkang University. UNESCO Chair in Futures Studies, Sejahtera Center for Sustainability and Humanity, Malaysia. Associate, Melbourne Business School. Researcher, Metafuture.org, https://www.metafutureschool.org/

Muamar Salameh, College of Law, Prince Mohammad Bin Fahd University, msalameh pmu.edu.sa

NOTES

[1] https://theconversation.com/how-coronavirus-challenges-muslims-faith-and-changes-their-lives-133925. Accessed 4 May 2020.

[2]https://www.dw.com/en/coronavirus-is-pakistan-taking-COVID-19-too-lightly/a-52824403.Accessed 4 April 2020.

[3]https://theconversation.com/how-coronavirus-challenges-muslims-faith-and-changes-their-lives-133925

REFERENCES

Al-Barghouti, T. (2016). *The Nation-State*. https://www.youtube.com/watch?v=v4Uy6FsAxno.

Al-Jakh, H. (2017). Joha. First Collection. *Dar Ajyal*, 63-67.

Cincotta, R. (2018, April 19). Age-structure and Intra-state Conflict: More or less than we imagined. *New Security Beat*. https://www.newsecuritybeat. org/2018/04/age-structure-intra-state-conflict-imagined/.

Financial Times Reporters. (2020). Middle East's Demographic Earthquake: the generation fueling protests. https://www.ft.com/content/03274532-21ce-11ea- b8a1-584213ee7b2b.

Inayatullah, S. (2016). Youth Bulge: Demographic Dividend, Time Bomb, and other Futures. *Journal of Futures Studies*. 21(2), 21-34.

Inayatullah, S. and Black, P. (2020, March 18)]. Neither Black Swan nor a Zombie Apocalypse. *Journal of Futures Studies*. https://jfsdigital.org/2020/03/18/neither-a-black-swan-nor-a- zombie-apocalypse-the-futures-of-a-world-with-the-COVID-19-coronavirus/.

Madsen, E. L., Daumerie, B., & Hardee, K. (2010). The effects of age structure on development. *Population Action International*. http://populationaction.org/wp-content/uploads/2013/01/Why-Population-Matters- to-Security.pdf.

Middle East Eye (2020, April 16). *Staying home is for the rich: Social distancing is a luxury Egypt's poor can't afford*. www.middleeasteye.net/ news/coronavirus-egypt-social-distancing-poor-cannot-afford.

Roy, A. (2020, April 4). The Pandemic is a portal. *Financial Times*. https://www.ft.com/content/10d8f5e8-74eb-11ea-95fe-fcd274e920ca.

Shakra, E (2020, April 9). *COVID-19 and the Conspiracy Theorists. Asharq Al-Awsat*. https://english.aawsat.com/home/article/2224911/eyad- abu-shakra/COVID-19-and-conspiracy-theorists.

Wordsworth, W. (2004). The Poetical Works of William Wordsworth. Vol. III. T*he Project of Gutenberg*. https://www.gutenberg.org/ files/12383/12383-h/12383-h.htm.

LOOKING FOR ALTERNATIVES UNDER COVID-19 CONDITIONS

Islamic Religious Education in Kazakhstan

Yelena V. Muzykin

FUTURES STUDIES AND FORESIGHT IN KAZAKHSTAN

Futures studies and foresight seem quite established disciplines in the global academic world. Some scholars even trace their origins as far as the futuristic novels by Jules Verne, a French writer publishing in the 1860s and 1870s (Bell, 1996, p. 7). Nevertheless, for Kazakhstan, this is a completely unknown field. The first steps were made in February 2019 when the Qazaq Research Institute for Futures Studies (QRIFS) launched its activities. Making connections with different local organizations, QRIFS established fruitful cooperation with creative companies and educational institutions, public and private sectors, governmental structures, and production industries. After some time, QRIFS work has overcome countries' boarders finding companions in the neighboring "stan" countries. Thus, in July 2020, Central Asian Futures & Foresight Association (CAFFA) came to life. Using the best of the futures and foresight theories and practices, CAFFA grounds its work on the principle of contextuality continually questioning what is done and paying particular attention to places and peoples around. Therefore, narrative foresight (Milojević and Inayatullah, 2015) seems to be an appropriate tool for building alternative perspectives in Central Asia for two reasons. Firstly, it resonates with breakthrough research of neurologists on humans in general, presenting them as symbolic species, i.e., using language to demonstrate a new mode of symbolic thinking (Deacon, 1998). Secondly, the narrative culture expressed in multiple epics and tales is a pivotal point of the nomadic culture in Central Asia (Chadwick and Žirmunskij, 2010).

That is why we are going to concentrate on the "seven questions" method (Milojević and Inayatullah, 2015, p.158) that includes

- What is the history of the issue?
- What is your forecast if current trends continue?
- What are the critical assumptions you used in your forecasts?
- What are some alternative futures based on different assumptions?
- What is your preferred future?
- Which strategies can be used in order to realize your preferred future?
- What is a new narrative or metaphor for your preferred future?

These questions will be applied to Islamic education in Kazakhstan. Its importance becomes evident if we take into account that 70.2 percent of the population considers themselves Muslims (Kazakhstan Demographics Profile, 2019) and 66 percent of the youth in the Republic, the generation of the future, use Islam as an integral component of their identity (Umbetalieva, Rakisheva, and Teschendorf, 2016, p.114). In this context, such questions as "who teaches them?" and "what they learn?" become paramount. Narrative foresight can help launch a more profound reflection on the past and present unleashing imagination to build futures alternatives and come up with a new narrative.

QUESTION 1: HISTORY OF THE PROBLEM

Legitimization of Islam in the Republic during the time of independence raised some urgent issues in religious education. Firstly, during the Soviet era, the system of religious education that existed before was almost destroyed (Derbissali, 2011, p.179). That led to the second problem, namely, the absence of the developed institution of the `ulamā´ or religious scholars. Researchers mention that in 1961, Kazakhstan had only twenty-five registered mosques, and none of the twenty-five imams had tertiary Islamic qualifications (Olcott 2009, 304-305). The lack of qualified Muslim clergy to nurture believers, edify them, and answer questions that naturally immerge during a spiritual quest was obvious.

In the 1990s, when the religious revival began as a reaction to the void after the collapse of the communist ideology, the number of officially registered mosques grew to one thousand. Extra four thousand operated without proper registration due to the almost unhindered religious freedom (Olcott 2009, 304-305). Kazakhstan held the status of the "least repressive post-Soviet Central Asian states with regard to freedom of religion or belief" (Kazakhstan: USCIRF, 2017, p.171). After October 13, 2011, the downward shift happened when President Nazarbayev signed the new legislation on registration requirements for religious organizations. As a result, the number of Islamic organizations and mosques dropped from 2,811 in 2011 to 2,229 in 2012 (Religious Conversions, 2017, p.154). If they were to continue their operation, mosques had to go under the jurisdiction of the Spiritual Administration of Muslims of Kazakhstan (SAMK), a semi-independent and heavily state-controlled body. In 2019 the SAMK had 2629 mosques and 4119 imams registered (Muzykina, 2019).

Where do imams receive formal education that makes them eligible for serving? Currently, Kazakhstan has a three-level structure of local Islamic institutions that focuses on nurturing Islamic clergy and prospective scholars. The first level includes *madrasahs*, a traditional form of education in the Muslim world since the 9th-10th centuries. In Kazakhstan, this form was re-launched in 2009 when the first *Abu Hanifa Madrasah* was opened after almost a hundred years of void in this realm (Derbissali, 2011, pp.194-195). Nowadays, there are nine of them, mostly concentrating in the country's southern regions. They are officially registered with the Ministry of Education of the RK, and their curriculum includes 60 percent of Islamic theological disciplines and 40 percent of general education subjects. Madrasahs' graduates receive a state diploma in Islamic Studies.

The second level includes the Republican Islamic Institute for Imams Advance Training in Almaty. Again, the institution's official state registration took place on April 10, 2002. Local and foreign professors from Turkey and Egypt lecture in Kazakh and Arabica variety of fundamental Islamic theology courses as well as Kazakh Language and History of Kazakhstan (Derbissali, 2011, p.192). Imams graduated with state-recognized certificates *(shahadah)*.

The first two levels' successful graduates can enter Nur-Mubarak Egyptian Islamic Culture University, the first and only one university of a kind in Kazakhstan that was open on September 1, 2001. It is a bilateral project launched and supported by Kazakhstani and Egyptian governments thorough the Board of Trustees supervising its activities (Derbissali, 2011, p.186). The main objective of Nur-Mubarak University is to prepare specialists in Islamic Studies, train imam-khatyb, and enhance the general level of Islamic theology in Kazakhstan.

However, the local research on the problem demonstrates that reform is highly required because 76 % of the experts acknowledged the need for changes (Models of Islamic Education, 2016, pp. 346-358). They argued that the faculty teaching Islamic courses has a low professional level and needs to comply with the world practices taking into account the Kazakhstani context. The latter means the affirmation of Hanafi Madhhab and its role in the Kazakh cultural tradition. This aspiration is a result of a top-down promotion of the "Hanafi Project" to safeguard Hanafi orthodoxy in Kazakhstan and secure the country from the intervention of "radical forces" (Karimov 2018, 300-312). The propaganda started in the early 2000s reflecting a reductionist plan of shrinking Islam to a nationalistic element of a secular doctrine when practicing believers face growing ostracism in society.

Moreover, the statistics also say that among more than 4,000 acting Muslim ministers, only 545 (13%) had higher education in 2016 (Religion Becomes a Required and Positive Factor 2016). No surprise that Kazakhstani secular authorities and ordinary people express concern about the educational and intellectual level of imams in mosques around Kazakhstan (Bondal 2019).

Summing up, ambivalence marks the history of the issue. On the one hand, Kazakhstan has built its Islamic educational system from scratch after the Soviet regime almost destroyed it. There are three levels of Islamic educational institutions functioning in the Republic. Before the COVID-19, the enrollment was growing, keeping the gender balance among the students.

On the other hand, the state is the main initiator of any change in the education system. It closely watches all religious educational programs through different Ministries and sets the standards for Islamic education. Only graduates with a state diploma from a state-accredited institution can get a job within the SAMK system that is entirely accountable to the state.

QUESTIONS 2&3: THE CURRENT STAGE AND ASSUMPTIONS

Therefore, from the perspective of narrative foresight, the metaphor that can describe the current situation with Islamic education in Kazakhstan can sound like this:

> In 2020, Islamic education in Kazakhstan looks like a prisoner bound hand and foot, forced to follow his taskmaster. He is poorly fed, has no perspective for freedom, and is frequently turned into a scapegoat whenever needed to switch public attention from economic or political downfalls and collapse.

Following up, if the trends described above continue, then by 2041, most of the imams in Kazakhstan can receive only local training, and we can assume the following:

1. The quality of that education will be quite low;

2. The curriculum will be narrowly focused that can lead to worldview dogmatization;

3. Restrictive measures and close control of religious educational institutions will grow;

4. A desire to go abroad and get an education there, e.g., in Turkey or Egypt will increase among potential students;

5. As a reaction, the so-called "foreign" Islam will gain the ground in the Republic, thus provoking counteractions from the government.

6. Nevertheless, let us think about some alternative perspectives and scenarios for Islamic education in Kazakhstan.

QUESTIONS 4: RECOUNTING ALTERNATIVE FUTURES

To imagine some possible scenarios of the Islamic education future, we will use the method developed by Jim Dator and his colleagues at the Manoa School (Dator, 2009). Instead of building scenarios from scratch, the approach suggests some context for integrating seven essential components (population, energy, economy, environment, culture, technology, and governance). Their quality leads to four types of generic futures (Foresight Manual, 2018, p.37):

1. "Continued Growth" (acceleration of the present);

2. "Collapse" (extinction or a lower stage of the present);

3. "Discipline" (highly controlled/regulated future);

4. "Transformation" (radical transformation of life, including humanity).

In addition to these four defined contexts, we will add the COVID-19 factor and see what alternative images can come up.

Reviving *Khalīfah* attitude. The global community has successfully won the battle against COVID-19, and the world now can unmask and breathe in deeply Students go back to their studies. The pandemic time triggered the revival of such a key Islamic concept as khalīfah or viceregency of humans on the Earth There were multiple voices in Muslim societies around the world that COVID-19 was a punishment from Allah because humans have forsaken their duties of the Earth stewards. Now Kazakhstani educators and researches are making a unique contribution to the revival of this concept. They launched a new international educational platform that unified all known works of Al-Farabi, a prominent Central Asian Muslim thinker of the 9th-10th centuries C.E., the author of *Mabādi´a ārā´ ahl al-madīnat al-fā´ilah (On the Perfect State)*. In that tract, he discussed many highly sought-after today ideas of building a society of happiness and prosperity based on Islamic principles. The *khalīfah* concept has become foundational not only for future imams but all Islamic professionals who receive their education at different universities around Kazakhstan.

Quest for *Karāmah*. Even the second lockdown and strict quarantine measures did not help Kazakhstan to overcome widespread COVID-19. After the country's economy sank into the deepest crisis, the society drowned in depression. People are looking for condolence and comforting. Mosques have become the primary centers for the spiritual-emotional help. Their nurturing and educational activity focuses on *karāmah* or a concept of dignity. It encompasses acknowledging themselves as Allah's creations, submitting to Him, following His commands, and striving for the restoration of social well-being. Though the attendance of religious places is still limited, the SAMK initiative group and some former professors of Nur-Mubarak University – they lost their jobs like many others – have developed and launched the educational platform *Hikmatan Wāsia*. It hosts Islamic courses of different complexity, and anyone can receive a state-accredited diploma in Islamic Studies upon passing online exams. Thus, helping others build their dignity, former public institutions professors found the way to keep their *karāmah*.

Revisiting ʻIlm Al-Akhlāk. The pandemic has seriously affected the economy of Kazakhstan. It did not collapse but barely survives. Therefore, the government imposed strong restrictions and control on all spheres of life. To legitimize Islam in the secular society, Kazakhstani Muslim scholars focus on the ethical norms of the religion, promoting them in teaching courses and public debates. A high interest arose in the society, especially among the youth, to a "science of virtues" [ʻilm al-akhlāk] that deals with proper conduct, personal character, and such qualities as self-mastery, justice, temperance, honesty, uprightness, and courage. Young people are not satisfied with the "traditional Islam" version promoted by government officials, state-controlled madrasahs, and universities. The underground movement is gradually emerging betting on *akhlāk* as a foundation for a new society to come. Members of that movement [akhlāqiyūn] are primarily known for reviving and popularizing the ancient art of calligraphy and miniature. Being denied access to printing and publishing facilities, they create handmade leaflets and posters that propagate their ideas.

Hi-tech *Mawāhib*. The pandemic COVID-19 served like a break time to reconsider the human-AI balance pushing tremendously the coming of the singularity era that Ray Kurzweil initially predicted for 2045. With its critical breakthroughs in biomedicine and AI technologies, Kazakhstan turned into a central AsiaEuro transit point linking South-East countries with the rest of the world. Now Muslim societies of Asia-Pacific are on the global frontline. Therefore, Islamic education in Kazakhstan focuses on Islamic Finance and Banking, Islamic Biomedicine, Chemistry, and Programming. Being integrated into the GlobalMuslimEdNet learning system, Kazakhstani Islamic institutions have access to all necessary resources that make their students top-level professionals. The system includes all the latest innovations, scientific projects, emerging technologies, and other things that come accompanied with legal judgments of the best Muslim *fuqaha* [jurists] who now widely use Big Data and AI in their work. The Al Sheikh Azamat_

KAZ that represents the Kazakhstani scholars' opinions, is highly respected for its consistency and progressive views. This systemic approach is a real *mawāhib*, the contribution to and of the Muslim world in this new transformed reality.

QUESTIONS 5-6: ENVISIONING THE PREFERRED AND MOVING THERE

Now, we have reached a crossroad with several options, and like an ancient knight-vityaz in Russian fairytales have to choose what route to take. In other words, we need to answer the question, "What will be preferable future?" Norman Henchey, a Canadian futurist, defines the preferable future as what we want to have happened (Henchey 1978). It does not yet exist and requires a clear vision that moves reality beyond the present toward the best possible. To make it speak to people's hearts, we can summarize it as a vision statement that will help move forward.

Therefore, the preferred future for Islamic education in Kazakhstan can sound like this:

> By 2041, Islamic education in Kazakhstan becomes a beacon of religious education in the Muslim world due to its critically innovative approach and radical reform in the education system. Graduates of this system are firmly rooted in the classical Islamic heritage yet actively contribute to the development of the contemporary Muslim thought that reflects the needs of a rapidly changing world, providing believers with a stronghold in times of turbulent uncertainties. A modern imam is a polymath that widely uses technology to fulfill God's will.

For someone, it might sound like a fiction introduction. However, specific steps can take place today to make the preferable future real using it and paving the path to it. Of course, the list of potential steps is not exhaustive, but include the paramount points:

- Kazakhstan establishes a genuine state-religion separation secured through the legislation and the Constitution, thus promoting the execution of authentic religious liberty;
- The Ministry of Education and the Ministry of Justice of the Republic

of Kazakhstan collaborate on developing new requirements for religious, educational institutions registration, thus ensuring their variety – from state-sponsored to private and independent;
- The curriculum of Islamic educational institutions includes futures literacy and futures studies that empower the youth to get ready for changes, generate them, and use the future to innovate the present;
- The SAMK system is reconsidered and changed; imams obtain a renewed status in the society that focuses on their personal, spiritual, professional, and civic traits and rights, not only duties.

CLOSING WITH QUESTION 7

Now, if things work right, a new metaphor for Islamic education can sound very inspiring:

> By 2041, Islamic education in Kazakhstan is like Ibn Battuta, the Space-Traveler that merges the best of the heritage and the most innovative of the present to create an unthinkable future.

This statement points out how the reform of Islamic religious education in Kazakhstan may go, thus bringing crucial changes to the spiritual life of the whole country in the long run. Through narrative foresight, the process can become more personalized and internalized, bring new perspectives and metaphors that will ensure the success of the endeavor. The very nature of narrative foresight can awake the creative component that Islamic educational organizations in the Republic and the Muslim world, in general, should promote in knowledge acquisition and production.

REFERENCES

Bell, W. (2004). *Foundations of futures studies: human science for a new era*. Transaction Publ.

Bizhanov A. (Ed.). (2017). *Religioznyye konversii v postsekulyarnom obshchestve: opyt fenomenologicheskoy rekonstruktsii [Religious Conversions in a Post-Secular Society: The Attempt of Phenomenological Reconstruction]*. Institute of Philosophy, Political Science, and Religious Studies.

Bondal, X. (2017, May 10). *Kazakhstantsy obespokoyeny urovnem religioznykh znaniy sredi imamov [Kazakhstanis are concerned with the level of religious knowledge among imams]*. KARAVANSARAI. http://central.asia-news.com/ru/articles/cnmi_ca/features/2017/05/10/feature-01

Chadwick, N. K., & Žirmunskij, V. M. (2010). *Oral Epics of Central Asia*. Cambridge University Press.

Dator, J. (2009). Alternative Futures at the Manoa School. *Journal of Futures Studies*, 14(2), 1-18.

Deacon, T. W. (1998). *The Symbolic Species: The Co-Evolution of Language and the Brain*. W.W. Norton & Company.

Derbissali, A. (2011). *Religious Educational Establishments of Kazakhstan*. Atamura.

Henchey, N. (1978). Making Sense of Future Studies. *Alternatives*, 7 (2), 24-27.

Index Mundi. (2019). *Kazakhstan Demographics Profile*. https://www.indexmundi.com/kazakhstan/demographics_profile.html

Karimov, N. (2018). A Contested Muslim Identity in Kazakhstan: Between Liberal Islam and the Hanafi Project. *Cultural and Religious Studies*, 6 (5), 300-312. DOI: 10.17265/2328-2177/2018.05.004

Milojević, I., Inayatullah, S. (2015). Narrative foresight. *Futures*, 73, 151-162. DOI: 10.1016/j.futures.2015.08.007

Muzykina, Y. (2019, September 05). *Private correspondence with the Spiritual Administration of Muslims of Kazakhstan*. E-mail letter.

Olcott, M. B. (2009). Kazakhstan. In J. Esposito (Ed.), *The Oxford Encyclopedia of the Islamic World* (Vol. 3, pp. 304-307). Oxford University Press.

Religiya Stanovitsya Neobkhodimym I, Bezuslovno, Pozitivnym Faktorom Razvitiya Gosudarstva [Religion becomes a required and certainly positive factor of state development]. (February, 2016). *INTERFAX Kazakhstan*. https://www.interfax.kz/?lang=rus&int_id=13&news_id=276

Smagulov M.N. (2017). Sotsiologicheskoye izmereniye islamskogo obrazovaniya v svetskom Kazakhstane: k voprosu modelirovaniya kachestvennoy modeli obrazovaniya [Sociological dimension of Islamic education in secular Kazakhstan: on the issue of modeling a qualitative educational model] In A. Bizhanov [Ed.] *Modeli islamskogo obrazovaniya v postsekulyarnom obshchestve: yevraziyskiye i yevropeyskiye trendy [Models of Islamic Education in a Postsecular Society: Eurasian and European Trends]* [pp. 345-360]. Institute of Philosophy, Political Science, and Religious Studies. http://iph.kz/doc/ru/1250.pdf

Umbetalieva, T. B., Rakisheva, B., & Teschendorf, P. [2016]. *Youth in Central Asia: Kazakhstan: Based on Sociological Survey.* Friedrich Ebert Stiftung [Kazakhstan]. https://library.fes.de/pdf-files/bueros/kasachstan/13343.pdf

UNDP Global Centre for Public Service Excellence. [2018, January]. *Foresight Manual. Empowered Futures for the 2030 Agenda.* United Nations Development Program. https://www.undp.org/publications/foresight-manual-empowered-futures

United States Commission on International Religious Freedom [2017]. Kazakhstan. *Annual Report of the United States Commission on International Religious Freedom.* U.S. Commission on International Religious Freedom, 170-175. www.uscirf.gov/sites/default/files/Kazakhstan.2017.pdf

THE SIGNIFICANCE OF FUTURES SCENARIO PLANNING IN ASSURING VIABILITY OF HIGHER EDUCATION IN DISRUPTIVE CRISES:

A Case Study of Universiti Teknikal Malaysia Melaka in Response to the COVID-19

Fazidah Ithn

The Novel Coronavirus or COVID-19 pandemic caught the world by surprise, even though many futurists and emerging infectious diseases experts had anticipated the 'seeds of the Corona', or the weak signals for a decade. What appeared impossible to the general comprehension, suddenly becomes plausible. The world is pushed towards a new normal that demands reeducation of norms.

The pandemic is catastrophic to humans and the whole ecosystem, in essence, the virus, may be invisible in nature but is extremely invincible to the politics, economics and social landscape of the world – henceforth, disrupting the otherwise operational future. For higher education providers, a new narrative ensues. The metaphor of universities as ivory towers has become a passé seriously challenged. Online learning which was delineated as one of the preferred futures in the beginning of the decade reigns supreme replacing the litany of face to face teaching and learning. Ensuring viability during the crisis period, Universiti Teknikal Malaysia Melaka (UTeM) reviewed the precision and significance of its scenario planning circa 2012.

In essence, substantial key outputs mapped through the CLA and integrated scenario approach, embedded in its Strategic Plan 2012-2020 had proven compelling in sustaining UTeM's operations. This testimony has resulted in the implementation of similar approach to the formulation of UTeM's Strategic Direction for the next decade.

Keywords: Higher education; Causal layered analysis; Scenario planning; Behavior; Science; Technology; Futures; Foresight

INTRODUCTION

Pandemics trigger radical changes in human behavior in all aspects. The COVID-19 pandemic is a catastrophic crisis of infinite magnitude for humanity.

Prospecting the futures of higher education, the immediate challenge is for institutions of higher learning worldwide to continue their relevance and operations within the learners status quo of where they are, within the infrastructure and setting they are in. This predicament requires hefty innovation and creativity that may not have been thought of. Remote learning tools, services and education surfaced at an exponential rate throughout the Movement Control Order as universities began to review their state of preparedness. Can universities remain relevant? Can remote learning or online learning parallel the conventional asynchronous learning? Are lecturers prepared with adequate knowledge and technical know-how to deliver classes online and offline while simultaneously providing students avenues for experiential learning? Are syllabi online-friendly? Can laboratory work and teaching-factory simulations be conducted virtually? Can administrative and academic staff be just as productive 'fishing from home'? As the future sees the importance of a balanced work and personal life as a catalyst to high- impact productivity and accelerated performance (Inayatullah & Ithnin, 2018), the foresighted future scenarios are not yet inclined towards this. Will the COVID-19 epitomize just as a pause button or will it kindle a justified norm towards a transformative shift in an organization's operations or will it return to business as usual, especially when states still do not support employees in this process as trust is a factor (Inayatullah & Black, 2020). The onset of the COVID-19 which has closed more than half of Malaysia's small and medium enterprises and almost certainly plunged the country into recession, is exacerbating the outlook for a university sector already in deep trouble (Hunter 2020).

This study is aimed at reviewing the salient outputs of the futures literacy and anticipatory foresight round table conducted by UTeM in 2012 and their omnipotence in ensuring the sustainability of university operations, specifically during the disruptive COVID-19 crisis. Analysis of pre and post scenario planning of UTeM as a higher technical and vocational education training provider were studied, the results of which became the determinant for the University to adopt a similar approach for its next decade's strategic planning direction.

The prelude to futures scenario planning in 2012 involved various levels of stakeholders, namely members of the Board of Directors, University senior management, deans and directors of faculties and offices, alumni and students. Images of the preferred technical university of the future were visualized, among others, through the causal layered analysis method which provided a platform in creating transformative spaces for the creation of alternative futures (Inayatullah, 2004). The consolidation of data and responses were documented into the University's 8-year Strategic Plan 2012-2020, which in essence would end in 2020. With the Strategic Plan's timeline culminating at the end of the year, UTeM had started the review process at the onset of 2020 and three months into the mapping of UTeM's next decade, the COVID-19 pandemic inundated. Embodying the intervention of a crisis, the COVID19 became a test-bed scenario for the predominance of foresight in ensuring a resilient strategy and providing a systematic framework towards the preferred future for UTeM.

The research process involved a review of the existing Strategic Plan followed by a comparative analysis of tangibles from the pre and post 2012 discourse and the canvassing of the University's way forward 2021-2025.

2. LITERATURE REVIEW

The capacity of a university in times of disruptive crises has been a cause for concern for higher education providers worldwide. University operations which include teaching, learning and assessment must be crisis-proof. Kernohan (2020) asserted that in the more specific context of universities, academics as higher education providers have been thrust headlong into providing for their students exclusively via a digital interface. Watermeyer et al (2020) pointed out that perhaps more than this, the experience of rapid online migration of learning, teaching and assessment has revealed much of the deficiencies of the higher education sector and much perhaps of what needs to change in universities. COVID-19 crisis, like nothing else before it, is articulating the severity of social and economic inequality and fomenting also a reconsideration, even refutation of the kinds of social stratification and democratic infringements (Zuboff, 2019) committed by global capitalism—and equally mobilizing the restitution and reclamation of the public sphere—so too is it magnifying the egregious faults and failures of universities (as explicitly, even now unapologetically neoliberalised organisations) and with such force that they may no longer be hidden or defended. Wang and M. Hutchins (2010) asserted that for administrators of educational institutions, it is crucial to develop an effective strategic plan that would likely prevent the occurrence of a crisis event or minimize the impact if one occurs. Inayatullah & Ithnin (2018) affirmed that it is imperative for organizations to envisage the future through the mapping of time – where we have come from and where we are heading next and in so doing, the unknowns are incorporated into decision making.

3. INCEPTING FUTURES THINKING IN THE HIGHER EDUCATION SETTING

Robert Greenleaf (1996, 170), who popularized the term "servant leader", esteemed foresight as "the 'lead' that a leader has, the possession of which is one of the bases of trust of followers, is that she or he cares more, prepares better, and foresees more clearly than others". Futures thinking, therefore, incites a future-oriented mindset, that challenges operational thinking through a systematic method of exploring alternative futures. In the case of UTeM, the need to catalyze new capabilities and incubate new possibilities resulted in the need to draft the Strategic Plan 2012-2020. Transformative leadership and breakthrough capacities were enabled through a 3-day foresight workshop which adopted the Six Pillars Approach Scenario Planning. The vision foresighted in the anticipatory futures planning workshop was for a preferred technical university of the future. The strategic directions then were skewed towards current trends in globalization, mobility, international collaborations, evolution in learning and teaching, optimum use of technology, global university best practices, student entrepreneurial attributes and community outreach (Inayatullah, S. & Ithnin, F., 2018).

While stakeholders concurred that UTeM will continue to offer market driven technical-based programmes, concerns of sustainable growth seeped in as the concept of a disowned future foreshadowed unto UTeM (Inayatullah & Ithnin, 2018). In search of alternative futures, the participants presented several preferred visioning and scenarios through the Causal Layered Analysis (CLA) (Inayatullah, 2020) which featured the four variables of litany, systemic, worldview and myth/metaphor. The futures approach has been about using the future to rethink and eventually re-create the present. The conviction is based on the assumption that while we live in a world of imperfect information and the future in particular is uncertain by using the views of many in the context of structured foresight methods, enhanced our ability to map and create desired futures.

CLA unpacks the future at four distinct levels. This method and theory of knowledge seeks to deepen the future [Inayatullah, 2007]. Understandably for UTeM, the futures included all four levels: data to measure the new desired future, systemic changes, mindset shifts, and new metaphors.

Table 1. Causal Layered Analysis [CLA] of UTeM's Futures 2012-2020

Causal Layered Analysis of UTeM's Futures			
	UTeM SOHO	UTeM@Apps University	University-Industry Integrated	UTeM Open University
Litany	UTeM staff spends more quality time with their family, resulting in savings of utilities and space.	Academic programmes offered by UTeM becomes available globally, functional and accredited internationally	UTeM leads in industry-driven and advanced technologies in collaboration with strategic industries in Malaysia.	UTeM offers higher education opportunities to all regardless of qualification, financial status, geographic location, age and abilities – indirectly promoting personal and professional growth in the society.
Systemic	Implementation of new policies, enforcing staff monitoring systems and discipline.	Programmes need to comply with needs of industries and duly accredited by international accreditation bodies.	Hosting industries within the university environment also known as the 'Teaching Factory' model. Industries providing factory-scale equipment for teaching and learning.	Advancement of technology & infrastructure. The need to establish a framework to support staff development.
Worldview	Out of sight, out of responsibility.	Globally recognized university and global graduate employability.	University educate; industry trains.	Internationalization of industry-based learning.
Myth/ Metaphor	Fishing from home	UTeM On-Deck	Partners for growth, 'Together as one'.	Mangrove Ecosystem
Strategy	Retain the dedicated staff and provide suitable incentives to encourage performance.	Attract top academics and students globally. Invest in latest technologies and teaching and learning facilities.	Organize structured collaborations with industries. Invite leaders of industries as academic programme advisory panels.	Introduce broad-based academic programmes alongside focused-based existing programmes. Invest in innovative teaching and learning infrastructure.

In essence, the CLA was aligned to the University's Strategic Plan 2012-2020 document. Resources were amalgamated towards prioritized sectors. UTeM Small Office Home Office (SOHO), UTeM@Apps University, University-Industry Integrated and UTeM Open University, all skewed towards an anomalous future. Ironically, these four visions have actualized as the best-case scenarios of higher education in the post COVID-19 which entails renewed norms in the daily operations of the university.

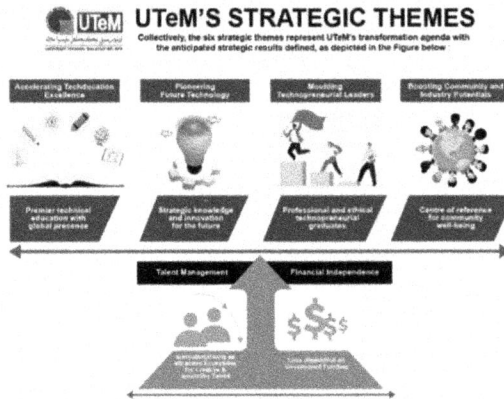

Figure 1. UTeM's Strategic Direction (2012-2020)

4. PUSHES FOR CHANGE: HIGHER EDUCATION IN THE POST COVID-19

As the globe revolves with pushes of uncertainties, the COVID-19 disrupted the higher education landscape like no other. Prior to the pandemic, intellectuals around the world identified various disruptors in the like of climate change, change due to digital age, disruptive technologies brought by industry 4.0, global competition due to globalization and global economic crisis. A lethal virus was the least likely factor.

On 31 December 2019, the Wuhan City Health Committee (2019) reported a cluster of 27 pneumonia cases stemming from an unknown etiology, with a preliminary source linking this to the now closed Wuhan Huanan Seafood Wholesale Market.

This was later determined to be a novel coronavirus (2019-nCoV) or COVID-19. Since then, there has been substantial growth across the globe. According to the World Health Organization (2020a), on 31 March 2020, there have been 697,244 confirmed cases with 33,257 deaths (4.77% mortality rate). The World Health Organization (2020b) has declared COVID-19 a pandemic. The top ten countries by reported cases are: China, Italy, United States of America, Spain, Germany, Iran, France, South Korea, Switzerland, and United Kingdom (World Health Organization, 2020a).

Malaysia was labelled "by far the worst-affected COVID-19 country in Southeast Asia" (New Straits Times, 2020b). In response to the alarming increase of infections in Malaysia, Prime Minister Muhyiddin banned all non-essential social activities (including religious, sport, social, and cultural events) from 18-31 March to combat the spread of COVID-19 under a nationwide Movement Control Order.

As of 16 March 2020, the response by most of Malaysia's 20 public universities was to encourage or mandate online learning (Lim, 2020), using live streaming on Facebook or YouTube, Light board Video Technology, Zoom, or in-house e learning platforms (Lim, 2020; Ramadan, 2020; Teoh, 2020; Universiti Malaysia Sarawak, 2020). This approach can be viewed as a fragmented approach to achieving higher education learning and teaching quality. This includes assessment strategies such as lab research continuing to be allowed at Universiti Kebangsaan Malaysia and Universiti Malaysia Terengganu; face-to-face lectures going on as usual at Universiti Utara Malaysia and International Islamic University Malaysia; or Universiti Malaysia Perlis banning their students from leaving campus without express permission (Lim, 2020).

After the nationwide closure of all public and private institutions of higher learning, Malaysia's Ministry of Higher Education took the unusual step to also prohibit all digital learning activities on 17 March (Asia Pacific University of Technology & Innovation, 2020). Both public universities and private higher education institutes are forbidden to conduct "any Teaching and Learning activities including in online mode, as well as examinations, vivas, student development and research activities" during the above-mentioned Restricted Movement Period (Asia Pacific University of Technology and Innovation, 2020).

Face-to-face classes at local universities were supported by online strategies, galvanizing a sudden EdTech boom. Universities use web-conferencing platforms such as Zoom, Webinar, and Panopto, partially as contingency measures, and partially integrated into their learning management systems. At UTeM, the alternative future of University@Apps parlayed in 2012 had aptly prepared the University towards this scenario. Structurally planned virtual or online-based programmes were designed; a full office to oversee e-learning was established on 26 April 2013. Massive Open Online Courses (MOOCs) were initiated and offered. Focused budget for expansion of information structure for online learning management system or U-Learn has since been prioritized.

5. COVID-19 PANDEMIC: THE WEIGHTS OF TECHNOLOGY-ENABLED EDUCATION

Higher Education worldwide has been in crisis since the onset of the COVID-19 due to the closure of schools and universities in over 188 countries which was aimed at "flattening the curve". This scenario took 91% (1.6 billion) of the world's students out of their classrooms of which 574 million of them are in the Commonwealth countries (UNESCO statistics, 2020). Funding dilemma hit universities exponentially especially the private universities of which depended highly on enrolment of international students.

The COVID-19 crisis confirmed the indispensability of technology-enabled education via distance and virtual learning. As Universities and schools moved from education in the classroom to education at home, Malaysia, as with many other countries were ill-prepared to do so. Enforcing the use of alternative technologies in areas without internet or electricity would be unfavorable. The pandemic has widened the inequalities of educational opportunities between the have and have nots. Teachers and lecturers are not adequately trained yet to do online learning and many countries were not adequately prepared to provide alternative technologies to educate students who do not have access to the internet (Ismail, 2020).

Online education is a complex issue. It is important to set realistic understandings and expectations of how it can support students affected by COVID-19 constraints.

Universities are not progressing strategic moves to online teaching. Rather, they are moving to emergency online delivery of in-person content (Crawford et al., 2020). On the contrary, UTeM had, by design, prepared for this digital shift earlier in 2012 through an intensive CLA discourse and was followed suit by a structured implementation plan. The setting up of the Centre for Instructional Resources and Technology (CIRT) which oversees the complete operations of online and remote learning enables consistent digitization of University courses. The table below presents the comparative data of UTeM's eLearning preparedness prior and post Futures Scenario Planning exercise

Table 2. Massive Open Online Courses (MOOCS) at UTeM (2015-2020)

2012-2014	2015	2016	2017	2018	2019	2020
Planning and Development of MOOCs post Scenario Planning Workshop	1) Critical & Creative Thinking (BLHC4032)	1) Technology Entrepreneurship (BTMW4012)	1) Japanese Language Studies (BLHL1312)	1) Numerical Methods (BEKG 2452)	1) Mechanical Vibration (BMCG 3233)	1) Arabic Language Studies (BLHL1112)
	2) Mandarin 1 (BLHL1212)	2) Programming Technique (BITP1113)	2) IT Security (BITP3433)	2) Motion Graphic (BITE3623)	2) Research Methodology (PPSW 6013)	2) Efficient Energy Management (UTeM Staff)
	3) Database (DITP1333)	3) Multimedia Systems (BITM1113)	3) Malaysia University English Test (MUET)	3) Principles of Electrical & Electronic (BETA1313)	3) Green Technology and Environment (BKKM 1931)	3) Green Sustainability Practices (BKKM 1911)

The data in Table 1 depicts the gradual shift from conventional teaching and learning to digitized learning; 2012 being the impetus of transformation with implementation of the first three courses in 2015, culminating to 18 MOOCs in 2020.

Blended Learning was introduced in 2016 at a meagre 2% implementation but sharply fortified through the years, eventually pitching at a strong execution of 84% in 2020.

Table 3. Percentage of Blended Learning at UTeM (2016-2020)

2016	2017	2018	2019	2020 (as at July 2020)
Sem. 2 15/16	Sem. 2 16/17	Sem. 2 17/18	Sem. 2 18/19	Sem. 2 19/20
2 %	61%	58%	80%	84%
Sem. 1 – 16/17	Sem. 1 17/18	Sem. 1 18/19	Sem. 1 19/20	
48 %	52%	76%	87%	

Publication of iBooks to complement the available physical resources at UTeM's libraries were also amplified. As students become more gadget-dependent during the pandemic-quarantined period, references too, as envisioned in the 2012 scenario exercise of the University, must be made apps-friendly. The process started with only four iBooks in 2014 and as at 2020, UTeM has since produced more than 35 iBooks which proved handy to the needs of the students who were logistically distant at their respective districts during the COVID-19 pandemic.

The significance of virtual learning had been projected through presentation of the CLA and the Integrated Scenario model, specifically, the Preferred scenario, Disowned scenario, Integrated scenario and Outlier scenario in the 2012 Futures Scenario Workshop. Through this Integrated Scenario model, the impossible can then become if not the plausible, at least the probable (Inayatullah, 2018).

Preferred	Disowned
-Number of preferred programs relevant to the global industry -Advanced infrastructure with global recognition -World Leading virtual technical university **Metaphor – global brain**	-Identity trade-off -Less hands-on -Lost human touch and soft skills, no physical assessment **Metaphor –brain drain**
Integrated	Outlier
-Competitive paid salary globally -Sharing resources globally/global franchise -Global Industrial based program with GLOCAL flavor. **Metaphor – networking brain**	-Limited programs meeting industry needs -Conventional way of delivery methods -Less presence felt **Metaphor – brain death**

Figure 2. Apps University (Virtual University)

Note. From Transformation 2050: The Alternative Futures of Malaysian Universities (p.43), by Sohail Inayatullah and Fazidah Ithnin, 2018, Malaysia, USIM Press.

The compelling image of the "university in a gadget" implies an "app-based university", similar to a mobile application of which UTeM is envisioned to be a university which is easily accessible and easy to use (Ithnin et al., 2017). The framework to reinforce the emergence of the nomadic, mobile learners who are dependent not on the teacher or formal education systems but on the network of knowledge and skills that are within reach - anywhere and anytime has been in place and continually developed since 2012.

6. DISCUSSION: THE PROCESS OF CHANGE (BEHAVIOR, SCIENCE AND TECHNOLOGY)

Deconstructing the normalcy of the past, scenario planning directs our thinking towards foreseeable alternative futures that remind us that while we cannot predict a particular future always accurately, by focusing on a range of alternatives, we can better prepare for uncertainty, indeed, to some extent embrace uncertainty (Inayatullah, S., 2007).

COVID-19 has, in its magnitude, forced an ultimatum for higher education to strategically embrace change with an ability to adapt to the changing landscape of the future (Inayatullah, S. & Ithnin, F., 2018). Higher Education in Malaysia has long pondered to such radical possibility. Various foresight-based planning at the organizational level had been carried out and post workshop reports submitted alas accepted with apprehension. According to Sardar, the post-normal times is a period of transition characterized by complexity, chaos and contradiction (Murray, D., 2020). The way forward for higher education now is to quickly adapt to a new age normalcy which requires sinew in behavior, science and technology. The new norm of physical distancing, digitalization of services and digitally-centered communications have challenged higher education to move to flexible education, lifelong learning and life-wide learning.

Critical of the present and anticipative of the future, academics must be proactive and aligned to clear foresights of the preferred future. In the case of UTeM, the metaphor, "Always A Pioneer, Always Ahead", calls for a mindset change – behaviorally, thinking needs to be strategized ahead of time or crisis. Visioning and creating alternative futures becomes a unifying factor for subsequent actions.

Transformation is a process of profound change with the tenacity to direct higher education in a new direction and places it on an entirely different level with little or no resemblance to the past configuration or structure. Entrenched ways of thinking and doing are idle barriers to change. A mere 'turnaround' which implies incremental progress on the same plane is not befitting and has a tendency of pushing an organization's thinking and actions towards a used future.

The best adoption of technology is a requisite to ensure that teaching and learning are sustained during the COVID-19 crisis. What was once a luxury, has now become a necessity. The alternative future of a virtual university or 'University Anywhere' has effectuated. The pandemic, in all its magnanimity, has provided an opportunity for the development of more flexible learning methods through ingenious use of distance learning and digital tools. With the Massive Open Online Courses (MOOCs), students are taught by the best faculty in the country.

Webinars created greater outreach for dialogues, discussions and conferences. The seamless learning scenario ignites global reawakening through the sharing of knowledge, solutions, expertise and the metaphor of a global brain is aptly depicted. Learning is no longer bound by traditional semesters, residential time spent in campus is no longer necessary. Travelling to campus is a passé. The sophistication of technology driven by urgency has enabled mass accessibility to learning at the comfort of home. "Education by Subscription" is the new metaphor for a preferred higher learning future in Malaysia and enrolment will soon become a luxury.

7. WAY FORWARD

In essence, UTeM garnered its strength to rise above the somber COVID19 through the methodical mapping of its 2012-2020 strategic planning; futures studies have provided UTeM with the "vision" in essence, the preconceptions of changes that will have occurred in the industry when its mission has been, or is being, accomplished (Curtis W., 2010).

The depiction of a virtual university or University Anywhere, University@Apps and the SOHO working environment which were crafted as imperative substances became highly feasible in times of crises, specifically the COVID19. The collective anticipatory scenario foresights had proven valuable and had become the principal basis for UTeM's next decade's strategic framework.

Leaving the analog era for the mainstream digital era of an unprecedented future, UTeM has started canvassing its next phase of relevance in the Malaysian Higher Education scenario. Intensive discussions and groundworks for the Strategic Plan 2021-2025 have been carried out. The series of engagements with the participation of key stakeholders of the university, encompassing the board of directors, top management, deans and directors of faculties and centers, student representatives and alumni, amalgamated valuable inputs. The University's next phase was triangulated into seven strategic goals as follows:

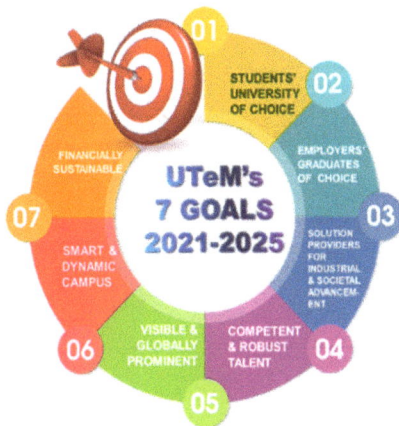

ure 3. UTeM's 7 Strategic Goals 2021-2025

sed on the 7 strategic goals, rigorous discourses and presentations were carried out. asuring on the success of the previous strategic plan, the CLA method of mapping the ure has been replicated for this next phase. Determinately, the stakeholders' CLA of M's next five years, is delineated as follows:

le 4. Causal Layered Analysis (CLA) of UTeM's Futures 2012-2025

GOALS	STUDENTS' UNIVERSITY OF CHOICE	EMPLOYERS' GRADUATES OF CHOICE @ TUAH*	SOLUTION PROVIDERS FOR INDUSTRIAL & SOCIETAL ADVANCEMENT	COMPETENT & ROBUST TALENT	VISIBLE & GLOBALLY PROMINENT	SMART & DYNAMIC CAMPUS	FINANCIAL SUSTAINABILITY
LITANY	UTeM as the best university in Higher TVET	Diversed future proof & employers' sought-after graduates.	Value creation through available expertise at university.	Technology scholars with pertinent knowledge and skills to support teaching and learning.	Positioning UTeM's visibility with the best among equals in the world.	Integrated, harmonious infrastructure within and outside campus	Anchored & sustainable financial growth.
SYSTEMIC	Specialised programmes locally approved & globally endorsed	Implementation of structured character-grooming programmes as graduates' added value elements.	Incorporation of TUNAI* in the university research, innovation and development initiatives.	Developing accomplished Researchers: Strengthening researchers' competencies to lead in strategic research fields that are highly relevant to the industry and societal needs.	Enhance initiatives towards global recognition and rankings.	Coordinated and connected campus planning.	Optimizing UTeM's Operating Expenditure
WORLDVIEW	Seamless and fluid recognition of programmes and accreditations.	Globally adaptive and holistic graduates imbued with the sound attributes of TUAH.	University as a wind tunnel for sustainable development.	Professional practitioners who are globally recognized, referred and respected by industry and society	World-ranked universities are well recognized and attract best students worldwide.	A dynamic and connected campus offers fulfilling student life-experience.	Financially sustainable operations increases confidence among stakeholders and investo
MYTH/ METAPHOR	UTeM UNO	UTeM TUAH*	UTeM TUNAI* PARK	UTeM R.I.S.E*	UTeM CHAMPS	UTeM CONNECTS	UTeM TREE OF LIFE
STRATEGY	Provide transformative and experiential learning environment through flexible industrial-based curriculum and latest technology. Enhance students' life experience. Intensify high impact marketing.	Position TUAH icons through leaderships, sports, entrepreneurship, volunteerism. Engage students with impactful TUAH Go! Programs .	Enhance industry driven based projects. Develop holistic and highly competent technology scholar. Strengthen strategic linkages between UTeM-Industry-Community. Promote Quadra-helix Engagement.	Inspired Educators: Elevating educators' talent and equipped with future ready teaching and learning innovative skills. Strengthen researchers' competencies to lead in strategic research fields.	Ensure UTeM's visibility in the world-ranking platform. Amplify strategic and dynamic technology scholars through affiliation with renowned global researchers. Empower Strategic collaboration with government, industry, academia, and community.	Enhance digital infrastructure & infostructure. Design and develop spaces/lands in-campus UTeM accordance to university physical development plan Provide high quality services to ensure on-campus facility are well maintained and up to the customer's expectations.	Increase student enrol Provide attractive programmes/activities which contribute to hig margins of profit. Strengthen asset monetization. Strengthen marketing initiatives.

8. CONCLUSION

Futures thinking is intrinsic to all decision-making. It is imperative that decisions are made upon meticulously weighted future consequences of such resolutions. Specifically, futures scenario planning and thinking empowers organizations to make definitive and to deconstruct deeply held assumptions of a used future, to examine signs of new contextual trends, to plan for feasible responses and to develop strategies of increasing an organization's capacity to adapt.

Futures scenario planning has played a substantial role in enabling UTeM to respond favorably to the disruptive COVID19 crisis. With all resolutions from the workshops factored in, the uncertain becomes apparent and the University realigns accordingly to the predicament of the pandemic while other universities had a lot more ground to cover. Scenario thinking had successfully generated awareness and enculturated literacy about future trends among the University senior management and policy makers, thus enhancing the robustness and complementing the far-reaching of the University's Strategic Plan 2021-2025.

AUTHOR

Fazidah Ithnin | Director, Chancellery Management and Relations Office,

Universiti Teknikal Malaysia Melaka (UTeM)

Email: fazidah@utem.edu.my

NOTES

• TUAH is an acronym of Tangkas (agile), Unggul (prominent), Adaptif (adaptive) and Holistik (holistic) which embodies the preferred attributes of UTeM graduates. TUAH is also an iconic symbol of a legendary Malay warrior famed during the Melaka Sultanate in the 1600's. The adoption of TUAH is symbolic and apt to UTeM's strategic location in Melaka.

• TUNAI is an acronym for Technology at University Advancing the Industry and Society. It is a commitment statement for UTeM's research and innovation and development initiatives that are aimed at aggrandizing UTeM's relevance and prospering the nation's development.

• RISE is an acronym for Responsibility, Integrity, Sustainability and Empathy. These are the attributes that UTeM aspires of its staff members.

REFERENCES

Berkhout, F., & Hertin, J. (2002). Foresight futures scenarios: Developing and applying aparticipative strategic planning tool. *Greener Management International*, 37–52. https://doi.org/10.9774/GLEAF.3062.2002.sp.00005

Crawford, J. (2020). COVID-19: 20 countries' higher education intra-period digital pedagogy responses. *Journal of Applied Learning & Teaching*, 3(1), 1-20.

Curtis W. R. (2010). Intersections of strategic planning and futures studies: Methodological Complementarities. *Journal of Futures Studies*, 15(2), 71 – 100.

Grapragasem, S., Krishnan, A. & Mansor, A. N. (2014). Current trends in Malaysian higher education and the effect on education policy and practice: An overview. International *Journal of Higher Education*, 3(1), 85-93.

Hunter, M. (2020). *The collapse of Malaysian Private Universities. COVID-19 just the latest problem*. http://www.asiasentinel.com/p/the-collapse-of-malaysian-private

Inayatullah, S. (2004). *The Causal Layered Analysis (CLA) Reader Theory and Case Studies of an Integrative and Transformative Methodology*. Tamkang University Press Graduate Institute of Futures Studies.

Inayatullah, S. (2007). Six pillars: futures thinking for transforming. Foresight, 10(1), 4-21, Emerald Group Publishing Limited.

Inayatullah, S. (2015). What Works: Case Studies in the Practice of Foresight. Tamkang University Press.

Inayatullah, S. (2018). Foresight in Challenging Environments. *Journal of Futures Studies*.

22(4), 15-24.

Inayatullah, S. (2020). *Conspiring to destroy or to create better futures*. UNESCO Futures of Education Ideas LAB. https://en.unesco.org/futuresofeducation/lab/inayatullah-conspiracy-theories-destroy-or-create-better-futures

Inayatullah, S. (2020). Scenarios for Teaching and Training: From Being "Kodaked" to Futures Literacy and Futures-Proofing*. *CSPS Strategy and Policy Journal*, 8, 31-48.

Inayatullah, S. & Black, P. (2020). Neither A Black Swan nor A Zombie Apocalypse: The Futures of A World with The Covid-19 Coronavirus. *Journal of Futures Studies*. https://www.jfsdigital.org

Inayatullah, S. & Ithnin, F. (2018). *Transformation 2050: Alternative Futures of Malaysian Universities*. USIM Press.

Ismail, A. (2020, June). *Executive Talk - Where is Higher Education Heading Post Covid-19?*. Executive Talk at Universiti Teknikal Malaysia Melaka.

Ithnin, F., Mohd Nor, M. J., & Yusoff, M. R. (2017). Futures Scenarios for Universiti Teknikal Malaysia Melaka (UTeM). *Journal of Futures Studies*, 21(4), 1-14.

Ithnin, F., Sahib, S., Mohd Nor, M.J., Raja Harun, R.S., Chong, K.E., & Sidek, S. (2018). Mapping the Futures of Malaysian Higher Education: A Meta – Analysis of Futures Studies in the Malaysian Higher Education Scenario. *Journal of Futures Studies*, 22(3), 1-18.

Kementerian Pengajian Tinggi Malaysia (2006). *Report of the Committee to Study, review and make recommendations on the development and direction of higher education in Malaysia: Steps towards excellence*. UiTM.

Kernohan, D. (2020) *Which universities are moving to remote teaching*. WONKHE: https://wonkhe.com/blogs/which-universities-are-moving-to-remote-teaching/

KPTM, K. P. T. (2007). *National higher education action plan 2007-2010* / Pelan Tindakan Pengajian Tinggi Negara 2007-2010, KPTM.

Lim, I. (2020). *COVID-19: What are Malaysia's public universities doing? Online Classes and more*. Malay Mail. https://www.malaymail.com/news/malaysia/2020/03/16/COVID-19-what-are-malaysias-public-universities-doing-online-classes-and-mo/1847071

Macquarie University. (2020). *Coronavirus (COVID-19) infection: latest information*. https://www.mq.edu.au/about/coronavirus-faqs MOHE, M. O. H. E. (2007). *The National Higher Education Action Plan*, Phase 2, 2011–2015.

New Straits Times. (2020b, March 16). *125 new COVID-19 cases in Malaysia, tally jumps to 553*. New Straits Times. https://www.nst.com.my/news/nation/2020/03/575121/125

new-COVID-19-cases-malaysia-tally-jumps-553

O'Brien, R. & Forbes, A. (2021). Speculative Futuring: Learners as the Experts On Their Own Futures (In-Press). *Journal of Futures Studies*.

Ramadan, S. (2020). *COVID-19: 9 universities are now conducting classes online.* Hype. https://hype.my/2020/184628/COVID-19-9-universities-are-now-conducting-classes-online/

Ramos, J., Uusikyla, I. & Nguyen, T.L (2020). Triple-A Governance: Anticipatory, Agile and Adaptive. *Journal of Futures Studies*. https://jfsdigital.org/2020/04/03/triple-a-governance-anticipatory-agile-and-adaptive/

Saniotis, A. (2020). Editor's Prelude to Special Issue: 'Coronaphobia and Fearscapes'. *Journal of Futures Studies*, 25(2), 1–2.

Sardar, Z. (2021). On the Nature of Time in Postnormal Times. *Journal of Futures Studies*. 25(4), 17-30. DOI: 10.6531/JFS.202106_25(4).0002

Sh Ahmad, S. (2012). Cairo ASIA Pacific International Conference on Environment-*Behaviour Studies*, Mercure Le Sphinx Cairo Hotel, Giza, Egypt.

Shariffuddin, S. A. (2017). Transformation of Higher Education Institutions in Malaysia: A Review, *Journal of Global Business and Social Entrepreneurship* (GBSE), 1(2), 126–136. http://gbse.com.my/v1no2jan17/Paper-32-.pdf

Sheriff, M.N., & Abdullah, N. (2017) Performance Indicators for the Advancement o Malaysian Research with Focus on Social Science and Humanities, *Asian Journal of University Education*, 13(2), 35-50.

Sirat, M. B. (2010). Strategic planning directions of Malaysia's higher education: University autonomy in the midst of political uncertainties. *Higher Education,* 59(4), 461-473.

Wang, J. & M. Hutchins, H., (2010). Crisis Management in Higher Education: What Have We Learned from Virginia Tech? *Advances in Developing Human Resources*, 12(5), 552–572, Sage Publications.

Watermeyer, R., Crick, T., & Knight, C. (2020). COVID-19 and digital disruption in UK universities: afflictions and affordances of emergency online migration. *Higher Education*, https://doi.org/10.1007/s10734-020-00561-y

World Health Organization Report, (2020). *Pneumonia of unknown cause – China Disease outbreak news.* https://www.who.int/csr/don/05-january-2020-pneumonia-of-unkown-cause-china/en/

World Health Organization Report, (2020). *Rolling updates on coronavirus disease (COVID-19).* https://www.who.int/emergencies/diseases/novel-coronavirus-2019/events-as-they-happen

Zuboff, S. (2019). *The age of surveillance capitalism: The fight for a human future at the new frontier of power.* Profile Books.

INFECTIOUS FUTURES:

A Conversation

INFECTIOUS FUTURES

328

his work aims not only to provide a snapshot of futures thinking during a time of crisis but also stimulate further reflections on how the pandemic exacts an influence upon possibilities for the future(s), both actual and perceptual. Authors were invited to attend an online session and share insights on the following areas:

- What is the role of futures and futurists in a time of infectious futures? Over the next 30 years?
- How can and/or might your practice/research/thinking/work evolve because of the pandemic?

In thinking through these two queries, some earlier insights were validated while new ones emerged. What follows is an edited transcript of the conversation on August 1st, 2021 followed with a very brief reflection on the project as whole. See you on the other side.

RAFEEQ BOSCH

So, three key ideas on the role of futurists now and over the next 30 years that I want to share. The first one that I want to exhort us to think about is the need to still keep pushing back the boundaries of this field. In the literature survey for my research, one of the components was to make sure that I've considered all the futures techniques that are available to futurists right now. My finding or commentary on that was that the academic literature of the past 4 years or so did not appear to contain anything radically new in the field of futures studies. It seems there was a

"Golden Age" that peaked around the year 2000, or thereabouts. And so that's why I think it's high time, especially over a 30-year horizon, to keep evolving the field. So that's my first point.

My second point is that, in this time of global infections, and infectious futures, and even moving forward, there is this constant need to highlight responsible futures practice. I still encounter, out in the world, a lot of stuff that feels weird to me from a futures point of view.. Stuff that seems designed mainly to be provocative (at best) or entertaining (at worst), rather than substantial. And while I know I run the risk of getting into territory that can come off as judgmental toward such work, I do want to advocate for this notion about responsible practice, in terms of futures. Because the pandemic shows us what the stakes are and why we have to be serious about the power and potential of our discipline.

And my third comment was that the pandemic, I guess, reminds us that as futurists, we possess this amazing toolset that allows us to really challenge predominant power structures within society. This was really the impetus for the article that we wrote that will appear in the book. When I think about that causal layered analysis work we were trying to do and the territory we ultimately found ourselves in... it was really an inspection of power structures that macro events like a pandemic tend to put into stark relief for us. So I will take a breather there on that first question. Those are my three comments on the role of futures now and over the next few years.

In terms of the insights the pandemic has delivered, I think there I have three core ideas as well. The pandemic is now a real, lived-experience example and the basis to tell stories about how to take a futures approach to other macro global phenomena. And I've got climate change on my mind here as I say that. I think sometimes these things live in quite a theoretical construct. But now, we're all living through this thing together and I think we can capture people's attention in a fundamentally more compelling way than we were able to three or four years ago. And I mean capture their attention to illustrate the ideas and approaches we stand for.

Second, the pandemic was a good illustration of systemic biases that are established by global systems and by global power structures. And so, again, we need to work on that to make sure justice features more in the systems that define our reality.

And I'm happy to talk more about that as we move through this conversation today. And my final insight I want to share goes back to some reading I did about how, after the horrors of World War II, there was sort of a post-war, societal reboot. And I feel very optimistic about something like that happening again as we free ourselves eventually from the grip of this pandemic. We may still struggle for a little bit.. Peter, to your point, I'm very mindful of the still very dire state of things all over the world. So the pandemic is by no means over, but I really look forward to that time where, having all suffered through this as a species, we ask ourselves those searching questions that can end up redefining how we organize ourselves around the world. I'm mindful of time now though, so let me stop there.

FAZIDAH ITHNIN

Alright, so on to the first question: the role of futures and futurists in a time of infectious futures. I've zoomed into three extremely important points here, with specific reference to Malaysia. Firstly, future studies is not new in Malaysia. But it has not seeped into most organizations yet, not expansively in the government sectors, not immersively either into the private sectors, as massively as it's supposed to be. Now, looking at the pulse of globalization, it's imperative to get future studies into the hearts, minds, and thinking of Malaysians. This is a tall order and this is something that I wish we could do more of. So this is where I got infected by it! From my perspective, the role of futures is significant in extending the map of strategic thinking and strategic planning. So, the role of futures in Malaysia, for me, is to have it 'educated' to the minds of the larger community, as an extension to the map of strategic planning.

Secondly, the role of futures should be pushed into transforming minds and shifting priorities. Transforming minds encapsulates the shift of thinking among the people about the futures - as something that is insurmountable. This mindset transformation is especially difficult in a multicultural setting where the perceptions of futures take multifarious assumptions - from Que Sera Sera to what's in it for me? Given a lucid understanding of how and why futures can work for all of us into getting to our preferred utopia or eutopia, then priorities will shift. We will see a more futures conscious community - people who want to be responsible citizens because they 'could see' the impacts of their present actions to their own futures and the futures of the world.

Thirdly, the role of futurists in a time of infectious futures is where we will see the return of the sage or the nuances of futurists, and more than ever, in times of infectious futures, the role of futurists in calibrating the futures of humanity as a whole is paramount. With acute knowledge, futurists assume the role of germinating the seeds of futures thinking in the development of younger generations so that they will become responsible citizens of tomorrow. Futurists will be playing a paramount role in enlightening people of the magnitude of foresight (wildcards and events) and by having as many narratives of plausible, probable, and possible futures, as well as the unknowns.

The role of futurists,to me, is best surmised in the words of PR Sarkar, "..the flame of a lamp lights up countless other lamps and the touch of the great personality wakes up innumerable sleeping hearts...". This is the time of the return of the sage or the futurists.

OTTO C. FROMMELT

I try to keep it short. For the first question, "the role of futures and futurist," I would like to contribute with my 20 years of scenario planning experiences mainly as a practitioner. My starting point is that having foresight and creating future worlds/visions, we know how to do, but it's not enough. What futurists should do is to contribute, and I really mean actively contribute, to make and bring foresight alive. When I saw what Joe Ravetz (future-wise conversations) is doing and what he presented is for me a little bit, the way to go. Hence, the futurist should play a truly active role in the following three main areas (BTW this is my practice approach): The first one is in having proactive engagement. I see that futures and scenario worlds should be discussed and debated more on a "strategic level" with government and all business actors concerned. I'm currently working in government. On top, I was working in small as well as big companies. Moreover, I have been practicing what Kees van der Heijden calls "holding a strategic conversation" for many years.

Based on holding strategic conversations about the future also allows to windtunnel (stress-test) scenarios and to regularly update them. (Note: The value of holding a strategic conversation with various stakeholders can also create new language and meaning etc.). Finally, scenarios should be checked, if there are any wildcard scenarios. If not, develop some to go beyond. My second point is to support the

*implementation journey. This means future worlds and visions should be "jointly"
translated into strategy (from strategy as is to strategy to be). Leaders should
be actively supported on their change journey to create and implement the new
strategy. My third and last point is the consideration of an xTeam approach. If you
have not heard about the notion of extended teams (short xTeams), I recommend
to read the published articles. Finally, support can be provided by utilizing an xTeam
approach, i.e., a kind of pop-up teams are constituted on an "expert of knowledge
basis" for a given context. These are my thoughts for the first question.*

In short: "from foresight to strategy to leadership driving change and transformation"

The second question with regards to "further insights and practice that work really
well", my main point is that collaboration among stakeholders, and co-creation of
the future, are needed. My practice and work can evolve in the following three
main areas: The first is via establishment of digital platforms and by driving
engagement. I mean establish a digital platform where futures are presented and
"specific" strategic dialogues can take place and can be initiated. I have tried it
too, with my website (https://ottocfrommelt.li/xLAB/) on a small scale. The second
point is, through dissemination of scenarios and visions to a "wider audience for
consultation and feedback". It is also suggested to publish more futures articles,
books, and create scenario animations such as videos. Dissemination of futures
at conferences and events drives further dialogue, too. My third and last point
of today: I believe the co-creation of the future by an xTeam approach could be
done more. It has worked very well for me so far. Based on foresight and visions,
to generate a "strategy for success and growth" is needed. Development of a new
strategy is key, but consider, of course in the implementation phase that is about
value creation and value capturing.

In short: "Foresight, strategy and leadership xLAB" (experience laboratory)

To conclude: you don't have to overthrow everything as Joe said: "You know, we
have a past, present and future". So what is good of the past and present, utilize,
but think about what and how to adapt for the future. Ladies and Gentlemen, these
are my two minutes reflections. Thank you very much.

JOE RAVETZ

Okay. So the role of futurists? Well, going back to 10,000 years of human civilization, we've always had futurists, they may be shamans, healers, priests, astronomers and so on. So I look at that word, with some little skepticism, okay, futurist, you know, are we professionals? Do we build things that might fall down, like an architect or something? So this is not to say that we should not use the word but just to say we have to place it in some kind of context. Anyway, through my recent decade or so of thinking and working, and experimentation, I began to realize there are different system modes, or system levels of organization. And we can roughly define about three and, depending on how you want to cut the cake, mode one is basically a linear change model where, you know, we know more or less how the present works, we adjust this and we have a forecast. The futurist is then a technical forecasting advisor. In mode two, it's all about evolution. And we know quite a bit about Darwinian evolution's "winner takes all," it's a competition, it's an innovation. And in that case, the futurist task is to elucidate or explore the winning strategy. And it's no accident that futurists usually get most of their money from consultancies for large corporations and governments.

So, we're all desperate to know the winning strategy. However, if we are, you know, eight or 10 billion people living on one small planet, we have to think not only about evolution, but co evolution, how to collaborate, how to generate synergy, how to learn together, and so on. So I've started to define this as a collective intelligence agenda. And in which case, futures thinkers, they are enablers, they're agents of transformation. And well, the pandemic has accelerated some of this, not everything, you know, we have had plagues in the last millennia, which were actually much more disastrous, but opened up some potential for transformative change in society and, everything else which is already going on. So futurists have much to play for. As for further insights, how could I help make this thing possible, I've, amongst other things, set up this online, global laboratory for collective intelligence. In fact, Peter, who's here on call, gave him an excellent contribution to that about six months ago. And roughly we have three main themes. One is about technology as an enabler of collective intelligence', and the notion of a CHAI or 'collective human artificial intelligence began to emerge. The next one is eco wise, so called climate resilience, sustainable cities, and so on. None of which is a done deal or a simple textbook answer, I can say from personal experience. And then the third one is foresight wise, which is basically where we turn the mirror back on to how we do all this stuff, futures methods, system transformations, and the overriding question, how to build the collective anticipatory intelligence. If I have a few seconds left, I would love to at least point to some of the cartoon series, which I use around the world, for instance this one is about deeper threats multipliers [Figure 1, p155].

And as you can see the COVID looks like a formless monster. And the point is that it is not only a pandemic, it then compounds with, you know, climate change, or civil unrest, with gross inequality, migration, financial collapse, and so on. And it's not hard to imagine how cities or whole nations will fall to pieces for a number of reasons, as some of them are already doing. But then we have to look at the other side of the coin and say: well, what are the positive synergies? How do we find those, work with them, understand them at least a little bit, and, and use these or positive transformation. A year ago when this was first proposed, as not only a futures task of, you know, stuff out there, but it's stuff in here, the unreality TV is, in everybody's minds, the viruses in the mind of the people. So what do we do them? So in this case, the futurist test then becomes something more about the personal, the personal, and the political, the liberation, or the empowerment of the person. And of course, that's the beginning of a very long story. Finally, we did some scenarios for the pandemic. Over a year ago, these were very popular at the time. And the point was interesting, because people were saying, Oh, I like that one on the top left. Let's do that one. You know, where everything's nice. And we party in the streets, and we've got the coat, the COVID under control. And, we have a social transition. And people say, Yeah, let's do that. And I was like, Yeah, sorry, guys. Life is not really that, just like that these are exogenous things for us to then grapple with whichever one it turns out to be. Well, that's the way you know, we'll have to learn to live. And let's talk about the lower right hand side, for example, which is the way that many countries have been going maybe. And so anyway, the rest is a long story, and I'm beyond my time, but I'll leave it there. And I welcome you into the Laboratory of collective intelligence, which just looks like that. More or less. And I'll send you all emails and hope to see you again. Thanks. Right.

PETER BLACK

I'm very interested in what I've heard from the other speakers. And it's got me thinking in other ways from what I originally was going to talk about. But in terms of the first question about the role of futures, I still think that at the most fundamental level— whatever techniques or methods or theories you're using— it's about expanding this range of strategic options for how we're going to deal with futures. But I think one of the things which has become more obvious for me is that we should be more explicit about what the realistic envelopes are about possible futures. This means accepting that some of the possible futures we might have talked about 10 or 15 years ago, have been cut off to some degree, because of our lack of action around some of the global limits (i.e., the planetary boundaries). Even though these boundaries were described over ten years ago, we have failed to act. So it doesn't mean that we can't have exciting and positive futures, but as futurists, we should be more explicit about what some of these things mean. For example, although we can't predict what the critical tipping points might be, we should be encouraging people to pay attention to them. In terms of our role around the modes of thinking, we should be acknowledging difference. There is a huge array of perspectives about what is desirable, what different cultures or people in different parts of the world might actually value in different ways. We need to be in touch with that. And that's part of the connection. In terms of theory and practice, we still need to work on acknowledging difference and making better connections.

We heard earlier that some of the Golden Age throughout the 2000s, with a lot of new foresight approaches happening has sort of dropped off a little bit. I'm not sure that's really true. There are definitely different ways that futurists are working. For example, with respect to practice, there's been a very big explosion in the way that futurists are interacting with communities and clients and what they're trying to achieve. From my perspective, it's not an academic sort of pursuit, but rather what we are all about is actually making a real difference in the world. That means that we have to be very flexible, and this issue around how we are connected, becomes critical. We should be working on better engagement and making connections with the parts of the world that have less options than the people who are talking tonight, because we are relatively privileged. We are simply not connecting well enough.

In terms of my practice, I have always seen my role as trying to infect other people with the perspectives that are possible within this field of foresight and futures. At the moment, the analogy I'd use is that I'd like to become a super spreader. So if I can actually get that happening (and in fact, wouldn't it be great if we all became super spreaders in a sense), we can infect a whole lot more people with this interest, and the capacity to be thinking differently. In order to keep this real, we actually need to keep evolving in the field. And we want to make sure that it *actually has impact. We should be talking about how we get through this pandemic, perhaps beyond it, and what we learn that can help us with the transformation that is required. That's a big part of how we can influence our practice for the future. There's a lot of opportunity here, and if we can keep this connection going in this community, we can really make a Big difference to the future of the planet. And isn't that a fantastic opportunity? And indeed, an obligation.*

ABRIL CHIMAL

Our role as future professionals and enthusiasts has been very important over the years. And now more than ever, the importance of developing this skill in a more mainstream way has been demonstrated. And we also have an unspoken duty of enabling openness to futures knowledge, and the pandemic has shown that futures thinking is a privilege, but it shouldn't be a privilege, it should be something that everyone can have access to. So, we need to change the way we communicate, not top-down from the expert to everyone but to share the knowledge in a more ecological way. So everyone can feel the perspective of a brighter future for all. And, I will say that we are not so narrowly human anymore. We cannot separate humanity from the rest of the planet. I think that the pandemic highlights the importance of our connections with the whole. We have been upcycling different knowledge during this time. And we are talking about technology, but not just high tech technology, but also we are going back to low tech: how past knowledge has been upcycled for this and the growth of minorities, and the importance of more people involved in these in this field and going back to the local on the importance of collectivity. And I think that we have to keep that in mind as an exploration for different industries, and not just for big organizations, or governments, corporations, etc. But, having a more individual way we can apply futures to be more connected with everything.

FAZIDAH ITHNIN

I think the only way of becoming a super spreader in infectious times is to spread the enthusiasm or the interest of futures consciousness among the next generation. The setting up of a structured futures social lab may be a potent agent. We want to embed futures and reinvigorate a futures-thinking society. As for my role here, I would like to initiate a futures social lab within my community first in Melaka and hen spread the 'futures thinking virus' further to the central states. This lab is going o be a research hub for futures studies and programmes. Through a consolidated and concerted effort from the futures community, I may need your help in this venture, we will be able to influence and infect more ministries and agencies to redirect and reinforce strategic planning into action foresight and futures scenario planning. The impacts of which will render disruptive uncertainties or threats or even X-events to be more pliable. This is especially because given the anticipated trajectory of the plausible, probable and possible alternative futures, resources can be reallocated, directions can be recalibrated and priorities can be optimized. And just for once, this is the 'virus' that we would be glad to spread and infect the wider population - the futures consciousness that is endemic!

JOHN A. SWEENEY

 have to say it's really been inspiring to listen to everyone and have a chance to absorb all of the extraordinary wisdom and insights. As I was thinking about what possibly to say that could add something, it was hard not to think of my personal journey, and over the last year and a half especially, and the morning of futures that seem lost. Of course, the grasping onto hope for futures that could be, but think I was really, really struck by something that repeated mentioned in his opening introduction around the community aspect, and it really has been the community that I think has, has felt like his staved off, you know, depression in many ways from what was a entirely forecasted and entirely in many ways, you know, absolutely probable crises. And to see, of course, the prolonging of the crises precisely because of the kinds of compounded issues that that Joe so eloquently pointed out to. And I think that, if anything, it really affirms this idea of the super spreader, or, as Joe mentioned, this super seer, but also the futurist in a role as the provocateur, and in some ways, maybe as the mortician of the futures that need to die, the systems that need to die, the things that aren't sustaining life. How do we shepherd and create spaces where we can actually transition into a new space? As we know, funerals aren't necessarily for the dead, but for the living to allow mourning and a sense of ritual to take place.

For me, it has been about trying to hold that space and to understand how this has had a profound effect on my practice. Certainly, there was a focus on participatory futures before, but I think, now more than ever, it's been an affirmation that we have to commit ourselves to the diffusion of futures in ways that might have been unimaginable a generation ago. And, of course, we know that we have amazing tools for this. But, there's still a lot, a lot more to be done, as Abril, Peter, and others have mentioned. I just want to affirm what a privilege it is to be able to share air with you in ways that we can nowadays. Jose, over to you for the last word.

JOSE RAMOS

Great, thank you. It's been really nice to hear people's thoughts and to bring a personal element to everything. So thanks to everyone. I'm going to start with a simpler idea. When I think of the role of futures over the next 30 years, what I really think about, of course, is to serve humanity. And I think when you take a step back, and you look at how we responded to the pandemic, and how prepared we were, I think it's fair to say that we were not prepared. I think it's fair to say that most governments and most communities were playing catch up. Of course, there were some that were. There were preparations within the pharmaceutical industry. There were some governments like Taiwan that already had the seeds, the DNA of responses, but by and large they weren't. And if you look at the influence that futures studies and strategic foresight has had, the impact was not there, unfortunately. So for me I think we have to look at that gap. And we have to imagine what that means for the next 30 years. For me, that means socializing futures thinking, that means futures literacy, that means anticipatory governance and participatory futures. That means futures seeping into many different aspects of life. I think a lot of people here have already spoken to the term collective intelligence: how do we harness diverse communities to think about the future together? The future not as a privilege, but as something that everyone has access to? I think a lot of people here are already sort of speaking that language. So for me the gap that needs to be addressed in the next 30 years is really how we're going to be of service to humanity, that our field actually has relevance for the next pandemic, or the next big problem, whether that's climate induced disruption, whether that's whatever technology is going to bring, so that we are prepared.

We have to help to socialize these ideas, and to socialize the responses in ways that are meaningful. I think that maybe that's a self critical lens to take. But I also see it as an opportunity. Because it means that there's a lot of creative work to be done, there's a lot of methodological hybridity to be plied into, if, if we're going to actually *be of service in this way. It also means that we're going to need to shift from being an inward looking community, to an outward looking community. I think that futures has been inward looking by necessity, because, when I came into futures, 20 years ago, people thought it was weird. And 10 years later, they thought it was cool. And five years ago, they thought it was necessary. And so we're inward because we need each other to survive, because it's a harsh world, because the scrutiny that people put on futures thinking and alternative futures is very tough. So we have needed each other, because we mutualize, we use a mutual support system, in order to be able to do what we do. But we're going to have to go from inwards to outward, I think. And we're going to have to take it to the world. And we're going to need to get beyond our fears, and our insecurities, and take the stage. This will require us to grow new selves. The future is asking us to grow and develop new selves.*

***

JOHN A. SWEENEY

Infectious futures can be understood in a few ways. Of course, and perhaps most obvious, we are living through a moment where the very threat of infection has proliferated some futures and collapsed others. Futures, as a practice, has become quite infectious, which is to say that the crisis has created a space for more futures dialogue, research, and work to be undertaken. This requires accountability, not to theory or method, but rather to the future itself: there is a need, as Jose eloquently outlines, to "lean into" the moment and "become who we are" as futurists (and to paraphrase Nietzsche). These new selves must, as Fazidah highlighted, be super spreaders whose enthusiasm, empowerment, and energy infects the world. This is what the future asks of us and is precisely what our present moment necessitates. It is the collective hope of the editorial team that this work contributes to infecting us all with dreams, analyses and experiments for the alternative futures that represent better places.

CONCLUSIONS

FROM MOURNING TO DREAMING...

John A. Sweeney

08 | 16 | 2021

It would be disingenuous not to stress that my personal experience of the pandemic has been one of immense privilege. There have been moments of despair, of course, but even when I was struggling with pneumonia, I had access to quality care. It is not lost on me in any way that many have not been so fortunate. In reflecting on the past year and a half, what strikes me the most is coming to grips with futures that will never be. I mourn for futures whose beauty, joy, and laughter will never be seen and heard. From those who abstained from the warm embrace of family to those who will never again express their love in person, the last year and a half has been a period of immense and daresay, incalculable, loss.

How can and might futures create a space for such mourning? Might we be able to utilize futures to process what we have lost without lapsing into nostalgia? What can futures (and futurists) truly do in times of crisis? These are the questions that I have been holding of late. And, to be fully transparent, I'm not sure that I have answers. In order to begin gleaming some solace from these mourned futures, I turn (as I have done many times before) to insights from two giants in the field: Ashis Nandy and Jim Dator.

It was the latter who introduced me to the former's work, particularly one piece that I read during my first semester in the PhD program at the University of Hawaii at Manoa in 2009.

Nandy's "Bearing Witness to the Future" remains as heartfelt and prescient today as it was then, and perhaps even more so than when it was originally published in 1996. There is a specific passage that I have returned to time and again, including during days spent in various forms of isolation/quarantine when the walls felt as if they were closing in. Nandy opines, "The challenge of futures studies [...] is to keep open the option of a plurality of dissent [...]" [Nandy 1996, 638]. At a time when many are seeking some sense of comfort and when many fingers are pointed squarely at futures in hopes of meaningful answers, I find Nandy's insistence upon holding a space where there can and might be a plurality of dissent affirming, if not comforting.

Of course, I would not go so far as to extend this plurality of dissent toward the various realms of mis- and disinformation that have wreaked havoc around the world, quite the contrary. Perhaps it is only through finding ways to facilitate spaces of dissent that the deleterious harm of such un-truths might be confronted and combated. Even as more are welcoming, if not wanting, futures/foresight, there continues to be a sense of being "on the other side of the fence" that is rooted within transformative foresight, which is the "collective caravan" approach to practice that mutates dissent into shared learning [Inayatullah and Sweeney 2021]. The actual "doing" of futures/foresight is never without its obstacles, especially during times of crisis, and I think that Nandy's charge to find and create the space to be and think otherwise is precisely what allows mourning to morph into something else, perhaps even hope.

I would not have a career as a futurist were it not for Jim Dator, so anything I say about him, despite my critical faculties, remains ensconced within an air of absolute awe and deep gratitude. And, I am far from alone in holding such feelings about him. Indeed, a quick review of this collection demonstrates the magnitude of Jim's impact, and infrequent email exchanges with him during the pandemic have been sources of joy, but I digress. While it might seem apt to quote Dator's 2nd Law of the Future, as others have done, my thinking has turned toward his fondness for aiglatson, which is a term that he credits to Gabriel Fackre. As the literal antithesis of nostalgia (it is merely the word spelled backwards), the term denotes:

the yearning for things to come; revering the future; without being disrespectful to the past (remembering that once it was all that was humanly possible), preferring the dreams of the future to the experiences of the past; always desiring to try something new; to go where no one has ever gone before in all areas of human—and non-human, and, soon, post-human—experience (Dator 2019, 14).

As my first degree was in history, I have always found the resonances between my mother discipline and futures quite strong, but I can also attest to the peculiarity of aiglatson as an affect, an embodied awareness that has washed over me many times since the start of the ongoing crisis and during specific moments where the weight of it all felt crushing. I revere the future as one who mourns, not seeking to recreate the past but cherishing what once was and feeling hope for what can and might lie beyond. One cannot be blind to the challenges all around and those just over the horizon, and Jose has elsewhere invoked the metaphor of the chrysalis (Ramos 2020). If this is gestation, then so be it.

I continue to prefer the dreams of the future, even though 2020 was the hottest year on record and, as it were, likely one of the coolest of the coming century (Teirstein 2021). It might seem foolhardy, if not irresponsible, to yearn for things to come given our current trajectory, but the alternative to aiglatson is not merely ignorance but a destructive force that consumes past, present, and future: an insatiable nostalgia that cannot mourn, which is always a letting go. As Nandy reminds us, there must always be an option-- alternatives where being and thinking otherwise can and might endure. It is my hope that this work enables dreaming of futures rather than merely mourning them.

REFERENCES

Inayatullah, S., & Sweeney, J. A. (2021). From Strategic to Transformative Foresight: Using Space to Transform Time. World Futures Review, 13(1), 27–33. https://doi.org/10.1177/1946756720971743

Nandy, A. (1996). Bearing witness to the future. Futures, 28(6–7), 636–639. https://doi.org/10.1016/0016-3287(96)84465-X

Sardar, Z. (6/2010b). Welcome to postnormal times. Futures, 42(5), 435–444. https://doi.org/10.1016/j.futures.2009.11.028

Teirstein, Z. (2021, January 16). 2020, the hottest year on record, will be one of the coldest this century. Grist. https://grist.org/climate/2020-was-the-hottest-year-on-record-well-remember-it-as-one-of-the-centurys-coldest/

COVID-19 IS HERE – 'IT'S JUST NOT EVENLY DISTRIBUTED'

Peter Black

As this COVID-19 pandemic continues to unfold, different parts of the world are at different stages in experiencing the impacts of this global disruption. Consequently—and not surprisingly—there are a number of elements from our analysis in March 2020 (Inayatullah and Black 2020) playing out across the globe with many possible outcomes. Different countries and even different areas within countries are being characterised as 'following the Indian path' (in 2020 it was the Italian path that people were worried about) –or 'not yet reaching peak cases' or 'still with a long way to go'. It is interesting that in mid 2020 there was commentary noting that for the first time in the post-war history of epidemics, more than 90% of all reported deaths at that stage had been in the world's richest countries (Cash and Patel 2020). This is now changing with the emergence of the COVID-19 Delta variant in combination with limited availability and access to vaccines in poorer countries. The mortality figures by say the end of 2022 will likely highlight yet again, the difference between the 'haves' and the 'have nots'. Of course, nothing is certain. New variants will emerge, vaccines will need to be modified in response to these variants and we may all suffer further surges in cases and deaths. Time will tell.

On a more personal level, I have found the explosion of information related to COVID-19 initially, absolutely overwhelming. The number of COVID-19 newsletters, or discussion groups or webinars that I could have signed up to or participated in has been staggering. I recognise most consciously my confirmation bias. I have tended to ignore information sources that I judge as low quality or misleading. Essentially, I was and continue to be very selective in allocating my time, effort and resources to those activities that make sense and allow me to maintain some control. I have certainly experienced feelings of tiredness, exhaustion and unexpectedly at times, disconnection. Many of the developments in other countries are distressing and I continue to recognise how fortunate I am to live where I do at this time on the planet. I have regular calls with colleagues and friends in South and Southeast Asia and hear first-hand how the situations have been evolving. In recent months it has been horrible and the near-term future is not at all comforting. I feel some guilt about being so fortunate, living where retreats into nature, a walk along the beach and a swim help me to keep balanced and maintain perspective. Communicating with people I trust and respect has also (I hope) kept me reasonably grounded. But how can I really tell?

One of the dominant themes of this pandemic concerns the power of disinformation and conspiracy theories swirling around the 'whom do I trust' metaphor. However, at a meta-perspective, interconnectedness rules. The economic fortunes of all countries are uncertain due to globalisation and interconnectedness. This is a complex world with brittle, fragile systems and clearly nonlinear relationships, but self-interest gives some clues about possible future scenarios.

With continual high levels of virus circulation in many parts of the globe and poor vaccination coverage, barriers in some form will likely continue. Nation states will understand the continuing threat from infection and borders will remain tightly controlled affecting both travel and trade. Countries classified as say 'tier one' or 'green' (i.e., low incidence of COVID-19 with relatively high vaccination rates) may trade and travel within regulated bubbles. Vaccine passports will be required. This again will accelerate the opening of the chasm between the 'haves' and 'have nots'. Countries having trouble with COVID-19 controls may shift the discourse so that health controls become less dominant and economic growth can once again take centre stage. Social transformations take on a lower priority.

Over the past year, there has been an increase in commentary about addressing the underlying drivers of disease emergence. At a broader level, the big questions about development models including the 'more, more, more' model of infinite economic growth are now being intertwined with another big challenge— climate change. Concerned citizens across the globe are calling for more holistic approaches to deal with civilisational challenges that are increasingly being recognised and described as truly interconnected. Scientists are pleading for policies that address the root cause of threatened planetary boundaries (including climate change)—not symptom relief. And the root cause is overexploitation of the Earth (Rockström et al. 2009). Increased focus on the root cause is not only desirable, but also a source of some inspiration and hope. However, in terms of postnormal futures and the three tomorrows' framework, the root cause is generally ignored—a black elephant (Sardar and Sweeney 2016).

Recently I have been asked as an epidemiologist and foresight practitioner to think about the next horizons, not as predictions, but as a simple personal exploratory exercise about possible futures. I am more comfortable within the extended present of the first tomorrow and although it is indeed a cliché, I do feel we are living through a time of transformation. COVID-19 has given us an opportunity to pause and reflect. It is weird that this 'gift' is built on the evolution of a virus on a microscopic scale that is playing out on the grand global scale. All of our successful and unsuccessful interventions, including the use of vaccines, will influence this evolutionary path and we will be complicit once again in the outcomes. These outcomes are likely to include many more COVID-19 virus variants, and it is possible that some will emerge that are more challenging than the Delta variant. Of course, the outcomes will also include a wide range of social, economic and environmental consequences that will initially reflect the dominant values across the planet.

With respect to COVID-19 specifically, over the second tomorrow of familiar futures, technological advances in developing pan-coronavirus vaccines (Saunders, Lee and Parks 2021) and pan-coronavirus treatments could keep the virus at bay as it continues to re-emerge from the ever-increasing global human population. The growing focus on identifying cheap and reliable therapeutics including vaccines will likely have 'flow-on benefits' in treating other emerging infectious diseases that will emerge as we continue to plunder the planet. Again, these benefits will not be equally distributed.

For the longer term, what are the unthought futures for the 50 to 100 year time period? Uncertainty and ignorance rule here and assumptions about human liveability on this planet would be very unwise. From my perspective, climate change, land-use change, biodiversity loss and emerging infectious diseases are black jellyfish which will interact in very chaotic and complex ways.

Of course, the opportunity for a global re-awakening exists in each of these tomorrows. It is a personal choice for each of us about how we will engage with any potential futures, individually and collectively. For me, I choose to keep the following words from Jim Dator in mind:

'The only way forward is through the imminent self-destruction of dominant values, behaviour and institutions, with the hope that a million phoenixes rise from the ashes … the countless tsunami that we must learn to surf with pleasure and pain.' (from Halal 2020)

REFERENCES

Cash, R and Patel, V. (2020). Has COVID-19 subverted Global Health, *The Lancet,* 395(10238), 1687-1688. https://doi.org/10.1016/ S0140-6736(20)31089-8

Halal, W. E. (2020, May 12) Collective Intelligence to solve the Megacrisis. *Journal of Futures Studies*. https://jfsdigital. org/2020/05/01/collective-intelligence-to-solve-the-megacrisis/

Inayatullah, S. and Black, P. F. (2020, March 18). Neither Black Swan nor a Zombie Apocalypse. *Journal of Futures Studies*. https://jfsdigital. org/2020/03/18/neither-a-black-swan-nor-a-zombie-apocalypse-the-futures-of-a-world-with-the-covid-19-coronavirus/

Rockström, J., Steffen, W., Noone, K., Persson, Å., Chapin III, F. S., Lambin, E., Lenton, T. M., Scheffer, M., Folke, C., Schellnhuber, H., Nykvist, B., De Wit, C. A., Hughes, T., van der Leeuw, S., Rodhe, H., Sörlin, S., Snyder, P. K., Costanza, R., Svedin, U.,.... Foley, J. (2009). Planetary boundaries: exploring the safe operating space for humanity. *Ecology and Society 14*(2), 32. URL: http://www.ecologyandsociety.org/vol14/iss2/art32/

Sardar, Z. & Sweeney, J.A. (2016) The Three Tomorrows of Postnormal Times, *Futures*, 75, 1-13. https://doi.org/10.1016/j.futures.2015.10.004

Saunders, K.O., Lee, E., Parks, R., Martinez, D.R., Dapeng.L., Chen,H., Edwards, R.J., Gobeil, S., Barr, M., Mansouri, K., Alam, S.M., Sutherland, L.L., Cai, F., Sanzone, A.M., Berry, M., Manne, K., Bock, K.W., Minai, M., Nagata, B.M....Haynes, B.F. (2021). Neutralizing antibody vaccine for pandemic and pre-emergent coronaviruses. *Nature*, 594, 553-559. https://doi.org/10.1038/s41586-021-03594-0

www.ingramcontent.com/pod-product-compliance
Lightning Source LLC
Chambersburg PA
CBHW051558030426
42334CB00031B/3251